F HEALTH & MEDICAL GUIDE

Contributing Writer: Rebecca Hughes
Consultants: Halina Brukner, M.D., Clinical Medicine
Ira J. Chasnoff, M.D., Pediatrics
Jeffery W. Ellis, M.D., Obstetrics and Gynecology
Zachary S. Fainman, M.D., Internal Medicine
Medical Illustrator: Teri J. McDermott, M.A.

TABLE OF CONTENTS

INTRODUCTION

This book is designed to help the person who is ultimately responsible for your health—you. After all, you are the one who can most closely monitor your physical well-being and regulate your personal health habits on a daily basis. You are the one who decides what you eat, how much you exercise, and where you go when a medical problem arises. You are the one who wishes to avoid expensive trips to the doctor while at the same time being prudent about obtaining medical advice when it is truly necessary. You are the one who is most directly concerned with preserving your good health and preventing illness.

The *Family Health & Medical Guide*, with its wide coverage of health and medical topics, will give you the information you need to protect your health and well-being.

To help you better understand disease, the *Family Health & Medical Guide* offers a survey of the human body and how it works in sickness and in health. Chapters are dedicated to different organ systems within the body as well as to such topics as child care and choosing a doctor. In those sections that describe a particular disease or disorder, the cause, the risk factors, the symptoms, the diagnosis, the treatment, and the prognosis are discussed, and preventive action (if available) is outlined. Each entry is as inclusive as possible, with language that is clear and easy to understand.

This book is intended as a home adviser about health and medical problems. It is not a substitute for your own doctor, however. If you suspect that you may need medical care, you should always consult a physician.

Remember that maintaining good health is a team effort between you and your doctor. With the help of the *Family Health & Medical Guide*, you can become a more active participant in protecting your health—and the health of your family.

YOU AND YOUR DOCTOR

Most people never think about how to choose a doctor until they need one in a hurry. When a person is injured or suddenly becomes ill, finding a good doctor is a necessity, and there is often no time to spare.

If a person does not have a family doctor or internist, injury or sudden illness often means a quick visit to the emergency room or outpatient section of the nearest hospital, where staff physicians who may know little about the patient's personal medical history must treat him symptomatically and, more often than not, on an urgent basis. This usually is not a good way to establish a lasting physician–patient relationship.

A better way to assure yourself of good medical care is to have a personal physician who is familiar with you and your family's medical history and who is available (or has associates who are available) when you need care. In this way, your health needs will be met by someone who knows you and whom you know.

The best time, then, to choose a doctor is when you don't need one. You should never wait until you have no choice about the doctor you see. How do you choose a doctor? Here are some guidelines for making an informed decision.

Choosing a Family Doctor

Many families want a doctor who is familiar both with family members as individuals and with the family as a group. Doctors who specialize in family medicine are called *family practitioners*. (An internist can also provide comprehensive care to adult patients. See Internal Medicine, page 14.) Their education and training enable them not only to provide medical care but also to recognize and handle the social, emotional, and psychological factors that affect the health and well-being of patients and their families. Whereas a physician

5

needs to have only one year of internship (postgraduate hospital training, usually divided among several branches of medicine) before entering general practice, today's family practitioner completes a one-year internship and a two-year residency in family practice. During that time, he or she receives more intensive training in general surgery, internal medicine, obstetrics/gynecology, and pediatrics, among other fields.

Family practitioners care for all the members of a family, so there is usually no need for a different specialist for each individual. A family practitioner is well equipped to handle most aspects of medical care, such as uncomplicated pregnancies, immunizations, and routine physicals. A family practitioner generally can diagnose and treat all of the common ailments, as well as many of the uncommon ones. A family practitioner can guide you to the right specialist when one is necessary.

In addition to providing comprehensive medical care for all family members, today's family practitioner is as interested in *maintaining* your good health as in curing or treating illness. The family practitioner's overall goal is to treat each family member as an individual with physical, emotional, and social needs, as well as medical requirements.

How can you find a family practitioner who is right for your family? You can call your county or state medical society. These organizations have uniform requirements for physicians to be admitted to their membership (for example, completion of appropriate training and board certification). They can also tell you where you can find a specialist. However, these societies do not offer an opinion on the overall quality of a physician. This is something you must assess for yourself. The questions listed below will help you make this assessment.

Another valuable source is the physician referral service of your local hospital. This service will give you the names of family physicians who are on staff and are accepting new patients.

You should also ask people in your neighborhood about their doctors. They may be able to offer suggestions based on personal experience with local physicians. In addition, if you live in a city, you may find that there is a local organization that evaluates the medical profession on behalf of the consumer. Neighborhood consumer groups will often make medical referral information available to you at no charge.

In the process of selecting a family physician, you should draw up a list of basic questions to ask the doctor and consider the following:

• Will the doctor treat all family members?
• Does the doctor provide care during pregnancy and perform deliveries?
• Does the doctor have staff privileges at a nearby accredited hospital?
• Does the doctor perform surgery? If so, what kind?
• Does the doctor encourage preventive medicine, such as routine checkups, immunizations, and follow-up tests?
• Does the doctor make emergency house calls for bedridden family members?
• Does the doctor have office hours that are convenient for your family, especially for those who work or attend school?
• What arrangement does the doctor have for a substitute when he or she is unavailable?
• What are the fees for the various services?
• Is the doctor certified by the American Board of Family Practice (or a specialty board of another area)?

The answers to these questions, along with the recommendations of friends and neighbors, will help you select the right doctor for you and your family.

How to Choose a Specialist

In approaching the problem of finding a specialist, you should remember that most specialists receive their patients through referrals from family doctors or from other specialists. Many have a policy of not accepting a patient who has not first been examined and referred by a family doctor. This is a method of making sure that those who really need specialists see them and that those who do not need them do not incur the expense that seeing a specialist entails.

Your family doctor or internist usually will decide whether your medical complaint needs the attention of a specialist. For example, if you have a mild inflammation of the ear canal, your family doctor is quite capable of treating it. If there is chronic inflammation of the ear canal, however, or if you have suffered a partial loss of hearing, your family doctor proba-

7

bly will refer you to an otorhinolaryngologist (ear, nose, and throat specialist).

Sometimes it may be difficult to determine the type of specialist needed to diagnose and treat a particular problem. For example, visual problems may be limited to abnormalities in the eye itself, but they may also be the result of a wide variety of causes, including diabetes, hardening of the arteries, a stroke, or a tumor in a part of the brain that controls vision. The human body is an organic system. Changes in one part of the system affect other parts, and no part of the system functions in isolation. Consequently, the first task in treating an illness is to discover the underlying primary cause of the ailment. When the culprit is found, you may then be referred to a specialist who deals with the specific area of the body most affected by that problem.

The first line of action in selecting a specialist is to follow the advice of your family doctor. Your family doctor will know whether you need a specialist. However, you always can ask for a second opinion or seek out a specialist on your own. If for no other reason than to know that you did all you were able to do, you should always try to get as much information as possible about your own or a family member's illness. You may even find something that one of the doctors missed.

If your family doctor refers you to a specialist, or if you seek one on your own, you should know what each specialty consists of and what to expect when you see a specialist. The following section gives you a brief description of more than 30 medical and surgical specialties. As you read about each one, remember that an internship is the period immediately after graduation from medical school, during which a doctor receives supervised practical experience in a hospital setting. A residency, also supervised in a hospital setting, follows an internship; it is a period of advanced training in a doctor's chosen medical specialty. The length of residency varies, depending on the specialty. Even within a specialty, the length of residency may vary from one medical center to another and may change with time. Board certification means that a doctor has been certified as meeting the professional standards of a medical specialty organization called a *board*, which requires completion of a residency at an accredited institution, acceptable performance on a rigorous set of examinations, and in some fields, a year or two of clinical experience as well.

Allergy and immunology

This branch of medicine is concerned with the study, diagnosis, and treatment of disorders related to immunity (the body's ability to resist disease or threatening substances). The body's immune system fights against the intrusion of outside forces, whether they are irritating substances that cause allergic reactions or microorganisms that cause infection. This is the system that helps us fight off illness every day of our lives. Modern immunologic research indicates that many infections can be as much a result of defects in a person's immune system as they are a result of exposure to viruses or bacteria.

Immunologists are also studying the role of the immune system in cancer growth. It someday may be possible to prevent cancer by modifying the immune system to reject cancerous growths in the body. Immunologists are also interested in the opposite effect of the immune system—the rejec-

tion of foreign substances that are actually beneficial (the most obvious example is an organ transplant). Immunologists are also seeking ways to make the immune system work selectively, so that the body would reject cancer cells but accept a new heart, kidney, or liver.

The best-known branch of immunology deals with allergies, which are responses of the body's immune system to irritating substances in the environment. Doctors who practice as allergists are involved in identifying environmental irritants that cause symptoms and in formulating a plan of treatment. Allergists may treat allergies by suggesting environmental modifications to eliminate the offending substance or by using drugs to relieve the symptoms. Another option is a program of desensitization, which involves injecting minute amounts of the offending agent into the patient's body to make the immune system less sensitive to it. Once such a program has been set up, your family doctor can often give the injections. Allergists also consult in the management of certain diseases, such as asthma.

An immunologist must complete a residency in internal medicine or pediatrics after

9

graduating from medical school. This residency is followed by a two-year fellowship program in allergy and immunology. Specialty board examinations are also required.

Anesthesiology

Thanks to the use of anesthetics, surgery can be performed without pain. Though many minor medical procedures can be done with a local anesthetic, more complex procedures require that the patient remain unconscious.

An anesthesiologist is a specialist in the use of those drugs that stop the experience of pain. Anesthesiologists must complete medical school, an internship, and a residency in their specialty before starting their practice.

An anesthesiologist also may receive some training in a field other than anesthesiology, such as internal medicine, pediatrics, or obstetrics. Some anesthesiologists may even complete tours of surgical residency in order to broaden their knowledge of the various surgical techniques and needs.

Bariatrics

Bariatrics is a relatively new field in medicine, brought into popularity by the public's keen interest in the problems of being overweight.

Bariatricians have been making advances in what is known about being overweight or underweight by dispelling myths and substituting hard scientific evidence. Their training usually includes an internship in internal medicine, with a special residency in bariatrics. Bariatricians are certified by their specialty group, the American Society of Bariatric Physicians.

Cardiology

Cardiology is a branch of internal medicine that deals with the diagnosis and treatment of disorders of the heart and circulatory system, including those that stem from birth abnormalities, childhood diseases, or advancing age. Cardiologists take care of a variety of heart conditions, such as rheumatic heart disease in children and congestive heart failure and heart attacks in adults.

Cardiology and cardiovascular surgery complement each other. Over the years, doctors in these fields have worked closely together in the treatment of heart diseases. For example, the cardiologist may determine that a child has been born with a hole between the chambers of the heart; the car-

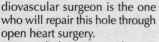

diovascular surgeon is the one who will repair this hole through open heart surgery.

A cardiologist must be acquainted not only with anatomy and physiology but also with modern computerized diagnostic equipment. One special diagnostic procedure performed by cardiologists is cardiac catheterization, in which a catheter (a long, thin, flexible tube) is inserted into the heart and adjacent blood vessels, allowing the injection of a special dye that affords a view of those structures. Angioplasty (the opening of a blocked artery by insertion of a balloon-tipped catheter) is a treatment procedure that is commonly performed by cardiologists.

Training in cardiology includes completion of a residency in internal medicine and at least two years of specialized training in cardiology.

Cardiovascular surgery

The cardiovascular surgeon performs many different types of surgery on the heart and blood vessels, including replacement of heart valves and bypasses of blocked coronary arteries. Open heart surgery came into its own during the 1950s and underwent further refinement in the 1960s and 1970s. Three decades have passed since the first heart transplant. In 1982, the first implantation of an artificial heart took place.

Training in cardiovascular surgery includes the completion of a general surgery residency, followed by two or three years of specialized training.

Dentistry

Dentistry is concerned with the prevention, diagnosis, and treatment of diseases, disorders, and malformations of the teeth, mouth, and jaws. Most people select a dentist with a general practice who can provide routine dental care and, if necessary, can recommend a dental specialist for those conditions needing specialized treatment. Some of the dental specialties include the following practices:
- Orthodontia (straightening of teeth)
- Periodontia (treatment of gums and underlying bone)
- Endodontia (root canal treatment)
- Exodontia (extraction of teeth)

A dentist planning to establish a general practice completes four years of dental school and perhaps an optional one-year general residency. Dental specialists have additional training in their chosen specialty.

11

Dermatology

Dermatology is the study of diseases and disorders of the skin, ranging from acne to psoriasis to skin cancer.

The dermatologist also must be knowledgeable about diseases that primarily affect other parts of the body but that may have some bearing on the condition of the skin. In addition, dermatologists have training in allergies, since over the years many skin conditions have been recognized as allergic reactions instead of skin diseases.

Dermatologists are required to do an internship, usually in internal medicine, followed by a three-year residency in dermatology.

Endocrinology

When we think of "messages" being sent throughout the body, we usually think of the nervous system. But there is another communication system in the body, called the *endocrine system*. It is made up of the ductless glands, including the pituitary gland, the adrenal glands, the thyroid gland, the parathyroid glands, the islet cells in the pancreas, the ovaries (in women), and the testes (in men). These glands secrete hormones that travel as messengers throughout the body to direct and integrate a vast number of bodily functions. Disorders of the endocrine system include diabetes, Cushing syndrome, and growth abnormalities.

An endocrinologist is a specialist in the diagnosis and treatment of disorders of the endocrine system. He or she must complete an internship and a residency in internal medicine, followed by two years of training in endocrinology.

Epidemiology

Specialists in this medical field study the outbreak, frequency, distribution, and control of communicable diseases. The unofficial headquarters of this activity is the Centers for Disease Control and Prevention in Atlanta, Georgia.

Epidemiology deals not only with communication of disease in general but also with the specific conditions under which certain diseases seem to flourish. For example, the relatively new field of urban epidemiology specifically addresses itself to those diseases and conditions peculiar to city settings. In addition, epidemiologists work to devise ways of preventing disease, such as developing vaccines.

Epidemiology also is concerned with causes of illness

other than infectious diseases. Epidemiologists have led the medical field in seeking environmental causes for a host of disorders once attributed to bacteria or other sources. Air and water pollution, toxic substances in foods, toxic substances used in the manufacture of various products—all have come under the scrutiny of the epidemiologist.

Epidemiology attracts physicians not only from internal medicine but also from other fields, such as immunology and pediatrics.

An epidemiologist usually has completed three years of specialized training and a year of independent research or teaching.

Gastroenterology

A gastroenterologist specializes in the diagnosis and treatment of diseases and disorders of the stomach and the intestines, as well as related organs that help in the digestive process, such as the esophagus, liver, and pancreas. Gastritis (inflammation of the stomach), enteritis (inflammation of the intestinal tract), ulcers, inability to digest certain foods, constipation, diarrhea, hyperacidity, and heartburn are among the disorders treated by the gastroenterologist.

Gastroenterologists often use a medical procedure called *endoscopy,* in which a flexible tubelike instrument is used to directly view hollow organs, such as the esophagus, stomach, and colon. Diagnosis and treatment of many conditions, such as ulcers and polyps, may be done with this procedure. Biopsies (in which tissue samples are gathered for testing) are also carried out with the endoscopy procedure.

These specialists are trained as internists or pediatricians with an additional two-year fellowship in gastroenterology.

Hematology

Hematology is the study of diseases and disorders of the blood and the blood-forming tissues, such as the bone marrow and the spleen. A hematologist is proficient in a range of diagnostic techniques in which blood and bone marrow samples are used to shed light on disease processes. Blood analyses can aid in developing treatment for a patient. The hematologist's primary concern, however, is the host of diseases and disorders related to the blood itself, including inability of the red blood cells to carry sufficient oxygen, inability of the white blood cells to fight against invading microorganisms, and inability of the bone marrow to manufacture enough red blood cells. The hematologist is also an expert on cancer of the blood (leukemia) and on blood clotting problems, such as hemophilia.

The hematologist must be firmly grounded not only in internal medicine, anatomy, and physiology but also in biochemistry. Knowledge of computerized diagnostic equipment and sophisticated biochemical analyses is also necessary.

A hematologist must complete an internship and a residency in internal medicine plus two years of training in hematology. Hematologists also are trained as oncologists (cancer specialists).

Internal medicine

Internal medicine is the branch of medicine that deals with the diagnosis and treatment of diseases of adults, except for those conditions that require management by a surgeon or an obstetrician. Like the family practitioner, the internist is trained to handle a wide range of illnesses; in fact, many people select an internist as their family doctor. The internist is specifically trained to deal with

chronic (long-term) illnesses, such as diabetes and high blood pressure, and acute (short-term) diseases, such as infections. In addition, an internist has both the range and the depth to diagnose illnesses that might escape detection by a specialist if they lie outside his or her special field.

After graduating from medical school, an internist completes one year of internship, followed by two years of residency in internal medicine. Internal medicine is also the basis for many other specialties, such as cardiology, endocrinology, gastroenterology, hematology, and nephrology. That is why these branches are often referred to as *subspecialties,* and the doctors who practice them as *subspecialists.* In order to become a subspecialist, an internist must complete at least two years of additional training, referred to as a *fellowship,* in his or her chosen subspecialty before becoming eligible for subspecialty board certification.

Nephrology

Nephrologists treat kidney disorders. Their patients usually are referred to them by internists when kidney problems are diagnosed as needing special care. In treating kidney disorders, the nephrologist may make use of medications or dialysis (removal of wastes and toxins from the blood by means of a special machine). Referral for surgery is initiated by a nephrologist. Nephrologists also perform kidney biopsies, which are used to diagnose a number of kidney diseases.

Nephrologists are thoroughly grounded in internal medicine, with special attention to the physiologic processes performed by the kidneys. They must be equally well grounded in biochemistry and the tools of modern biochemical analysis. A nephrologist also must be familiar with all of the latest computerized diagnostic equipment, as well as the latest in kidney dialysis machines.

Training in nephrology includes internship and a residency in internal medicine, followed by a two-year fellowship in nephrology, after which specialty board examinations may be taken.

Neurology

Neurology is the field of medical science that is concerned with the nervous system—the brain, the spinal cord, and the complex network of nerves. Clinical neurology concerns itself specifically with the diagnosis and treatment of diseases of the nervous system, but the neurologist must be familiar with the total functioning of the body, because disorders of other systems can affect the nervous system and vice versa.

Training in this field includes a one-year internship in internal medicine, followed by a three-year residency in neurology.

Obstetrics/gynecology

The fields of obstetrics and gynecology are closely related, and physicians generally practice these specialties together. While gynecology focuses on the diagnosis and treatment of a variety of disorders of the female reproductive system, obstetrics deals specifically with pregnancy, childbirth, and related conditions.

Many obstetricians are members of a group practice. Most obstetric groups make sure that every doctor in the group either has seen or is familiar with each patient during her pregnancy. Thus, when it comes time for delivery, the mother will generally be taken care of by a doctor whom she knows.

After medical school, an obstetrician/gynecologist completes a four-year residency. During this time, he or she also will receive some training in internal medicine, general surgery, and care of the newborn infant.

The obstetrician/gynecologist often acts as the primary caregiver for women. He or she also will work closely with other medical specialists if specific problems occur that do not directly involve the reproductive system.

Occupational medicine

Occupational medicine began with industrial and business clinics, which were usually staffed by a physician and an industrial nurse (one who has specialized in the care of patients within a working environment). Occupational medicine has grown to include the study, diagnosis, and treatment of a vast range of illnesses caused by the industrial environment itself. Asbestos-induced cancer, "black lung" (in which coal dust literally turns the inside of the lungs black), allergic reactions to industrial fibers, and injury to the feet from jobs that require standing are but a few of the hundreds of disorders treated by physicians that practice occupational medicine.

Specialists in occupational medicine generally have a strong background in internal medicine, with special training in the causes of industry-related illnesses. Often these doctors complete a public health program before going on to their specialty residency.

Oncology

Oncology is the study of tumors, particularly cancer. This relatively new field is often associated with hematology (the study of the blood). Strictly speaking, oncology deals only with solid tumors and not with cancers of the blood. Today, however, hematologist/oncologists are certified to deal with both types of cancer.

Oncology requires expertise in a large number of medical and technical disciplines, from surgery to nutrition, from immunology to biochemistry, from diagnosis of symptoms to the treatment of tumors with nuclear radiation.

There are subspecialties within the field of oncology. The medical oncologist primarily is responsible for prescribing and implementing chemotherapy, along with diagnosing and treating complications unique to cancer and coordinating the total treatment plan for cancer patients. Surgical oncologists perform cancer surgery. Pediatric oncologists diagnose and treat cancer in children. Gynecologic oncologists deal with cancer that occurs in the female reproductive system. Radiation oncology is concerned with the application of radiation in the treatment of cancer.

After graduating from medical school, a medical oncologist completes an internship and residency in internal medicine, followed by an additional training program in oncology, which includes training in hematology and chemotherapy. Surgical oncologists usually are general surgeons who have completed a fellowship in cancer surgery. Pediatric and gynecologic oncologists are first certified in their respective fields and then go on to oncology fellowships.

A specialist in radiation oncology must complete a one-year internship, either rotating among specialties or in internal medicine, followed by a three-year residency in the specialty.

Ophthalmology

An ophthalmologist is a doctor who diagnoses and treats diseases and injuries of the eyes. Most ophthalmologists are also eye surgeons. They perform a variety of operations, such as reattaching retinas, removing cataracts, relieving pressure caused by glaucoma, and repairing blood vessel ruptures and other injuries.

Ophthalmologists have a background in both internal medicine and surgery. This specialty requires an additional three- or four-year residency in ophthalmology after a one-year general internship before specialty board examinations may be taken.

There are allied health-care workers who are often referred to as "eye doctors" but who are not medical doctors and therefore are not permitted to treat diseases of the eyes or to prescribe medication. An optometrist tests the eyes for the purpose of fitting a person with glasses or contact lenses. An optician makes and fits glasses according to the ophthalmologist's or the optometrist's specifications. An ocularist performs the task of fitting artificial eyes.

Orthopedics

Orthopedics is the branch of surgery that is concerned with the diagnosis and treatment of disorders of the bones and joints. The orthopedist treats broken bones, disorders of the bones and joints that can be corrected surgically, and bone tumors, as well as other problems of the skeletal system. Because of his or her knowledge of the functioning of the musculoskeletal system, the ortho-

YOU AND YOUR DOCTOR

pedist often treats sports injuries and may serve as the physician for athletic teams.

The orthopedist is required to complete a one-year internship in general surgery, four years of training in orthopedic surgery, and a year of medical practice before taking specialty board examinations.

Otolaryngology

This specialty combines the study of the ear, nose, and throat into a single discipline commonly referred to as *ENT*.

The ears and throat are connected by the eustachian tubes, which lead from the middle ear to the throat. The nose leads directly into the part of the throat referred to as the *nasopharynx*. Inflammations of the nose may spread to the throat, and vice versa. Inflammations of the throat often spread through the eustachian tubes to the ears. Consequently, infection in any of these areas could result in infection in all of them.

Ear, nose, and throat specialists primarily are surgeons who perform such varied procedures as rhinoplasty (reconstructive nose surgery); removal of tumors from the oral, nasal, and neck areas; reconstructive ear surgery; and sinus surgery. Ear, nose, and throat specialists also

diagnose diseases of the head and neck, excluding the brain and eyes.

Ear, nose, and throat specialists must complete a one-year residency in general surgery and a four-year residency in otolaryngology.

Pathology

Pathology is the study of the changes in body tissues brought about by disease and the ways in which these changes provide clues not only to the causes of disease and death but also to ways in which the spread of disease may be checked.

There are a variety of subspecialties within pathology, including the following:

- Cellular pathology, in which cells are the focus of study
- Clinical pathology, in which laboratory methods are used to aid clinical diagnoses
- General pathology, which is the study of the processes that occur in various diseases
- Forensic pathology, in which the results of pathologic examinations (such as autopsies) are used as evidence in legal proceedings

Much of the pathologist's work is done with a microscope, preparing and examining biopsy specimens (tissue samples). Pathologists are charged with deciding whether a tissue specimen indicates the presence of a disease. They also perform autopsies to determine the cause or causes of death. The pathologist must be knowledgeable about both the cause and the course of disease processes.

Pathologists ordinarily do work in both internal medicine and surgery during their training. A strong laboratory background is a necessity, with extensive training in modern instrumentation. Three- to four-year residencies in pathology are required, depending on the subspecialty.

Pediatrics

Pediatricians often serve as primary care physicians for children; they specialize in the diagnosis and treatment of diseases of children from birth through adolescence. They administer the appropriate immunizations to prevent disease and watch for any abnormalities during the growth of the child. They also advise parents about the child's social and psychological needs.

After completion of medical school, pediatricians must have at least three years of training in general pediatrics. This is followed by an examination by the specialty board.

Peripheral vascular diseases

While cardiovascular surgeons treat disorders that affect the heart and its blood vessels specifically, surgeons who specialize in peripheral vascular diseases treat conditions that affect the rest of the circulatory system. Included among these conditions are

- Arteriosclerosis, in which the artery walls become abnormally thickened or hardened
- Arterial occlusion and embolism, in which undissolved material in the bloodstream (such as clumps of clotted blood or tissue fragments) blocks the flow of blood in the artery, causing a loss of blood to tissue beyond the blockade
- Carotid occlusive disease, in which the carotid arteries (the arteries in the neck that supply the brain with blood) become blocked
- Aortic or femoral artery occlusive disease, in which the aorta (the main artery going through the chest and abdomen) or one of the femoral arteries (the main arteries that carry blood to the legs) becomes blocked
- Pulmonary embolism, in which blood clots travel to the lungs

Specialists in peripheral vascular diseases can be internists with extensive cardiovascular training. For the most part, however, they are surgeons.

Physical medicine and rehabilitation

The field of physical medicine and rehabilitation is concerned with the diseases and disorders of the neuromuscular system (the nerves and muscles). Specialists in this field are skilled in using heat, cold, water, electricity, massage, and exercise to help patients regain use and function of parts of the body that have been damaged by stroke, severe arthritis, or other injury.

After completion of medical school, the physical medicine and rehabilitation specialist is required to complete at least three additional years of training, followed by two years of specialty practice. Specialty board examinations are required.

Podiatry

Podiatrists treat diseases and injuries of the feet. (Only recently have all the states recognized podiatry as a legitimate healing field.) Doctors in this area have degrees in podiatric medicine but not M.D. degrees and they have not attended medical school. Many podiatrists have

joined the ranks of sports medicine practitioners, since many foot injuries result from sports activities.

Some podiatrists are qualified to perform surgery on the feet when it is indicated. They also fit a variety of orthotic devices (inserted into shoes) to correct foot problems. The boom in jogging and walking for fitness has increased the demand for podiatric services.

Preventive medicine

Specialists in this relatively new field of medicine seek to prevent illnesses. In addition, preventive medicine is concerned with reviewing present health services and anticipating and planning to meet future medical needs. Physicians from every field have made contributions to preventive medicine. Practitioners range from immunologists (who seek to prevent illness with inoculations) to urban epidemiologists (who search out the causes of widespread illnesses, such as childhood lead poisoning, and try to alter the environment so that illnesses can be prevented).

Preventive medicine advocates often recommend regular or periodic physical examinations, prescribe certain regimens, and warn against toxic environments. Critics of the field claim that there are no safeguards against some types of illnesses. Advocates of the field point out that the same was said of infections before antibiotics.

Preventive medicine specialists complete at least three years of specialized training, one year of research or teaching, and examinations by their specialty board.

Psychiatry
A psychiatrist is a medical doctor—with the authority to prescribe medications and make medical decisions—who deals with mental disorders. (Psychologists do not have a medical degree and, therefore, cannot prescribe drugs.) Many psychiatrists use psychoanalysis as part of their therapeutic or diagnostic method, and all psychiatrists have intensive training in psychology.

There are four chief branches of psychiatry: (1) descriptive psychiatry, which is based on the observation of external factors that may be the cause of mental illness; (2) dynamic psychiatry, which is the study of the processes, origins, and mechanisms of emotional states; (3) forensic psychiatry, which deals with the legal aspects of mental

illness; and (4) orthomolecular psychiatry, which is the study of the molecular bases of mental illnesses. Areas such as psychopharmacology (the study of the effects of drugs on a person's emotional and mental state) and psychophysiology (the study of the physiology of mental illness) are offshoots of orthomolecular psychiatry.

Psychiatrists go through the usual medical sequence: medical school, internship, and residency. The psychiatrist may spend five years or more in specialized training in psychiatry and neurology.

Pulmonary medicine
This field deals with the study, diagnosis, and treatment of diseases and disorders of the lungs and related passageways. These diseases can include
- Lung cancer
- Tuberculosis
- Pneumonia (inflammation of the lungs)
- Bronchitis (inflammation of the passageways from the windpipe into the lungs)
- Tracheitis (inflammation of the windpipe)
- Pleurisy (inflammation of the lining of the lungs and the chest cavity)
- Emphysema (in which lung tissue is destroyed, causing air

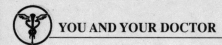

to become trapped within the lungs, often accompanied by severe breathing problems)

Specialists in pulmonary medicine also perform bronchoscopy (direct examination of the trachea and bronchial passages with a flexible, lighted, tubelike instrument) and specialize in managing ventilators (artificial breathing machines).

The pulmonary specialist's training is in internal medicine, followed by two years of specialized training in the diagnosis and treatment of pulmonary diseases and disorders.

Radiology/radiation oncology/nuclear medicine

A radiologist is a physician who uses X rays to diagnose and treat disorders. Radiologists have training in physics and instrumentation, as well as in biochemistry and the effects of radiation on human tissues.

Diagnostic radiology is primarily concerned with the administration of radiation to produce images of the body and the interpretation of the resultant X-ray films. Some procedures involve the injection of special dyes, called *contrast media*.

Other procedures also performed by radiologists use sound waves or magnetic impulses, rather than radiation, to create images.

A specialist in diagnostic radiology must complete a four-year residency in that field, which is often preceded by a year of internship in another medical field. Some diagnostic radiologists then subspecialize by completing a fellowship in a branch of radiology, such as neuroradiology (imaging of the nervous system) or uroradiology (imaging of the urinary tract).

Nuclear medicine is the field in which radioactive substances, called *isotopes,* are used to diagnose and treat diseases, such as an overactive thyroid gland. A nuclear medicine specialist must complete a three-year residency in diagnostic radiology in addition to a one-year residency in nuclear medicine.

Rheumatology

Rheumatology is the field of medicine concerned with the study, diagnosis, and medical treatment of diseases and disorders of bones, joints, and muscles. These disorders often are characterized by inflammation or degeneration and include such conditions as arthritis, gout, and other diseases of the connective tissue.

A rheumatologist has completed an internship and residency in internal medicine, followed by two or more years of training and experience in rheumatology.

Sports medicine
This is one of the newest fields in medicine and is largely a result of two factors: the training and rehabilitation needs of amateur and professional athletes and the tremendous growth in fitness and sports-related activities among the public. Doctors from a variety of fields now list themselves as sports medicine practitioners. Many of them have trained as orthopedists, since that specialty field is concerned with the mechanics of muscular and skeletal function. Orthopedists are surgeons and thus are qualified to diagnose and surgically treat many sports injuries. They also apply casts, splints, and many other aids. Since most sprains, fractures, and muscle strains do not require surgery, many nonsurgical physicians also practice sports medicine. Exercise physiology is an integral part of medical and sports training programs.

Sports medicine has made great contributions to the general public welfare by producing hard evidence of the benefits of healthful exercise. As a consequence, information about subjects such as nutrition, kinesiology (the study of body movement), and biomechanics (the study of lever systems and their effect on performance) has become available to the average weekend athlete.

Surgery
Surgery is the branch of medicine that uses surgical operations to treat disease, injury, or deformity. Surgeons go into the human body by way of incisions through the skin and muscles to alter, correct, remove, or replace the offending organ or tissue. The various surgical specialties include
• General surgery (including surgery of the abdomen)
• Thoracic (chest) surgery
• Cardiac (heart) surgery
• Oral (mouth) surgery
• Neurosurgery (surgery of the nervous system, particularly the brain and spinal cord)
• Plastic surgery (to correct damage caused by injury or to improve appearance)
• Orthopedic surgery (to correct disorders of the bones, joints, ligaments, and tendons)

Surgeons work closely with internists, pathologists, radiologists, anesthesiologists, and other specialists.

After the usual four years of medical school, surgeons complete a general surgery internship and a general surgery residency, followed by additional training in their specific field of surgery.

Urology

Urology deals with diseases and disorders of the kidneys, urinary tract, prostate gland, and male sex organs. (Gynecologic urology is a specialty that focuses on female problems such as incontinence.)

After completion of medical school, the urologist has two years of training in general surgery, followed by a three-year training period in urology and urologic surgery and an 18-month period of clinical practice before taking specialty board examinations.

A Note About Managed Care

The term "managed care" describes a more formally structured relationship between health care providers and patients. The concept offers more efficient service and lower cost.

At the heart of managed care is the relationship between the patient and the primary care physician, who provides immediate care for most medical situations and provides preventive care in the form of checkups and advice. The primary care physician also provides referrals to specialists and hospitals as necessary.

Managed care offers several advantages. First, because the patient always deals directly with the same doctor, his or her medical history is always up to date, and continuity of care is guaranteed. Second, the guesswork of choosing a specialist is removed; your primary care physician is your own referral service. Third, the preventive care that the primary care provider can give holds down the costs of providing medical service.

Certainly, managed care plans are not without their drawbacks. Much has been made about the limits such plans place on the patient's choice of doctors and facilities. There are trade-offs, but for most people, managed care may offer more effective health care at a lower cost.

INFECTIOUS DISEASES

The human body is both surrounded and inhabited by billions of microorganisms (living organisms that are so small that they can be seen only with a microscope). Most microorganisms are harmless or even beneficial; for example, bacteria that normally live in the digestive system help digest food. Occasionally, however, a microorganism capable of causing a disease invades the body. Diseases caused by such microorganisms are called *infectious diseases*.

Infectious diseases are contagious; that is, they can be passed from one person to another. They can be transmitted by skin contact, through body fluids, in contaminated food or drink, or via airborne particles containing the microorganisms. Animal or insect bites are another means of transmission. (If an insect, for example, bites an infected person, the insect can carry the microorganism and pass the disease by biting another person.) The two most common types of infectious diseases are bacterial infections and viral infections.

Disease-causing, or pathogenic, bacteria either attack the body's tissues directly or cause damage by secreting poisonous substances called toxins. Fortunately, bacterial infections frequently are curable. Certain bacteria can be killed by drugs; other bacterial diseases can be prevented by vaccination.

Viruses are the smallest known microorganisms. They are responsible for diseases as relatively harmless as the common cold and as serious as meningitis. Viruses live and reproduce only within living cells, and only certain cells are susceptible to a specific virus. You can be host to many viruses without suffering any adverse effects, but if enough cells are attacked, you will become sick.

There is no effective medical treatment for most viral infections. Because a virus lives inside a cell, any treatment designed to kill the virus is also likely to harm the cell. In addition, there are thousands of different viruses—each with different properties—and an agent effective against one virus probably will not affect the others. Although there are vaccinations for some viral diseases, therapy for most viral diseases is limited to treating the symptoms.

The body's defenses
Despite the prevalence of disease-causing microorganisms, the body is not defenseless against these invaders. The body fights infections in three ways: by preventing the organisms from entering the body, by attacking those that do manage to enter, and by inactivating those organisms it cannot kill. Sometimes, too, the body fights disease by developing defensive symptoms. Fever is an example. During an illness, the body's temperature regulator may respond to the illness by raising the body's temperature. Some researchers believe that this is an effective response because the microorganisms causing the disease may not be able to survive the higher body temperature.

The skin is the first barrier that guards the underlying tissues of the body. Where there are natural openings in the skin, there are also defenses. For example, tear glands in the eyes secrete and bathe the eyes with fluid that contains bacteria-fighting components. The salivary glands in the mouth and the tonsils in the throat help prevent microorganisms from attacking the mouth and throat. Many openings, as well as internal passages, in the body are lined with mucous membranes. These delicate layers produce mucus, a slippery secretion that moistens and protects by repelling or trapping microorganisms.

Internally, certain body organs fight infection. For instance, the liver and the spleen (a large glandlike organ located in the abdomen) filter out harmful substances from the blood flowing through them. The lining of the stomach produces acids that attack germs in food that has been eaten. The body's lymph system manufactures white blood cells, which attack and kill invading organisms.

The lymph system
The lymph system is a network of vessels that carry lymph, a watery fluid containing white blood cells, throughout the body. Lymph drains from the blood vessels and body tissues, carrying away waste products. The waste products are filtered out of the lymph by small struc-

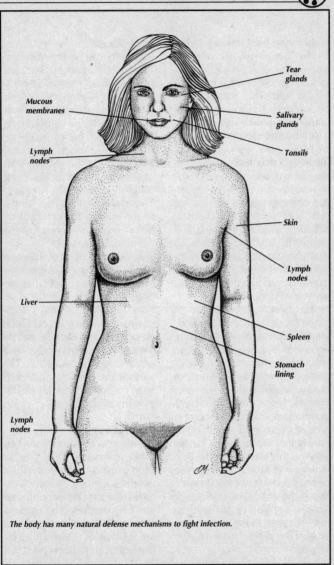

Tear
glands

Salivary
glands

Mucous
membranes

Tonsils

Lymph
nodes

Skin

Lymph
nodes

Liver

Spleen

Stomach
lining

Lymph
nodes

The body has many natural defense mechanisms to fight infection.

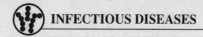

tures called *lymph nodes*. Within the lymph nodes, harmful microorganisms are trapped, attacked, and destroyed by white blood cells. This is one of the body's primary and most efficient lines of defense.

Antibodies are manufactured in the lymph system. Antibodies are protective substances that the body produces in response to invasion by a hostile organism or the presence of a foreign substance. Antibodies counteract some invading bacteria and viruses by inactivating them so that they are powerless. Antibodies that neutralize toxins (poisons) produced by bacteria are called *antitoxins*.

The body's production of white blood cells and antibodies in response to an invading organism is called the *immune reaction*. Immunity is the body's ability to resist an invasion of disease-causing bacteria and viruses. Once antibodies have been made to fight a certain type of microorganism, that microorganism usually no longer poses a threat to the body. That is why one attack of a disease often prevents its recurrence down the road. The first attack causes antibodies to be produced, and these antibodies protect the system against future attacks.

Immunization

Immunity can be provided artificially by vaccination and other forms of immunization. A vaccine is a preparation containing the offending organism—usually in a weakened form that will not cause the actual disease. When introduced into the body, the vaccine stimulates the body to produce antibodies against the disease. These antibodies often remain in the system for life, and the body is thus prepared to resist the actual disease.

A number of viral diseases can be prevented by immunization. There are vaccines for polio, measles, rubella (German measles), mumps, some strains of influenza, and chicken pox. A new vaccine against the organism *Hemophilus influenzae* also is available. This vaccine prevents the most common cause of bacterial meningitis in children.

Medications

Besides vaccination, there are other measures that can be used to help the body's natural defenses fight off infectious diseases. Bacterial infections often can be conquered by medications called antibiotics. These are substances derived from living microorganisms that kill

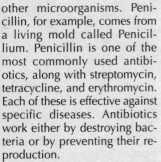

other microorganisms. Penicillin, for example, comes from a living mold called Penicillium. Penicillin is one of the most commonly used antibiotics, along with streptomycin, tetracycline, and erythromycin. Each of these is effective against specific diseases. Antibiotics work either by destroying bacteria or by preventing their reproduction.

Sulfonamides, or sulfa drugs, are synthetic antibiotic drugs that also are effective against infections. This type of drug often is prescribed for localized infections in the urinary tract.

Unfortunately, these medications do not attack viruses. Viruses, therefore, are responsible for many of the serious or fatal infectious illnesses today because no generally effective cures have been developed. The virus that causes acquired immunodeficiency syndrome (AIDS) is an example of a particularly lethal virus for which there is no cure.

Researchers are continually searching for new ways to help the body combat infectious diseases. Medical advances against these diseases have already been dramatic; not too many years ago infectious diseases were uncontrollable and thus a constant danger. The control of

many infections has been one of medicine's greatest accomplishments.

The more common infectious diseases are discussed in greater detail in the following pages.

AIDS

Acquired immunodeficiency syndrome (AIDS) is a disease in which the body's natural defense system is disabled, allowing organisms that are normally fought off to become deadly.

Causes

This disease, discovered in 1979, is caused by a microorganism called the human immunodeficiency virus (HIV). This virus is carried and transmitted in bodily fluids (mainly blood, semen, and vaginal secretions). Sexual intercourse (heterosexual or homosexual), use of nonsterile hypodermic needles (a common practice among drug addicts), and infected blood transfusions have all been implicated as a means of transmission. Transmission from a pregnant woman to her infant or from a mother to her nursing infant may also occur. An infected physician or dentist can infect a patient if proper precautions aren't taken.

In Western countries, prostitutes, people who inject drugs, and hemophiliacs who receive multiple blood transfusions for their disorder are all at high risk of developing AIDS. In Africa and Asia, heterosexual intercourse is apparently the most common route of transmission.

A widespread misconception has been that AIDS can be contracted by *giving* blood—this is not true. In addition, since the introduction of a blood screening test for use in blood banks and hospital laboratories, acquisition of HIV by *receiving* blood transfusions is now extremely unlikely.

Symptoms
Clinical illness from AIDS can have its onset as long as ten years after initial infection with the virus. Initial symptoms include low-grade fever, swollen lymph nodes, weight loss, fatigue, night sweats, and persistent diarrhea. (It is important to note that these symptoms can also be present in a large number of less serious illnesses.)

Because of impairment of the immune system, people with AIDS easily fall prey to many diseases, including various types of cancer, skin infections, fungal infections, and tuberculosis. About one third of people with AIDS develop a previously rare cancer known as Kaposi sarcoma, which often appears as purplish bumps on the skin. Many suffer *Pneumocystis carinii* pneumonia (a serious and often fatal lung infection).

Diagnosis
The blood of people with AIDS contains an abnormally small number of specialized white blood cells called lymphocytes. Lymphocytes play an important role in combating infectious diseases and may also be instrumental in destroying malignant growths in their early stages. There are two types of lymphocytes actively engaged in coping with infection: T cells, which directly kill invaders, and B cells, which are involved in the production of infection-fighting antibodies. The finding that people with AIDS have decreased numbers of T cells, particularly a subtype called helper T cells, has proved useful in diagnosis.

A person may be a carrier of the virus without being aware of the fact and without having any of the symptoms. For this reason, blood tests for the detection of antibodies to HIV have been developed. The implications of a positive blood test are controversial, however.

Although a positive blood test definitely indicates exposure to the virus, it is not known whether all individuals with positive test results will subsequently develop AIDS. Newborns whose mothers are infected with the virus will initially test positive for the antibody to HIV. However, in only about half of those infants will this positive test persist after 15 to 18 months of age, and these are the infants who may eventually develop the disease.

Treatment

No cure for AIDS has yet been found. The drug zidovudine (formerly called azidothymidine or AZT) acts by preventing replication of HIV in cells. In some studies, this drug has been shown to prolong survival and improve the quality of life for people with AIDS, but it cannot be considered a cure. New drugs are being studied as well—some to be used in combination with AZT.

Until a cure for AIDS is discovered, treatment is limited to countering the effects of the disease.

Prevention

Since there is no cure for AIDS, prevention is critical. Limiting the number of one's sexual partners and using condoms decrease the risk of sexual exposure to the AIDS virus. Avoiding contact with potentially contaminated hypodermic needles and with blood and blood products is also important.

If a person has tested positive for the presence of the HIV antibody, there are a number of precautions that should be taken to promote the effectiveness of the immune system and to prevent the possible spread of infection. Substances that will burden the immune system should be avoided. These include live-virus vaccines, such as those against measles, mumps, rubella, and polio; alcohol, tobacco products, and illicit drugs, such as marijuana and heroin; and possible sources of salmonella and other food-borne infections, such as unpasteurized milk and inadequately cooked meats. A physician may also recommend avoidance of immunosuppressive drugs, such as corticosteroids, some antibiotics, and certain anticancer drugs.

Among the activities that may increase risk of infections in a person with HIV infection are changing cat litter (cats transmit toxoplasmosis), cleaning bird cages (birds transmit histoplasmosis and psittacosis), sharing razor blades and toothbrushes,

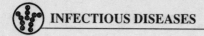

and engaging in sexual activity without a condom or with a partner who might transmit cytomegalovirus, Epstein-Barr virus, or syphilis. Pregnancy is also somewhat immunosuppressive. It is important that the immune system be bolstered by maintaining general health—the person should choose a balanced diet, get regular exercise and adequate rest, and avoid stress as much as possible.

Needless to say, the infected person should inform all sex partners and medical and dental personnel with whom he or she comes into contact and should not donate blood, sperm, organs, or body tissues.

Bacteria

Bacteria are one-celled microscopic organisms. Some kinds of bacteria cause disease in humans and animals, but many others are beneficial. Bacteria dispose of organic waste, enrich the soil, and are used to make wine, beer, vinegar, cheese, and yogurt. In human beings, certain beneficial bacteria live in the intestines, where they assist in digestion.

Bacteria are different from viruses in that they are able to multiply outside a living cell, whereas viruses can grow and multiply only in living cells. Bacteria are different from other causes of infection—protozoa (one-celled animals) and fungi (plantlike organisms)—in two ways: They have a primitive nucleus (center where genetic material is located), rather than a well-defined one with an enclosing membrane and chromosomes; and they reproduce simply by splitting in two (binary fission), rather than by means of the more complex process, called mitosis, that is seen in higher organisms.

Types

One way of classifying bacteria is by shape:

Rod-shaped bacteria are known as *bacilli*. They often have waving projections known as *flagella*, which they use to propel themselves. Some bacilli form thick-walled cells known as spores, which can survive for long periods even after the parent bacteria have been killed by freezing, disinfectants, or other forces. When conditions are favorable, the spores are able to generate new bacteria. Typhoid fever is caused by bacilli.

Round or egg-shaped bacteria are known as *cocci*. They occur singly (micrococci), in chains (streptococci—the cause

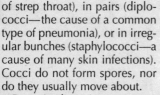

of strep throat), in pairs (diplo-cocci—the cause of a common type of pneumonia), or in irregular bunches (staphylococci—a cause of many skin infections). Cocci do not form spores, nor do they usually move about.

Bacteria also exist as comma-shaped organisms called *vibrios*—the organisms responsible for cholera. Spiral-shaped organisms are called *spirochetes*; one such organism causes syphilis.

Another way to classify bacteria is by whether they can live in the presence of air. Those that can are called *aerobic*; those that cannot are called *anaerobic*. Some can live either with or without air and are called *facultative anaerobes*. Tetanus (lockjaw) is an example of a disease caused by anaerobic bacteria that are commonly found in the soil. They pose no danger to humans unless they enter the body through a wound, particularly a puncture wound (such as one made by a nail). The air then cannot get to the organisms to destroy them, and so they multiply within the body, unless the infected person has been vaccinated against tetanus.

How bacteria are transmitted

Disease-causing bacteria enter the body in many different ways. Those that cause pneumonia and sore throat are carried in droplets that an infected person sneezes or coughs into the air. The bacteria are then inhaled and deposited on the mucous membranes of the throat or lungs of a healthy person, where they multiply and eventually cause disease, unless checked by the body's immune system. The bacteria that cause intestinal diseases like cholera and typhoid can be transmitted in foods that have been handled by an infected person or in water tainted by body wastes from an infected individual. Another important route for infection is any break in the skin, which is why it is important to clean cuts as soon as possible.

Bacteria and the body

Once inside the body, bacteria do their damage in two main ways: by direct destruction of tissue and by producing toxins. Certain white blood cells, known as *lymphocytes*, produce antitoxins (which neutralize the toxins of the bacteria) and antibodies (which destroy the invading bacteria themselves). Once created, the antibodies against a specific disease can persist in the body or be reproduced when needed, providing continuous immunity—sometimes for

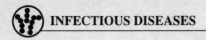

life. Still other white blood cells, known as *phagocytes*, entrap and destroy bacteria.

Candida albicans

Candida albicans is a fungus that is normally present on the skin and on membranes of the mouth, throat, intestines, and vagina. *Candida albicans* becomes an infecting agent only when there is some change in the body environment that allows the fungus to grow out of control.

Causes
The most common cause of infection may be the use of antibiotics that destroy beneficial as well as harmful microorganisms in the body and permit *Candida* organisms to multiply in their place. The resulting condition is known as *candidiasis, candidosis, moniliasis*, or a "yeast" infection. In the mouth, a yeast infection is known as thrush; on the skin, its appearance resembles that of a rash (such as diaper rash); in the vagina, it is vaginitis, moniliasis, or yeast infection; and in or next to the nails, candidal onychomycosis or paronychia, respectively. Candidal infection can also affect the esophagus

(food tube) and the digestive tract. When body resistance is low, *Candida albicans* can enter the bloodstream and causes infection of the vital organs.

Those at risk
Drug addicts, people with diabetes or HIV infection, and patients receiving chemotherapy are especially at risk of developing a yeast infection. Also at risk are those whose natural defenses are weakened by drugs used to suppress the immune system (such as recipients of organ transplants and asthmatics who are taking corticosteroid drugs).

Pregnant women are often susceptible to moniliasis, and thrush may develop in babies who passed through an infected birth canal. As a result, breast-feeding mothers may also contract a yeast infection of the nipples. If left untreated, she and her infant can pass the infection back and forth. Babies may also contract a yeast infection of the diaper area because of the constant wetness.

Symptoms and treatment
The symptoms and treatment for the various forms of *Candida* infection are as follows:
• Vaginitis is characterized by a white or yellow discharge,

with inflammation of the walls of the vagina and of the vulva (external genital area). A white, curdlike substance may cling to the walls of the vagina. Treatment is with an antifungal drug, such as nystatin, which is inserted deep in the vagina and, if necessary, applied to the entire region around the entrance to the vagina. The infection is often passed to the woman's sexual partner, causing irritation, redness, and soreness of the head of the penis. Recurrent *Candida* vaginitis or vaginitis that does not respond to treatment may indicate that another illness, such as diabetes, is present or that a different microorganism is responsible for the infection.

• Thrush appears as creamy-white or bluish-white patches on the tongue (which is inflamed and sometimes beefy red), on the lining of the mouth, or in the throat. This is especially common in young infants. Treatment is usually with nystatin oral solution or drops.

• Diaper rash caused by *Candida* infection can be treated by keeping the baby as dry as possible by frequent diaper changes. An antifungal ointment may be prescribed.

• Infections of the fingernails and toenails appear as red, painful swelling around the nail; later, pus develops. After the area has been treated with hot compresses and drainage (if necessary), and the nail has been cut back, an antifungal lotion is applied. The nail itself may be involved (appearing hard, yellow, and dull), making treatment more difficult and perhaps necessitating long-term use of oral drugs. Newer oral drugs, such as fluconazole, are reserved for treatment of more severe or resistant infections.

• Systemic infection (infection that enters the bloodstream and affects the kidneys, heart, lungs, eyes, or other organs) can result in high fever, chills, anemia, and sometimes a rash or shock. Disease in the lungs can cause bloody sputum; in the kidneys, blood in the urine; in the brain, seizures; in the heart, murmurs and valve damage; and in the eye, pain and blurred vision. An antifungal medicine is usually given intravenously.

In all cases, the underlying condition that caused the outbreak of *Candida* infection must be removed. This may mean stopping the use of antibiotics or controlling conditions such as diabetes. The

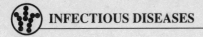

same approach is used to prevent future infections.

Chicken pox

Chicken pox is an extremely contagious disease that is characterized by a blistery rash. It occurs most frequently in children between the ages of five and eight; less than 20 percent of the cases in the United States affect people over 15 years old. Chicken pox is transmitted so easily that almost everyone gets the disease at some time.

Causes
Chicken pox is caused by infection with the varicella zoster virus.

Chicken pox is contracted by touching an infected person's blisters or anything that has been contaminated by contact with them. The virus is also thought by some researchers to be airborne, since an infected person can transmit it before the rash develops. Another way to get chicken pox is by exposure to shingles, which is a localized rash caused by the same virus.

The incubation period (the time between exposure to the virus and the appearance of symptoms) of chicken pox is 10 to 21 days. It is contagious for about six to eight days after the rash appears or until all of the blisters have dried out.

Symptoms
The first symptom of chicken pox is usually a rash, which can be very itchy. It begins as small, red spots on the trunk. Within hours, the spots become larger, fluid-filled blisters on a red base that begin to spread out from the trunk to the face, scalp, arms, and legs. Over the next few days, the blisters continue to fill with pus, burst, and then form a scab or crust. New spots appear periodically during a two- to six-day period. They may spread to the soles and palms. The rash may even affect the eyes, mouth, throat, vagina, and rectum.

Another main symptom is a mild fever (101°F to 103°F) that rises and disappears as the rash comes and goes. Some children have a slight fever and feel sluggish a few days before the rash begins; however, this warning is more common in adults.

Adults usually have higher fevers, a more severe rash, headaches, and muscle aches, and they take longer to recuperate than children. Recovery from all symptoms takes ten days to two weeks.

Complications

Complications of chicken pox seldom develop in otherwise healthy people. The most common complication is bacterial infection of the blisters, which can occur if a blister is scratched and the skin is broken. In some instances, the rash spreads to the eyes, causing pain and possible damage. Generally, the chicken pox rash heals without leaving scars, unless the blisters have been scratched and become infected.

Treatment

Since there is no known cure for chicken pox, treatment consists of reducing the effects of the symptoms. A soothing lotion, such as calamine lotion, lessens itchiness. Baths in warm (not hot) water sometimes mixed with a special oatmeal solution keep the skin clean, reduce the risk of infection in the rash, and reduce itching. It is important to gently yet thoroughly dry the skin after bathing. If itching is severe, fingernails should be trimmed and gloves should be worn at night to minimize scratching. Children may need to wear mittens and socks all day for the duration of the rash.

Since an association has been established between aspirin use during a viral infection and Reye syndrome in children, it is recommended that aspirin not be given to a child or teenager with chicken pox. A doctor can suggest an aspirin substitute if needed for discomfort or fever.

Prevention

Although almost everyone contracts chicken pox once, most people do not get it again because the body manufactures antibodies to combat the virus. Nevertheless, the same virus may cause shingles later in life.

The American Academy of Pediatrics recommends the varicella (chicken pox) vaccine for all children, adolescents, and young adults who have not already been infected with chicken pox. A single dose should routinely be given between 12 and 18 months of age. This immunization can be given at the same time as the child's first MMR (measles, mumps, rubella) vaccination. Older children may be immunized at the earliest convenient opportunity, also with a single dose. Individuals over the age of 13 who have not been immunized previously and have no history of varicella infection should receive two doses of the vaccine four to eight weeks apart. Once immunized, most

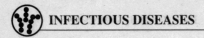

individuals are protected from chicken pox for life.

Diphtheria

Diphtheria is a sudden, severe, and highly contagious disease that primarily affects the tonsils, upper airways, and larynx (voice box). Diphtheria bacteria destroy the outer layer of the mucous membrane of the throat or larynx; the slush of dead cells, bacteria, and white blood cells that remains forms the grayish membrane covering the tonsils and throat that is the chief sign of the disease. Complications may include inflammation of the heart muscle (myocarditis), which sometimes results in heart failure, and temporary neuritis (nerve inflammation).

Cause

Diphtheria is caused by the bacteria known as *Corynebacterium diphtheriae*, which are transmitted via droplets of moisture from the throat and nose of an infected person. The infection is most common during the colder months, when schools are in session and people are in closer contact. The bacteria can be transmitted by carriers—people who have no symptoms

and do not even know that they harbor the disease. The incubation period (the time between exposure to the bacteria and appearance of the first symptom) is one to seven days.

Symptoms

Early symptoms include a mild sore throat, hoarseness, a rasping croupy cough, pain when swallowing, and a mild fever. Children may experience nausea, vomiting, chills, headache, and fever. The membrane that forms typically is tough, adheres tightly, and causes bleeding if removed. It appears in patches and can vary from yellowish to grayish green or dirty gray (the most common color). Some people have little or no characteristic membrane. If the membrane extends from the throat to the trachea (windpipe), larynx, or bronchi (air tubes in the lungs), it can become detached and obstruct the passage partially or completely, choking off the air supply. Signs of this life-threatening emergency are rapid breathing, high-pitched breathing sounds, and blue lips and fingertips. Narrowing of the air passage may also be caused by edema (swelling of fluid-filled tissue) of the lining of the larynx and throat.

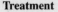

Treatment

Treatment is with diphtheria antitoxin (a solution of refined and concentrated protective antibodies obtained from the blood of horses that have been immunized against the poisons created by the diphtheria bacteria). The treatment should be given at once, after a skin test to determine that the patient is not allergic to horse serum. (A patient who is found to be allergic is desensitized with a series of diluted doses of the antitoxin.) After the antitoxin has been administered, antibiotics, such as penicillin or erythromycin, are given for at least a week to eliminate the diphtheria organisms. The patient is isolated until two cultures obtained 24 hours apart indicate that the infection is gone.

Because of the possible severe or even fatal complications of diphtheria, patients with symptoms need to be placed in a hospital intensive care unit for complete rest and careful observation. If signs of airway obstruction occur, a tracheotomy (surgical creation of a hole in the neck) is performed immediately so that a tube can be passed into the lungs to supply oxygen. Frequent checking of the heart and nervous system is needed to identify complications. In severe cases, these can include heart irregularities, cardiac arrest (heart stoppage), and nervous system disorders, such as swallowing difficulty caused by paralysis of swallowing muscles.

Those who have been in close contact with the patient and who have not been immunized should receive throat cultures and be immunized with vaccine. These people should be watched carefully for the development of symptoms and be given antitoxin should symptoms occur. Another approach is to give antitoxin immediately (after allergy has been ruled out). In people who have been immunized, a booster of vaccine will be sufficient. Cultures of the nose, throat, and any open wounds should be obtained from all contacts of patients with diphtheria. Carriers of diphtheria should be given seven to ten days of treatment with an appropriate antibiotic (usually erythromycin). If the organism is still present, another course of drug therapy should be given. If this fails, tonsillectomy may be needed.

Prevention

Fortunately, widespread immunization has made diphtheria a rare disease. To maintain this status, children should be immunized beginning in infancy. The diphtheria vaccine is usually given in combination with the vaccines against tetanus and pertussis (whooping cough)— the DTP immunization. After age 20, adults should receive the diphtheria tetanus booster every 10 years.

Enteroviral infections

The enteroviruses are a group of viruses that cause a wide variety of usually brief, but occasionally serious, illnesses that are particularly common in children. Included in the group are the coxsackieviruses, the echoviruses, and the polioviruses.

Enteroviral infections occur most often in the summer and fall and can be spread by contact with infected human feces or respiratory secretions. Although they produce a great deal of temporary discomfort, most of the enteroviral infections generally do not cause lasting illness. Often, the only treatment possible is to make the patient comfortable, with plenty of liquids, bed rest, lukewarm sponge baths, and non-aspirin pain relievers to control fever until the illness has run its course. Careful hand washing and proper disposal of human wastes can help prevent the spread of infection.

The following diseases are among those caused by the enteroviruses.

Aseptic meningitis
This inflammation of the membrane covering the brain causes headache, pain and stiffness in the neck and back, fever, nausea, vomiting, drowsiness, and a general sick feeling. Most patients recover from aseptic meningitis in a week or so, but the disease may be fatal for newborns.

Hand, foot, and mouth disease
In this disease, which is common in young children, little blisters erupt all over the mucous membranes in the mouth, on the hands and feet (including the palms and soles), and sometimes in the diaper area. A low-grade fever is also somewhat common.

Herpangina
An epidemic disease in infants and young children, herpangina is marked by sudden high fever, headache, sore throat, vomiting, and the appearance

of grayish spots on the soft palate (rear roof of the mouth), tonsils, or throat. The spots become shallow ulcers and heal in three to six days.

Myocarditis and pericarditis
Possibly fatal heart failure in newborns may result from myocarditis (inflammation of the heart muscle) caused by coxsackieviruses or echoviruses transmitted to the baby by the mother. Myocarditis and pericarditis (inflammation of the sac around the heart) in older children and in adults may also be caused by a coxsackievirus; patients usually make a complete recovery, although congestive heart failure can occur.

Paralytic disease
Various echoviruses, coxsackieviruses, and polioviruses produce muscle weakness or paralysis that is similar to the paralysis of poliomyelitis and is treated in the same manner.

Pleurodynia
Sudden, recurrent pains in the lower chest or abdomen signal the onset of this illness, which is often accompanied by fever, headache, nausea, abdominal tenderness, and sore throat. The disease may spread to cause pleuritis (inflammation of the membrane sac surrounding the lungs and the lining of the chest cavity), pericarditis, or aseptic meningitis.

Poliomyelitis
Poliomyelitis (also known as *polio* and *infantile paralysis*), caused by the three types of polioviruses, is a serious infection of the spinal cord, which can result in paralysis of all of the muscles. The symptoms of poliomyelitis include muscle soreness and stiffness of the neck and spine.

With the development of the polio vaccine, polio has been virtually eradicated in the United States, but the threat remains if children are not routinely immunized.

Respiratory disease
The enteroviruses can cause respiratory illnesses accompanied by head cold, fever, sore throat, and sometimes vomiting and diarrhea.

Rubellalike rash
A mild rash like that of rubella (German measles), but lasting longer, usually occurs in epidemic form and only on the face, neck, and chest. Fever is common, and meningitis can develop, but usually this is a mild disease.

Hepatitis

Hepatitis is an inflammation of the liver, usually caused by a viral infection, which is characterized by jaundice (yellowing of the skin and whites of the eyes).

Causes and types

The disease is caused by several viruses, but the most common are those that cause hepatitis A (infectious hepatitis), hepatitis B (serum hepatitis), and hepatitis C (non-A, non-B hepatitis).

Hepatitis A is transmitted from person to person via contaminated food or water or contact with the stools of an infected person. This disease may occur in epidemics where sanitation is poor and the water supply is contaminated. The incubation period (the time between exposure and the appearance of symptoms) is between 14 and 40 days. Sometimes, hepatitis A is so mild that symptoms never appear, but the infected person can still be a carrier and can transmit the disease to others.

In hepatitis B, the virus enters the bloodstream through contact with contaminated blood or other body fluids, such as semen, or with stool or through the use of contaminated hypodermic needles. Hepatitis B begins more gradually than does hepatitis A, so the disease may be present 40 to 180 days before the onset of symptoms. Because the virus can live in almost all body fluids, including saliva, semen, stool, and tears, hepatitis B can be transmitted by sexual contact or, rarely, by casual contact.

Hepatitis C virus is presumed to be a major cause of what was previously known as "non-A, non-B hepatitis." The incubation period of the virus is somewhere between that of A and B, and its mode of transmission is similar to B. It's the most common cause of post-transfusion hepatitis.

Chronic hepatitis is a condition of persistent (more than six months) inflammation of the liver. It is most frequently due to infection with hepatitis B or C virus. Although some forms of chronic hepatitis can be mild, others can lead to severe liver damage and cirrhosis. Cirrhosis is a condition where the liver is so scarred and distorted that it is no longer able to perform its functions normally. The diagnosis of chronic hepatitis is usually confirmed by liver biopsy. In this procedure, a local anesthetic is injected into the right upper abdomen. A thin needle is inserted into the liver, and a

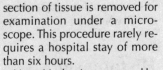
section of tissue is removed for examination under a microscope. This procedure rarely requires a hospital stay of more than six hours.

Hepatitis that is not caused by any of the above viruses can be associated with mononucleosis and other viral illnesses as well as side effects of certain medications.

Symptoms

Early signs of hepatitis include general fatigue, joint and muscle pain, and loss of appetite. Nausea, vomiting, and diarrhea or constipation may follow, with a low-grade fever of 101°F or less. As the disease develops, the liver enlarges and becomes tender. Chills, weight loss, and a change in taste sensations appear along with the characteristic jaundice. Jaundice results from an accumulation of yellow bile pigment in the blood, which turns the skin and whites of the eyes yellow.

In hepatitis A, the disappearance of jaundice generally signals the beginning of recovery. However, in hepatitis B or C, the virus may persist for years or even a lifetime.

Diagnosis

To determine the extent and severity of hepatitis, a physician analyzes blood specimens from the patient. Usually, over the course of several weeks, the liver function tests (blood tests sometimes called *liver enzymes*) return to normal. Most individuals recover completely and are immune to reinfection with the particular virus they had.

Treatment

There is no cure for viral hepatitis, and treatment is limited, especially for acute hepatitis. Once the virus attacks, recovery is usually up to the body's natural defense mechanisms.

To encourage the healing process, physicians advise patients to avoid strenuous activity. Bed rest is important during the acute phase of hepatitis. More serious cases may require hospitalization to ensure adequate nutrition.

All hepatitis patients must avoid alcoholic beverages, because processing alcohol puts a tremendous strain on the liver. All drugs taken, including over-the-counter preparations, must first be approved by the physician, because the liver is responsible for clearing most drugs from the body. Inflammation of the liver may lessen its ability to do this and thus lead to increased levels of the drugs in the body, which can cause

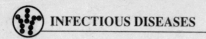

toxic effects. The treatment of chronic hepatitis depends on its form and severity.

Prevention

Persons exposed to hepatitis A or traveling to areas in which it is common will probably benefit from an injection of gamma globulin. This substance contains antibodies to the virus. Although it will not cure the disease, it can prevent it from occurring in an exposed individual, or it can minimize the severity of the symptoms in an infected person. A vaccine is also available, but it must be administered at least two weeks before travel begins.

Hepatitis B can be effectively prevented by a vaccine as well. A special type of globulin with a high concentration of hepatitis B antibody may be used in conjunction with the vaccine in acute exposures such as a needle stick from an infected person, in the hope of preventing or mitigating the illness. The vaccine consists of three injections: right away, one month later, and six months later. The hepatitis B vaccine is recommended for all individuals at high risk of hepatitis, and recently, the vaccine has been recommended for all children as well. There is, as yet, no vaccine available for the prevention of hepatitis C.

Histoplasmosis

Most common in the midwestern United States, histoplasmosis is an infection that follows the inhalation of spores from the fungus *Histoplasma capsulatum*. The parts of the body principally affected are the lungs, the liver, and the spleen.

Cause

The *Histoplasma capsulatum* spore is found in soil and in the air. There is no practical defense against breathing the spores. Development of symptoms seems to be a matter of individual immune system response.

Symptoms

In most instances, histoplasmosis does not reach the point at which symptoms appear. People may have the disease but, because of the action of their immune system, never have enough damage to make the symptoms noticeable. However, if symptoms do appear, they can be serious, especially when left untreated. The most common symptoms are
• Acute pneumonia (inflammation of the lungs)

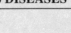
- Influenzalike illnesses, with lethargy, cough, fever, and lung involvement
- Enlargement of the liver and the spleen, with accompanying interruption of normal function
- The development of fibrous scar tissue in affected organs, particularly the lungs

Histoplasmosis can become inactive and then be reactivated at a later date. In cases of reactivated histoplasmosis, the lungs, meninges (covering of the brain and spinal cord), heart, peritoneum (lining of the abdominal cavity), and adrenal glands can be involved.

Diagnosis

Treatment for histoplasmosis begins with diagnosis. The best procedure is to cultivate growths of *Histoplasma capsulatum* organisms from tissue or fluid samples. Another method is to note the rise in the body's production of antibodies (the protective substances produced by the body).

Treatment

An antifungal medication, such as ketoconazole or amphotericin B, is usually used to treat chronic cases. These drugs help control the disease but appear to have little effect on the fibrous scarring that often occurs in advanced cases.

Influenza

Influenza, more commonly called the *flu*, is a contagious disease that is accompanied by respiratory problems and fever.

Causes

Two types of viruses cause influenza: influenza A virus and influenza B virus. Each type encompasses several different strains, which are named for the place where they were first identified (for example, Hong Kong flu virus and Russian flu virus).

The unusual characteristic of the flu viruses is that once a strain has spread throughout a population, it changes in structure, becoming capable of causing a new form of influenza. The antibodies produced by the body to combat the virus are no longer effective because the virus has taken on different qualities. Scientists are generally able to predict what type of altered virus to expect each year, but about every ten years an entirely new strain of the virus appears.

Because influenza is thought to be transmitted by airborne

particles from an infected person's respiratory tract, large numbers of people can easily contract the disease in a short period of time. Overcrowded living conditions promote the transmission of the virus. Since the flu spreads most easily when temperatures and humidity are low, most cases of influenza occur in the fall and winter.

Symptoms

Flu symptoms usually develop one to three days after exposure to the virus. Some people experience symptoms in as short a time as 18 hours. Fever, chills, headache, muscle aches, and total exhaustion can occur suddenly. Fevers generally do not exceed 104°F, but they can rise to 106°F.

Frequently, people experience a dry cough and a runny or congested nose as their initial symptoms begin to subside. These respiratory symptoms worsen and remain for three to four days. The cough and fatigue may persist for two weeks or more after the other symptoms have disappeared.

Complications

The most common complications of the flu are those that involve parts of the respiratory system—for example, pneumonia (infection of the lungs), which affects both adults and children, and croup (infection of the larynx), which affects young children. If the patient has extreme difficulty breathing, blood in coughed-up mucus, bluish skin, or a bark-like cough, a physician should be consulted immediately.

One life-threatening complication of influenza that affects children and adolescents between the ages of 2 and 16 years is Reye syndrome. It is a type of encephalitis (inflammation of the brain) that is accompanied by deterioration of the liver.

Treatment

In most cases, influenza cannot be cured and is treated only by relieving symptoms. Amantadine, a drug used in the treatment of Parkinson disease, can be used to prevent and ameliorate some forms of influenza A infection. This drug can produce serious side effects, however, so physicians usually prescribe it only when a patient is susceptible to additional complications or during a severe epidemic.

Treatment for flu is generally the same as treatment for a bad cold or fever. Physicians recommend bed rest, extra fluids, and an aspirin substitute to reduce fever and muscle aches. Because an association has been established between aspirin use during a viral infection and Reye syndrome in children, it is recommended that aspirin not be given to a child with influenza. Acetaminophen, however, has not been linked to Reye syndrome and can be used.

Nasal sprays or drops (when used sparingly so that nasal tissues are not damaged) and cough medicines can help relieve coldlike symptoms. Using a vaporizer in the patient's room to add moisture to the air relieves congestion.

Prevention

Each year, researchers prepare an influenza vaccine in an attempt to prevent spread of the virus. The vaccine is composed of inactivated organisms from several virus strains and provides protection against influenza caused by these strains. Unfortunately, protection is not necessarily afforded against new or different strains. Vaccines are typically between 67 and 92 percent effective. It is important for the elderly; people with lung disease, heart disease, or other chronic diseases; and those with immune system disorders to have this vaccine. Influenza can be devastating in these individuals.

Some people have reactions to the vaccine that range from inflammation at the injection site to mild flu symptoms. On very rare occasions, nervous system disorders result.

Influenza vaccines are commonly prepared using eggs. Therefore, individuals with known allergies to eggs should inform their physician before receiving the vaccine. Influenza vaccination is not usually recommended or necessary for children or young adults.

Measles

Measles (also called *rubeola*) is a contagious disease that mainly affects the respiratory system, skin, and eyes. It was once considered one of the more dangerous childhood diseases because the threat of serious complications was so great. Development of a vaccine to prevent measles has drastically reduced its occurrence.

Causes

Measles is caused by a virus. The virus is transmitted via droplets of moisture from the

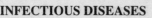

respiratory tract of an infected person that travel through the air. Some researchers contend that the virus enters the body through the eyes.

The incubation period (the time between being exposed to the infectious organism and actually showing symptoms) for measles is 8 to 12 days. An infected person is considered contagious for up to four days before symptoms appear and for up to six days after the rash develops.

Symptoms

Measles usually begins much like a cold, with a runny nose, nasal congestion, sneezing, a dry cough, and a fever of 102°F to 104°F. After three or four days, the eyes may become red and swollen and sensitive to bright light. The fever drops, and red spots with tiny white centers (called *Koplik spots* after the physician who first identified them) appear in the cheek pouches of the mouth.

By the fourth or fifth day, the fever increases again, and a rash appears. The rash usually starts on the face and neck and behind the ears, and then spreads to the rest of the body. As the spots multiply, they grow larger, become raised, and sometimes blend together. They turn dark red and then brown before the skin begins to peel in small flakes. This process takes about one week after the rash first emerges, although skin discoloration can last as long as two weeks. Other symptoms usually disappear within seven to ten days after the appearance of the first symptoms.

Complications

Breathing problems, increased coughing, earache, or extreme drowsiness may indicate complications that warrant consulting a doctor immediately.

The more serious complications are pneumonia (inflammation of the lungs) and encephalitis (inflammation of the brain). Subacute sclerosing panencephalitis, a rare but often fatal brain disease, has also been linked to measles. Severe ear infections can occur, particularly in young children. Bronchitis, laryngitis, and swelling of the lymph nodes in the neck can prolong the course of the illness.

Diagnosis

Generally, physicians diagnose measles by the initial symptoms. To confirm diagnosis, nasal discharge, blood, or urine can be tested for signs of the virus.

Treatment

Since measles is caused by a virus, it does not respond to antibiotics, and treatment must focus on relieving the patient's discomfort. A vaporizer in the patient's room will ease cold-like symptoms by adding moisture to the air. If the eyes are irritated, warm compresses may relieve the inflammation. Also, dim lights are easier on the eyes. Soaps that irritate the skin should not be used. The doctor may suggest adding baking soda to bath water or applying a soothing lotion, such as calamine lotion, to the rash to help relieve itching.

An association has been established between aspirin use during or immediately after a viral infection and Reye syndrome (inflammation of the brain accompanied by deterioration of the liver). It is recommended that aspirin not be given to a child with measles. A doctor can suggest an aspirin substitute, such as acetaminophen, for relief of discomfort or fever.

Prevention

Until recently, measles had been almost eliminated through childhood immunization. Unfortunately, over the last few years, the number of measles cases in the United States has increased dramatically due to low rates of immunization. This new epidemic tends to occur in young children and older adolescents. The newest recommendation is that children receive the initial measles vaccine by injection at 15 months of age; a measles booster vaccine should be given at 11 or 12 years of age. If a measles outbreak occurs, anyone between 4 years and 21 years of age should receive a measles booster. If measles or vaccine history is unknown in an adult, it is best to check with your doctor. Blood tests that can show immunity to the disease are available. The vaccine, which is prepared from measles virus, stimulates production of antibodies (protective substances) in the body. Because the vaccine effectiveness rate is very low in young infants, babies are not vaccinated before 15 months of age unless measles cases have been reported in the area. The infants of women who are immune to measles (either because they have had measles or have been immunized against it) acquire temporary natural immunity that lasts for about the first six months of life. If a baby is exposed to measles, however, a doctor should be consulted. Measles is dangerous for anyone under three years of age and for anyone with a chronic (long-term) illness.

Mononucleosis

Infectious mononucleosis, or "mono," is a contagious viral illness that initially attacks the lymph nodes in the neck and the throat. When these tissues become less effective in fighting infection, sore throat, swelling of the lymph nodes, and fever result.

Cause

Mono is caused by the Epstein-Barr virus, which is named after the scientists who first identified it in the mid-1960s. The virus enters the lymph nodes and attacks the lymphocytes (the white blood cells manufactured there). As the white blood cells come into contact with the virus, they change shape and multiply. At first there are no symptoms, because it takes several weeks before enough of the altered cells can accumulate to generate a reaction. Gradually, however, symptoms appear. First, there is a mild sore throat, sluggishness, and fever. The symptoms worsen as the body tries to fight the infection by creating more white blood cells. The symptoms usually disappear about six to eight weeks later.

Mono spreads by contact with moisture from the mouth and throat of an infected person. Kissing, sharing drinking glasses, or touching anything that has been near the mouth of an infected person may result in transmission of the disease.

Those at risk

Teenagers and young adults seem most susceptible to mono. However, even children less than one year old can contract mono. The disease is uncommon in persons over the age of 35.

Symptoms

In all cases, the infection develops so slowly with such mild symptoms that it may be initially indistinguishable from a cold or the flu. However, a sore throat that lasts two weeks or more; swollen lymph nodes in the neck, throat, armpits, and groin; a persistent fever (usually about 102°F); and tiredness and malaise (a vague feeling of discomfort) may indicate mono. Mono symptoms can be so severe that throat pain impedes swallowing and fever reaches

105°F. Some people also experience a rash, eye pain, and discomfort in bright light.

Complications

Most cases of mono run an uncomplicated course. Occasionally, however, the infection spreads to other parts of the body besides the throat and lymph nodes. For example, mono may lead to monohepatitis (an inflammation of the liver that is not the same as hepatitis A, B, or non-A, non-B). Jaundice, a symptom of this complication, appears as a yellow discoloration of the skin and whites of the eyes. A much more serious problem is pain or tenderness in the abdomen. This discomfort may mean a swollen spleen (an organ in the lymph system), which could burst. Any of these symptoms should be reported to a physician for immediate medical attention.

Diagnosis

To diagnose infectious mononucleosis, blood samples are analyzed to detect the presence of antibodies to the Epstein-Barr virus and to determine overall blood cell count. Inflammation of the liver can also be detected and followed up with blood tests.

Treatment

As long as there are no complications, the best treatment for mononucleosis is to rest, drink plenty of liquids until the temperature returns to normal, and then gradually resume normal activities as strength returns. If the patient feels well enough, complete bed rest is probably not necessary.

Antibiotics are ineffective against mono, since it is a viral infection and viruses do not respond to antibiotics. However, mono can be accompanied by a streptococcal infection of the throat, in which case an antibiotic will be prescribed to treat that condition. In severe cases, corticosteroid drugs that reduce swelling of the throat are prescribed. If the spleen is swollen, the doctor may recommend avoiding strenuous activities, such as lifting and pushing, that can cause sudden rupture of the spleen. Hospitalization is necessary if a serious complication, such as rupture of the spleen, occurs.

Most people recover in six to eight weeks, but some cases take as long as six months for complete recovery. A tired feeling, which may include depression, is the last symptom to disappear. Mono may return in a milder form within a few

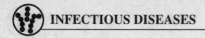

months. Fortunately, mononucleosis almost never reappears in its full-blown form after a year.

Mumps

Mumps is a contagious viral disease that is usually contracted during childhood. More than 85 percent of the cases occur before the age of 15, most often between the ages of 6 and 10 years.

Cause
Mumps is caused by a virus that attacks cells of the parotid salivary glands. This invasion results in painful swelling of the face beneath the ear along the jawline. Mumps virus spreads by contact with airborne moisture from an infected person's nose or throat. Sometimes, the infection comes from someone who has the disease without symptoms or who is not yet aware of the symptoms. The disease occurs most often during the spring months, although it can happen at any time of the year.

Symptoms
Symptoms can be so mild that they are almost nonexistent, or they can be very severe. Fever (101°F to 103°F), headache, and loss of appetite usually develop first, followed by earache; then the characteristic swelling of the salivary glands appears. Swelling may start on one side of the face and then appear on the other side of the face within a few days. Sometimes, however, only one side swells. The inflammation may cause soreness and difficulty in eating or swallowing.

The sex glands may become swollen as well. Orchitis (inflammation of one or both testes) can cause considerable pain. Affected testes may shrink somewhat, but contrary to popular belief, it is not common for mumps to lead to sterility. Girls may have swelling in the ovaries, but there is seldom any severe discomfort. In addition, swelling may occur in other glands and organs, including the breasts, the liver, and the brain.

Complications
Although mumps can be unpleasant, it rarely has long-term complications. Encephalitis (inflammation of the brain) is the most dangerous complication of mumps, because it carries the risk of death. Another possible consequence of encephalitis is hearing loss or

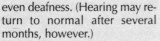

even deafness. (Hearing may return to normal after several months, however.)

A milder complication of mumps is meningoencephalitis (inflammation of the brain and its covering, the meninges). This disease causes a stiff neck, headache, high fever, drowsiness, sensitivity to bright light, and sometimes delirium. The symptoms of meningoencephalitis usually disappear without causing permanent damage to the brain.

Pancreatitis (inflammation of the pancreas) can also result from mumps. Symptoms of pancreatitis include stomach pain, vomiting, chills, fever, and extreme weakness. Although these signs usually vanish and leave no damage, diabetes can result in rare cases.

Other complications include nerve inflammation, heart problems, and nervous system disorders. Symptoms of any of these conditions should be immediately brought to the attention of a physician.

Diagnosis

A doctor diagnoses mumps on the basis of the characteristic form and texture of the swollen parotid glands. Boys may have swelling and tenderness in the testes.

Exposure to the disease is also a clue. The incubation time (the time between exposure to the virus and the appearance of signs and symptoms) is 14 to 21 days. If your physician suspects mumps, secretions from the salivary glands can be tested for mumps virus.

Treatment

Treatment for mumps involves relieving the discomfort of the symptoms, since there is no cure for the disease. Depending on the patient, bed rest may or may not be necessary. A diet of soft foods and liquids is recommended. (Fruit juices with a high acid content may sting the mouth, however, and should be avoided.)

If the glands are severely swollen, a physician may prescribe painkilling drugs. Steroid drugs may be recommended for men or boys with extremely swollen testes. Warm or cold compresses or an ice pack may relieve some pain. Most mumps symptoms disappear within about ten days.

Prevention

There is a vaccine that is 95 percent effective in preventing mumps. The vaccine stimulates the production of antibodies to resist the disease.

Mumps vaccine is usually combined with measles and rubella (German measles) vaccines and given to children by injection when they are 15 months of age.

Rubella

Rubella, or German measles, is a relatively mild viral infection with coldlike symptoms and a short-lived rash. The disease is contagious; however, rubella outbreaks have become infrequent since the development of a vaccine to prevent the illness. Rubella is usually not dangerous, unless it occurs during pregnancy, when it can cause serious birth defects.

Cause
Rubella is caused by a virus. The virus spreads from one person to another via airborne droplets from an infected person's respiratory system. The incubation period (the time between exposure to the virus and appearance of symptoms) is usually 14 to 21 days. An infected person can spread the virus as early as one week before the rash appears and as late as five days after the rash has faded. A child with congenital (present at birth) rubella syndrome can transmit the virus until he is about 12 to 18 months old. Second infections have been reported, but they are uncommon.

Complications
Although rubella is generally a mild infection, some complications can arise. Encephalitis (inflammation of the brain) occurs in 1 in 5,000 cases. Thrombocytopenic purpura, a blood disease characterized by a lowered platelet count, can prove fatal when it accompanies rubella. High or prolonged fever and extreme fatigue should be reported to a physician to prevent further complications.

Congenital rubella syndrome occurs when the disease is transmitted to the fetus during pregnancy. Rubella virus may cause one or more serious organic and growth disorders of the fetus. The most common problems include congenital heart defects, hearing and vision problems, blood disorders, and mental retardation and other brain disorders.

Symptoms
The first symptoms of rubella are a runny nose, swollen lymph nodes in the neck, and a low-grade fever (up to 101°F).

About two days later, a rash of very small red or pink spots appears on the face and neck. The spots are flat initially. They then become slightly raised and fade within a day or two. As the first spots fade, more spots develop until the rash has spread over most of the body. The rash lasts only two to three days, but swelling of the lymph nodes may persist for a week. All other symptoms have usually disappeared by then. When there is joint pain, as is common with older women, discomfort may last another week.

Diagnosis

Under normal circumstances, rubella is difficult to diagnose because the symptoms are so mild and variable. Sometimes there is no rash, and the disease resembles a cold. Other cases may be so severe that the infection may be confused with measles. A doctor can identify the virus by testing a blood sample. Tracing a history of exposure to the disease also helps to establish the diagnosis.

Treatment

Most patients require little or no treatment for rubella, because the symptoms are so mild. An aspirin substitute may afford relief from joint pain. Otherwise, drugs are not usually necessary to treat rubella.

Prevention

Rubella is now rare because children routinely receive rubella vaccine at about 15 months of age. The vaccine is usually combined with measles and mumps vaccines in one injection, but it can be given alone. The rubella vaccine can cause some mild muscle or joint aches, but they are rarely significant. The rubella vaccine works in the body to stimulate the production of antibodies that fight the disease.

Women who want to become pregnant should have a blood test to determine whether they are already immune to rubella; if not, they can be vaccinated. Vaccination is not recommended during pregnancy because of the possible risk to the fetus. Doctors also caution women to wait at least three months after rubella vaccination before trying to become pregnant.

Scarlet fever

Scarlet fever (also known as *scarlatina*) is a highly contagious illness caused by Streptococcus bacteria and is almost always accompanied by strep throat.

Symptoms
The symptoms of scarlet fever include fever; sore throat; widespread scarlet rash beginning in the armpits and groin and spreading to the neck, chest, back, extremities, and even the tongue; and peeling and scaling of the skin, even on the palms of the hands and the soles of the feet. The incubation period (the time between exposure to the disease and the appearance of symptoms) is two to four days.

Treatment
In the past, scarlet fever was often fatal, but today it is easily treated with penicillin, and complications are rare. Bed rest and a nourishing diet with plenty of fluids can help speed recuperation.

Shingles

Shingles, or herpes zoster, is a painful viral infection of one or more nerves. The infection produces a blistery, itchy skin rash on the area of skin supplied by the affected nerve.

The shingles rash looks identical to the rash of chicken pox, which should not be surprising, because shingles and chicken pox are both caused by the same virus, the varicella zoster virus.

Causes
Shingles usually occurs only in persons who have already had chicken pox. Some scientists believe that after a case of chicken pox has run its course, the varicella zoster virus lies dormant in the body but can be reactivated by injury to the affected area or by emotional or physical upset. Others believe that the number and strength of antibodies produced by the body to fight the varicella zoster virus diminish with time, making the person susceptible to another attack of the virus; because some antibodies endure, the person gets shingles rather than chicken pox. If an adult who has not had chicken pox is exposed to the virus, he will get chicken pox, not shingles.

The incidence of shingles increases with age. More than 50 percent of those who get shingles are over 45 years of age.

Symptoms
Shingles begins with prickling or tenderness in the skin over the affected nerve. Burning or shooting pain in the same area

is also an early symptom. Within two to four days, a rash of small, red spots appears over the affected part of the body. As the spots enlarge, they blister and sometimes blend together. Eventually they fill with pus, burst, and crust over, much the same as a chicken pox rash.

The shingles rash is very itchy. Pain increases as the area beneath the rash becomes redder and more swollen. Shingles most often attacks nerves of the chest, back, neck, arms, and legs; however, facial nerves are frequently involved. The rash appears in a band or strip following the distribution of the nerve, usually on one side of the body. The rash persists for two to three weeks before clearing; the pain continues for about three or four weeks.

In persons over age 60, pain may persist for months to years after the rash has disappeared; this condition is called *postherpetic neuralgia*. This condition is difficult to treat. Antidepressants, antiseizure medications, electrical stimulation of the affected areas, and analgesics have been helpful in reducing the pain.

Complications

Occasionally, the shingles rash spreads over the entire body. This develops most often in people who have some underlying disease, such as Hodgkin disease (cancer of the lymph system) or leukemia (cancer of the blood). When these serious disorders already exist, shingles can cause death. A signal that another illness may be present is recurrence of shingles, since the condition seldom occurs more than once.

The most common complication of shingles is bacterial infection of the rash. Less common complications may follow a shingles attack on facial nerves. Eye disorders and Bell palsy (a disorder that temporarily paralyzes one side of the face) can result. Shingles in other parts of the body can cause similar temporary paralysis of the area over the affected nerve.

Treatment

Since there is no known cure for shingles, treatment focuses on reducing pain. An analgesic may relieve the burning sensation. Acyclovir, an antiviral drug given orally has been shown to shorten the course and decrease the severity of the illness in many cases.

Some physicians prescribe steroid drugs to reduce nerve inflammation. To be effective,

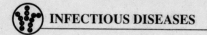

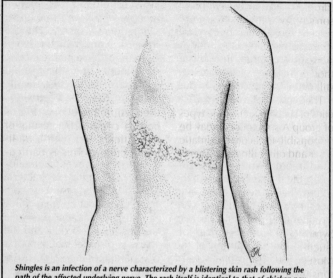

Shingles is an infection of a nerve characterized by a blistering skin rash following the path of the affected underlying nerve. The rash itself is identical to that of chicken pox, since both diseases are caused by the same virus.

steroids must be taken soon after shingles begins. Steroid treatment is usually not recommended for those with underlying disease, because steroids can interfere with resistance to infection.

Preventing infection is also important. Baths in warm (not hot) water help soothe and clean the skin. If itching is severe, patients should cut their fingernails and wear gloves when asleep to control unconscious scratching.

Strep throat

Strep throat is a contagious bacterial illness that is most common in children aged 5 to 15 years.

Cause
Strep throat is caused by *Streptococcus* bacteria, or streptococci, that attack the mucous membranes of the throat and other body systems. The most common source of infection is contact with airborne moisture

(droplets) from an infected person's nose or throat. "Carriers" are individuals that harbor the streptococci but do not exhibit symptoms of the illness. Even though they are not ill, they can still transmit the bacteria.

There are many different varieties of streptococci. Some types of group A streptococci may be responsible for acute rheumatic fever and other illnesses. Therefore, it is important to recognize and treat group A strep throat promptly.

Symptoms

Symptoms may be nonexistent (such as in carriers) or severe. Most commonly, swelling of the tonsils or redness and pain in the throat develop about two to four days after exposure. Fever, chills, and fatigue are also common symptoms.

Complications

Group A strep can cause anything from otitis media (ear infection) and sinusitis to acute rheumatic fever and glomerulonephritis. Treatment with antibiotics will probably prevent most complications.

Diagnosis

The diagnosis of group A strep infection involves the patient's medical history and physical examination and is confirmed by taking a culture. The results are usually available within 24 to 48 hours. Rapid strep identification, where swabbed specimens are treated immediately and results are available within an hour, are now commonly used. Although accurate, it is best to confirm the results of this quicker test with a traditional culture. This is particularly true where the rapid test is negative and the physician is highly suspicious of group A strep infection.

Treatment

Treatment of group A strep throat is aimed at preventing rheumatic fever and other complications and at relieving symptoms. Eradicating the strep is the goal of treatment. Penicillin has become the drug of choice for treatment. It can be administered by mouth or injection. If given by mouth, a full ten-day course must be taken in order to ensure eradication of the bacteria.

Penicillin-like drugs or erythromycin also are effective. Family contacts of the patient who develop symptoms are also treated. (Culture and treatment of asymptomatic individuals is usually reserved for certain circumstances.)

Prevention

There is no specific means of prevention of strep throat. Good hygiene, diligent hand washing, and avoiding close contact with infected individuals are all helpful. The role of tonsillectomy in the prevention of recurrent strep infection remains a controversial topic.

Tetanus

Tetanus is a potentially fatal bacterial infection that causes severe muscle contractions. Tetanus is commonly associated with improperly cleaned wounds.

Cause

Tetanus is caused by toxins (poisonous substances) that are produced by *Clostridium tetani* bacteria. These bacteria may be present on the skin at the time of the injury or may enter the body through a wound caused by an object that has been in contact with material, such as soil, in which bacterial spores are present.

Puncture wounds and animal bites, on account of their depth, are especially vulnerable to tetanus infection because they are often difficult to clean and medicate.

Symptoms

Tetanus symptoms vary, depending on the extent of the infection and the body part that is affected. A common symptom is lockjaw, in which the muscles of the jaw go into severe, continuous contraction, thus rendering the jaw immobile.

Other symptoms include bowing or arching of the body (a rare occurrence) because of contraction of lower back muscles, back muscle spasms, and throat spasms, which can cause blockage of the airway. The affected body parts become immobile because of the simultaneous and continuous contraction of opposing muscles.

In severe cases, the contractions involve most of the fibers in an affected muscle, similar to what would be required to lift a heavy weight or to marshal all the potential force of a muscle against a great resistance. Such violent and prolonged muscle contractions can be very painful.

Treatment

Treatment includes muscle relaxant drugs, such as diazepam, to ease the contractions. Antimicrobial drugs, such as penicillin, are used to fight the infection. Tetanus antitoxin is injected into a muscle in the

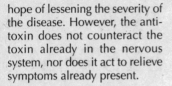

hope of lessening the severity of the disease. However, the antitoxin does not counteract the toxin already in the nervous system, nor does it act to relieve symptoms already present.

Prevention
Immunization with the tetanus vaccine is the best preventive medicine against the disease. Infants begin at two months of age to receive the initial series of tetanus shots combined with diphtheria and whooping cough. Boosters are given at 18 months and five years and then every ten years after that through adulthood.

Wounds should be attended to and cleaned immediately. An individual with a hard-to-clean wound often requires an additional tetanus booster, especially if the individual has not received a tetanus shot in more than five years. If small skin wounds are a common occurrence in the course of the workday, it is important that the tetanus booster be administered periodically.

ALLERGIES AND THE IMMUNE SYSTEM

Immunity is the body's ability to defend itself against harmful organisms and substances. Essentially, immunity is a resistance to infection that may be inherited or acquired naturally or artificially.

Immunity develops when foreign organisms or substances, called antigens, enter the body, causing particular specialized cells to react either by attacking the antigen directly or by producing special proteins that neutralize the foreign agents. The most common types of antigens are forms of bacteria (one-celled organisms that have the potential to attack body tissues or secrete poisonous substances called toxins) and viruses (the smallest infective agents, responsible for a variety of diseases).

Lymph system

The lymph system is the body's drainage system. It is composed of a network of vessels and small structures called lymph nodes. The lymph vessels convey excess fluid collected from all over the body back into the blood circulation. Along the way, however, these fluids are forced to percolate through the lymph nodes so that they can be filtered. Harmful organisms are trapped and destroyed by the specialized white blood cells, called lymphocytes, that are present in these nodes. Lymphocytes are also added to the lymph that flows out of nodes and back to the bloodstream.

Antibodies

Antibodies are manufactured by the lymph system. Antibodies are specialized proteins that the body produces in response to invasion by a foreign substance. The process of antibody formation begins when an antigen stimulates specialized lymphocytes, called B cells, into action. Antibodies then counteract invading antigens by combining with the antigen to render it harmless to the body. Some antibodies coat the harm-

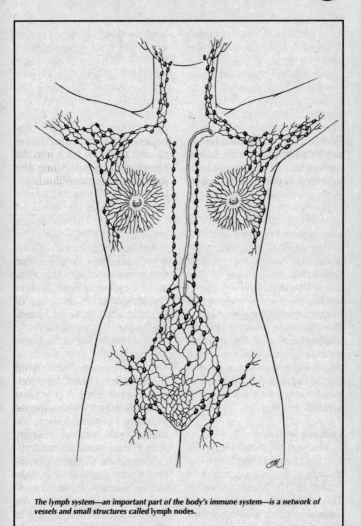

The lymph system—an important part of the body's immune system—is a network of vessels and small structures called lymph nodes.

ful organisms so that the body's scavenger cells can recognize and destroy them more easily. The antibody molecule combines with the antigen molecule by matching combining sites; they fit together like the pieces of a jigsaw puzzle. Other antibodies that neutralize toxins produced by bacteria are called *antitoxins.*

During periods of active antibody production, lymph nodes often enlarge and become tender to the touch. For example, a vaccination (injection of a natural or artificial antigen to stimulate the body to produce protective antibodies) in the arm can cause swelling of the nodes in the armpit, while mononucleosis causes enlargement of nodes that can be felt under the skin of the armpits, groin, and neck. The spleen (an organ located in the upper left part of the abdomen) is also important in the production of antibodies.

Immune response
Production of white blood cells and antibodies in reaction to an invading disease organism is called an *immune response.* This response is one of the body's primary and most efficient lines of defense. In most cases, once antibodies have been produced to fight a certain organism, it no longer poses a great threat to the body. That is why one attack of a disease often prevents that same disease from infecting the body again—the first attack causes production of antibodies that protect the body against subsequent attacks. With measles, for example, antibodies are produced as a result of having the disease or of being immunized with the measles vaccine. These antibodies are able to resist a second attack of the disease.

Antibodies are not always beneficial. For example, when tissue from another body, such as a transplanted heart, is introduced, antibodies are produced to destroy the "invader." Transplants usually are made possible only by means of drugs that act against the body's natural immune response. Also, when blood is transfused from one person to another, it must be of a matching type; otherwise, the recipient's immune system will manufacture antibodies to destroy the transfused blood.

Sometimes, the immune system causes reactions that make the body unusually sensitive to foreign material. When the immune response is disruptive to the body in this way, it is called an *allergic reaction.*

Allergic reaction

An allergy is a state of special sensitivity to a particular environmental substance, or allergen. An allergic reaction is the body's response to exposure to an allergen.

Although an allergy can be present almost immediately after exposure to an allergen, it usually develops over time, as the immune system forms antibodies against the foreign substance. Under normal conditions, such antibodies work to protect the body from further attack. In the case of an allergy, however, the antibodies and other specialized cells involved in this protective function trigger an unusual sensitivity, or overreaction, to the foreign substance. The antibodies stimulate specialized cells to produce histamine, a powerful chemical. Histamine causes the small blood vessels to enlarge and the smooth muscles (such as those in the airways and the digestive tract) to constrict. Histamine release can also cause other reactions, such as hives.

No one knows why allergies develop, but it is known that an allergy can appear, disappear, or reappear at any time and at any age. Allergic reactions rarely occur during the first encounter with the troublesome allergen because the body needs time to accumulate the antibodies. Also, an individual's sensitivity to certain allergens seems to be related to a family history of allergies. People who have a tendency to develop allergies are referred to as *atopic*.

An allergic reaction can be so mild that it is barely noticeable or so severe that it is life-threatening. Common symptoms of allergy are watery eyes, runny nose, itching or inflamed skin, and a swollen mouth or throat. Some allergic reactions may be accompanied by headaches, sinus stuffiness, a reduced sense of taste or smell, or difficulty breathing.

An extremely severe allergic reaction, called *anaphylactic shock*, is characterized by breathing difficulties (caused by swelling of the throat and larynx and narrowing of the bronchial tubes), itching skin, hives, and collapse of the blood vessels, as well as by vomiting, diarrhea, and cramps. This condition can be fatal if not treated immediately.

Types of allergens

There are four categories of allergens: inhalants, contactants, ingestants, and injectants.

Inhalant allergens are those that are breathed in, including

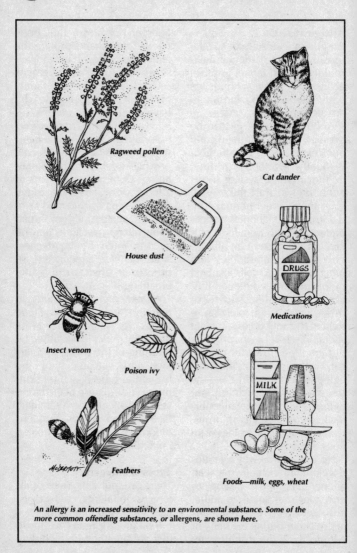

Ragweed pollen

Cat dander

House dust

Medications

Insect venom

Poison ivy

Feathers

Foods—milk, eggs, wheat

An allergy is an increased sensitivity to an environmental substance. Some of the more common offending substances, or allergens, are shown here.

such substances as dust, pollen, feathers, and animal dander (small scales from an animal's skin). Hay fever is an inhalant allergy in which the mucous membranes react to various inhaled substances, usually the pollens associated with the changing seasons. Year-round "hay fever" may actually be a reaction to pet dander, feathers, mold, or dust. (For additional information on hay fever, see page 73.)

Substances you come in contact with that irritate the skin—such as poison ivy, poison oak, cosmetics, detergents, fabrics, and dyes—are called *contact dermatitis.*

Ingestant allergens are those that are swallowed. A variety of foods and medications can act as ingestant allergens. Food allergies occur more frequently in children than in adults. Common ingestant allergens are milk, eggs, shellfish, fish, peanuts, chocolate, strawberries, tomatoes, and citrus fruits. (For additional information on food allergies, see page 71.)

Injectant allergens are substances that penetrate the skin, such as insect venom and drugs that are injected. For example, people who have severe allergic reactions to insect bites or stings are suffering from a reaction to an injectant allergen. (For additional information on insect bites and stings, see page 76.)

Diagnosis

Identifying an offending allergen may be uncomfortable, time-consuming, and expensive, but it is sometimes necessary in order to avoid future allergic reactions. A medical history, a record of any recent changes in daily habits, skin-scratch tests (in which small amounts of suspected allergens are applied to tiny scratches in the skin), and intracutaneous skin tests (in which allergens are injected under the skin) are used to help identify the troublesome foreign substance. A special study called *radioallergosorbent testing (RAST)* is sometimes performed to detect and measure antibodies in the blood that have been manufactured in response to invading substances.

Treatment

Once the allergen has been identified, half the battle is won. Avoiding the troublesome substance is the first step toward relieving an allergy problem. If the allergen cannot be avoided or removed, medication or immunotherapy may be recommended. Three types of medications are commonly prescribed: antihistamines, which combat the effect of the histamines in the body; corticosteroids, which reduce inflammation and swelling; and bronchodilators, which ease breathing by opening bronchial tubes.

Allergy immunotherapy, or desensitization, consists of injections of an allergen in gradually increasing quantities. This allows the body to build up a tolerance to the offending substance. Immunotherapy works best in controlling allergies to pollen, insect venom, and house dust.

A little common sense goes a long way toward controlling allergies. Obviously, the offending allergen needs to be avoided. Keep windows shut during pollen season. Bathe your pet frequently if you are allergic to animal dander. Replace natural fibers in the home with synthetics. Air conditioners or air filters can be installed for hay fever sufferers. Those susceptible to insect bites can wear protective clothes and avoid wearing bright clothing and perfumes, both of which attract insects. Babies born into allergy-prone families should be breast-fed as long as possible to delay exposure to cow's milk, eggs, and citrus fruits.

Prevention
In most cases, allergies cannot be prevented, but much can be done to help control or diminish their effects on overly sensitive individuals.

Anaphylaxis

Anaphylaxis is said to be present if a person is extremely sensitive to a substance on first exposure. If the person is exposed to the substance again, the result may be anaphylactic shock, an explosive overreaction of the body's immune system. Anaphylactic shock is a violent allergic reaction characterized by itching skin, hives, breathing trouble, collapse of the circulatory system, and sometimes vomiting, diarrhea, and cramps in the abdomen.

Causes
Anaphylaxis may be triggered by an insect sting; a food allergy; by animal serum used in a vaccine; by desensitizing injections; or by one of various drugs. The allergen (the substance that sets off the reaction) is usually a protein, called an *antigen*. When it first enters the

body, certain body cells treat it like an invading microorganism and create antibodies, which are protective substances that fight infection. On subsequent exposures to the same antigen, the antibodies are ready for the "invader" and stimulate the release of certain chemicals. One of these chemicals, histamine, causes contraction of muscles in the digestive and respiratory tracts, resulting in abdominal cramps and wheezing. Histamine also causes the small blood vessels to enlarge and lose plasma (blood fluid) to surrounding tissues. The decrease in the volume of blood in the vessels results in a drop in blood pressure, which can lead to shock (collapse of the circulatory system).

Symptoms

Symptoms of anaphylactic shock develop rapidly. Within 15 minutes, the victim becomes uneasy, upset, and red in the face. Rapid heartbeat, prickling and itching sensations in the skin, throbbing in the ears, sneezing, coughing, and breathing difficulty are also likely. Vomiting, incontinence, and even convulsions may occur. Shock may result, in which blood vessels collapse, the pulse becomes weak and rapid, and the person becomes cold, clammy, and faint. Without immediate medical aid, anaphylactic shock may result in death.

Treatment

In cases of anaphylactic shock, medical aid should be obtained as quickly as possible—call an emergency squad. Keep the patient's airway open. Have the patient lie down, with his legs elevated.

Immediate treatment with the drug epinephrine is critical. It counteracts the action of the histamine released in the blood, which is causing the symptoms of anaphylactic shock. In extreme cases, especially when shock has occurred or there is great breathing difficulty, intravenous solutions are given to restore blood volume and raise blood pressure. Anyone with a severe reaction is usually hospitalized for at least 24 hours.

Prevention

A preventive measure against anaphylactic shock is routine allergy skin testing. In addition, anyone who has had an allergic reaction to an insect sting should carry a kit containing a syringe of epinephrine and an epinephrine-filled nasal sprayer for prompt self-treatment. Desensitizing injections of the insect venom should also be considered to allow the body to build up a resistance to the venom.

Anaphylactoid reactions

Similar to anaphylaxis in effect (but not in cause) are anaphylactoid reactions, which can occur on the first injection of certain drugs, such as morphine, and of contrast media (special solutions used when performing certain X-ray studies). These are not allergic reactions in the pure sense, but they are serious nevertheless.

Autoimmune diseases

Autoimmune diseases are disorders in which the body's immune system reacts against some of its own tissue and produces antibodies to it.

Examples

Ailments believed to be autoimmune diseases include Hashimoto thyroiditis and Graves disease, which are disorders of the thyroid gland; systemic lupus erythematosus, which attacks multiple organ systems; myasthenia gravis, a neuromuscular disease; and autoimmune

hemolytic anemia, in which red blood cells are destroyed.

Diseases that are, at least in part, autoimmune disorders include rheumatoid arthritis, a connective tissue disease; pernicious anemia, a serious blood disorder; glomerulonephritis, a disorder that affects the kidneys; and Addison disease, which attacks the adrenal glands. Other diseases that have autoimmune features are chronic active hepatitis (a liver disorder) and some forms of vasculitis (inflammation of blood vessel walls).

Causes

An autoimmune disease can begin in several ways:

• A body substance that ordinarily never enters the bloodstream may do so because of injury. For example, a disease known as *sympathetic ophthalmia* occurs when tissue from the inside of an injured eye is released into the bloodstream. The tissue is recognized as "out of place" or "foreign" by the body's own immune system, and antibodies attack it, causing irritation in both the injured eye and in the noninjured eye.

• A body substance may be altered by chemicals, sunlight, or a virus so that it seems for-

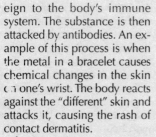
eign to the body's immune system. The substance is then attacked by antibodies. An example of this process is when the metal in a bracelet causes chemical changes in the skin on one's wrist. The body reacts against the "different" skin and attacks it, causing the rash of contact dermatitis.

- Infection may cause an immune response so strong that the body reacts against some of its own normal tissues.
- Genetic factors may play a role.

Treatment

Treatment is dependent on the particular autoimmune disease present. Many treatments involve decreasing the patient's immune response. Other cases require more aggressive therapy to allow repair of damage caused by the body's attack on itself.

Food allergy

A food allergy is an unusual sensitivity to a specific food. A food allergy is not a food intolerance, which exists when the body lacks the enzymes that are needed to digest a certain food. A food allergy exists when the body's immune system manufactures antibodies as a reaction to the food. This food then becomes an ingestant allergen (an allergy-causing substance that is swallowed or eaten). Any food can become an allergen, but the foods most commonly found to cause allergic reactions are milk, eggs, shellfish, fish, peanuts, chocolate, tomatoes, strawberries, and citrus fruits.

Symptoms

The symptoms of a food allergy most commonly arise in the digestive tract and include cramps, nausea, vomiting, and diarrhea. Other signs that may also be present include hives, rash, headache, nasal congestion, and anaphylactic shock (a very serious reaction that can be fatal). Food allergies occur more often in children than in adults.

Diagnosis

Food allergy is diagnosed by having the patient maintain a detailed record of all foods eaten, as well as of the times when symptoms appear. Elimination trials may also help identify the allergen; the patient eliminates one food at a time from the diet to see if the symptoms disappear. In addition, several tests are used to detect various types of allergens: scratch tests, in which a small amount of the suspected allergen is applied to a scratch on the skin; intracutaneous tests, in which a small amount of the allergen is injected under the skin; and RAST, in which antibodies developed in response to specific allergens are measured.

Treatment

There is no way to treat a food allergy other than to avoid eating the offending food and to treat the symptoms of a reaction should one develop. Fortunately, children usually outgrow these allergies.

Gamma globulin

Gamma globulin preparations are derived from the blood of a person or animal and contain antibodies made by that person or animal in response to invasion by harmful agents, such as bacteria and viruses.

Gamma globulin preparations are widely used for the prevention, modification, diagnosis, and treatment of many different kinds of infectious diseases.

Gamma globulin is usually injected. Since it contains almost all the antibodies circulating in the blood, it can provide passive (borrowed) immunity that lasts for about six weeks.

Gamma globulin injections may be useful in preventing infectious hepatitis when given—within two weeks of exposure—to individuals who have been in intimate contact with someone with hepatitis A. Many physicians recommend that persons traveling to underdeveloped countries, particularly rural areas, receive doses of gamma globulin before departure. (Individuals can opt for the hepatitis A vaccine instead, but it must be taken two weeks before beginning travel.)

If injections of gamma globulin are received within five days of exposure, measles can often be prevented. The injections are especially important for children under three years of age, for pregnant women, for tuberculosis patients, and for those with impaired immune mechanisms. Even if measles is not prevented by gamma globulin injections, a less serious case may result, however.

Gamma globulin level in the body can also be used as a diagnostic tool. For example, one symptom of multiple sclerosis is an elevated level of gamma globulin in the cerebrospinal fluid.

Hay fever

Hay fever is an acute (short-lived), seasonal attack that is an allergic reaction to pollen. Most often, spring attacks are reactions to tree pollen; summer attacks are reactions to grass pollen; and autumn attacks are reactions to weed pollen.

Symptoms
The symptoms of hay fever are usually the same, regardless of the allergen. Common symptoms include itching of the nose and roof of the mouth; itchy, watery eyes; sneezing; headache; irritability; insomnia; loss of appetite; and in advanced cases, coughing and wheezing may occur.

Diagnosis
Hay fever, as with other allergies, is diagnosed by identifying the allergen. This is done by reviewing the patient's medical history, environment, daily habits, and recent changes in lifestyle. Skin tests and blood tests may also be performed.

Treatment
A severe case of hay fever may be best treated by changing the environment, that is, by removing the allergen causing the reaction or reducing the patient's exposure to it. Many hay fever sufferers will benefit from using an air conditioner, which filters the air and thus keeps pollen levels in the home to a minimum.

Several medications are available for the hay fever sufferer: oral antihistamines, which counteract the histamine that is released by the body in reaction to the allergen; corticosteroids, which reduce inflammation; eyedrops, which relieve itching and redness of the eyes; and desensitization shots, which cause the body to develop tolerance to the allergen.

Prevention
There is no way to prevent hay fever, but avoiding the allergen as much as possible may at least help to relieve some of the discomfort.

Immunization

Immunization is the means of producing immunity to a specific disease. Immunization can protect against diphtheria, measles, mumps, pertussis (whooping cough), polio, chicken pox, rubella (German measles), and tetanus. There are two types of immunization—active and passive.

73

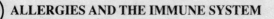

Active immunization

Active immunization is accomplished by injecting weakened or killed viruses or bacteria into the body. This stimulates the body's natural defense system. Certain specialized white blood cells produce antibodies, which are carried in the bloodstream and are tailor-made to fight the specific invading organisms. These antibodies remain in the body for years—sometimes a lifetime—to protect it against that particular disease.

Passive immunization

Passive immunization involves injecting ready-made antibodies into the body. These antibodies are usually extracted from the blood of humans who are immune to a certain disease or of animals that have been immunized solely for the purpose of producing antibodies to be used in passive immunization. Passive immunization is borrowed immunity and is only temporary, but it serves to protect a person who may already be infected until the body has time to create sufficient quantities of its own antibodies.

Children's immunizations

Every child should receive injections of the diphtheria-tetanus-pertussis (DTP) vaccine at 2, 4, 6, and 18 months of age. The child should also receive a dose of the oral polio vaccine (OPV) at 2, 4, and 18 months of age. Every child should also receive injections of the vaccine against *Hemophilus influenzae* type B (Hib), the most common cause of bacterial meningitis in children.

The recommended schedule for Hib vaccination depends upon the brand of vaccine used. For example, one brand of the vaccine should be given at 2, 4, and 12 months of age; another should be given at 2, 4, 6, and 15 months of age. The physician who performs the initial vaccination can tell you which schedule applies to your child.

At 15 months, a child should receive the combined measles, mumps, and rubella (MMR) vaccine and a test for tuberculosis (TB). DTP and OPV boosters should be given when your child is four to six years old. A measles booster should be given when your child is 11 or 12 years of age, and anyone between 4 and 21 years of age should receive a measles booster during a measles outbreak. A diphtheria and tetanus toxoids (DT) booster shot should be given between 14 and 16 years of age.

The American Academy of Pediatrics recommends the varicella (chicken pox) vaccine for all children, adolescents, and young adults who have not already been infected with chicken pox. A single dose should routinely be given between 12 and 18 months of age. This immunization can be given at the same time as the child's first MMR (measles, mumps, and rubella) vaccination.

Older children may be immunized at the earliest convenient opportunity, also with a single dose of the varicella vaccine. Individuals over the age of 13 who have not been immunized previously and have no history of varicella infection should receive two doses of the vaccine spaced four to eight weeks apart. Once immunized, most individuals are protected from the chicken pox for life.

Adult immunizations
After age 20, adults need a diphtheria and tetanus toxoids (DT) booster shot once every ten years. Otherwise, there are no routine immunizations necessary for adults in the United States, with the possible exception of influenza shots given annually (usually in the fall) to the aged and to patients with heart, lung, or other chronic diseases. A vaccine that would protect against 80 percent of serious cases of pneumonia is available; it should be given to individuals over the age of 65 and those with chronic health conditions. Immunization against rabies is possible both before and after exposure. Immunizations should not be given routinely to pregnant women, nor in general to anyone whose immune system has been weakened by leukemia, cancer, AIDS, or prolonged X-ray or corticosteroid treatment.

Vaccinations for foreign travel
Most persons traveling abroad in developed countries need no additional vaccinations. In general, in the United States, Canada, Australia, Japan, New Zealand, and Europe, the traveler is safe without vaccinations. Travel in Mexico and the less-developed countries of Africa, Asia, South America, Central America, the South Pacific, the Middle East, and the Far East may hold more risks, particularly in small villages and rural areas not usually visited by tourists.

In recent years, no vaccination has been necessary for direct travel from the United States to most countries or for return to the United States. However, some countries require proof of vaccination from travelers who have passed through infected areas, and it is best to get the necessary vaccinations before leaving home.

Any physician can give immunizations except for yellow fever vaccinations, which must be given at an official "Yellow Fever Vaccination Center." Months before you plan to leave on your trip, call your local health department for information about vaccination requirements and recommendations for all the countries you plan to visit.

Insect bites and stings

Insect bites and stings are minor inconveniences to most people, but to those who have an allergy to insect venom, the consequences can be serious.

Symptoms

Reactions to insect venom show themselves in various symptoms—shortness of breath, rapid heartbeat, coughing, wheezing, and light-headedness. The affected area swells and becomes tender or numb. In extreme cases, anaphylaxis (see page 68) can occur.

Treatment

Serious reactions to bites and stings are treated by slowing the spread of the venom throughout the body and getting emergency medical treatment as soon as possible. The progress of the venom can be slowed somewhat by applying an ice pack to the affected area to slow the blood flow. Emergency medical treatment will usually consist of an epinephrine injection and an injection of antihistamine. In some cases, a corticosteroid may be given in addition to the injections.

Prevention

Prevention of recurrent reactions may be accomplished with desensitization shots; starting with an initially weak solution of insect extract, doses are gradually increased with each shot. This allows the body to build up tolerance to the effects of the insect venom.

People who know that they have a sensitivity to insect bites should carry kits with injectable epinephrine (available by prescription).

THE BRAIN AND NERVOUS SYSTEM

The nervous system is a complex network of specialized tissues that regulates thoughts, emotions, actions, sensations, and basic body functions.

Nerve cells

The basic element of the nervous system is the nerve cell, or neuron. In combination, neurons form nerves, which transmit impulses throughout the body. A protective covering of myelin, a fatty substance, insulates parts of those fibers.

The action of nerve cells is both electrical and chemical. At the ends of each nerve cell there are specialized regions called *synaptic terminals,* which contain large numbers of tiny membranous sacs that hold neurotransmitter chemicals. These chemicals transmit nerve impulses from one nerve cell to another. After an electrical nerve impulse has traveled along a neuron, it reaches the terminal and stimulates the release of neurotransmitters from their sacs. The neurotransmitters travel across the synapse (the junction between the neighboring neurons) and stimulate the production of an electrical charge, which carries the nerve impulse forward. This process is repeated over and over again until a muscle is moved or relaxed or a sensory impression is noted by the brain. These electrochemical events can be considered the "language" of the nervous system, by which information is transmitted from one part of the body to another.

Nervous system

There are two major divisions of the nervous system: the central nervous system and the peripheral nervous system. The central nervous system consists of the brain and the spinal cord. The brain lies within the skull and governs body functions by sending and receiving messages through the spinal cord. Protecting the brain and spinal cord are bones, layers of tissue, and cerebrospinal fluid.

Once messages leave the central nervous system, they

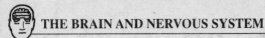

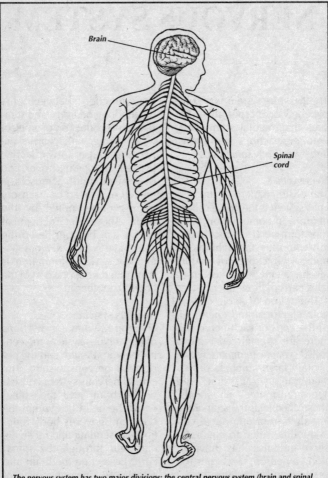

The nervous system has two major divisions: the central nervous system (brain and spinal cord) and the peripheral nervous system (nerves that branch out from the spinal cord).

are carried by the peripheral nervous system. The peripheral system includes the cranial nerves (nerves branching from the brain) and the spinal nerves (nerves branching from the spinal cord). These nerves convey sensory messages from receptor cells in the body to the central nervous system. They also transport motor impulses from the central system out to the body, where muscles and glands can respond to the impulses.

The autonomic nervous system, which is part of the peripheral nervous system, regulates all activity that is involuntary but necessary for life, including activity of the internal organs and glands.

Working together, these divisions coordinate adjustment and reaction of the body to internal and external environmental conditions.

Brain

The brain is the body's control center. The brain sends messages to and receives stimulation from all parts of the body. More than 10 billion interlinked brain cells regulate the functioning of the body during sleep and wakefulness.

Different areas of the brain control different body functions. At the back of the skull is

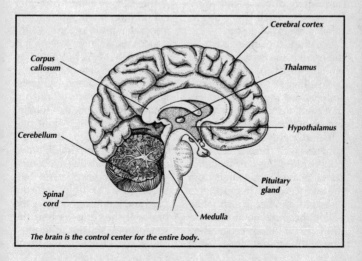

The brain is the control center for the entire body.

79

the cerebellum, which controls coordination of movements, balance, and posture. Deep inside the brain is the thalamus, which is the relay station for incoming impulses from the rest of the body, conveying sensations of pain, touch, and temperature to other parts of the brain. Around the thalamus is the hypothalamus, which governs involuntary (automatic) body operations, such as heartbeat and blood circulation. The pituitary gland is attached to the hypothalamus by a thin stalk. Because the pituitary gland controls most of the hormones in the body, the hypothalamus is considered a major influence on primary drives governed by hormones, such as hunger, thirst, and sexual desire.

Covering the inner parts of the brain is the cerebral cortex, which consists of two cerebral hemispheres. In these hemispheres are the nerve centers that regulate thought and voluntary action. Connecting the left and right cerebral hemispheres is a broad band of fibers called the *corpus callosum.* Because nerve fibers from the two cerebral hemispheres cross one another in a structure called the *medulla* at the base of the brain before progressing down the spinal cord, each hemisphere generally controls functions in the opposite side of the body. For example, a region in the left hemisphere governs movement of the right arm.

The brain is the most complex organ in the body. Although research has identified many of its capabilities in memory, reasoning, and creative thought processes, many functions of the brain continue to remain a mystery.

Cerebrospinal fluid

Cerebrospinal fluid (CSF) is a clear, colorless fluid that surrounds the brain and spinal cord, cushioning them against injury.

The CSF is made of water containing small amounts of minerals and organic substances (especially protein). It is continually being produced by a specialized network of capillaries (tiny blood vessels) known as the *choroid plexus,* located in the ventricles (chambers) of the brain. About one pint is produced every 24 hours, and approximately five ounces is circulating at any one time. From the two lateral ventricles, the CSF flows into the third and fourth ventricles of the brain. It then passes into the space between the innermost and second layers of the tissue covering the brain, bathing the entire outer surface of the brain in fluid before passing downward around the spinal cord. Eventually the fluid returns upward, is absorbed into special tissue between the linings of the brain, and passes into the blood vessels.

Samples of CSF (drawn from around the spinal cord with a needle inserted in the lower back—a procedure known as a *lumbar puncture*) can be valuable in diagnosing disorders of the brain and spinal cord. The samples may indicate a hemorrhage or blood clot in the brain, various types of meningitis, a brain abscess, or a tumor of the brain or spinal cord.

Alzheimer disease

Alzheimer disease is a disorder in which there is a steady deterioration of brain function, resulting in progressive loss of memory, recognition, personality, and mental powers. Although Alzheimer disease may begin as early as age 40, it is most prevalent in the elderly. It accounts for about half of all serious mental impairment in persons over age 65.

Changes in the brain

In Alzheimer disease, as in any senile mental disorder, there is atrophy (shrinkage or wasting) of the cerebral cortex (the outer layer of the brain, which is mostly concerned with intellectual and social functioning).

There are also more specific abnormalities, such as the presence of tangles of fibers within the nerve cells and of senile plaques, which are probably deposits of amyloid (a semisolid protein complex seen in many degenerative diseases). These abnormalities are scattered throughout the cortex of a person with Alzheimer disease; they distinguish the disease from other forms of senility. Because brain biopsy specimens (tissue samples taken from the brain for laboratory examination) are not obtained without very specific reasons and without intention of specific treatment, these abnormalities are usually discovered only after death.

Causes

Theories abound as to the possible causes of Alzheimer disease. So-called slow viruses (viruses acquired early in life that take many years to do their damage) have been considered, as have environmental factors and damage from previous diseases. Recently, a diminished amount of the enzyme cholineacetyltransferase (which is necessary to manufacture the neurotransmitter acetylcholine) has been found in some patients, and theories about replacement of the enzyme or the neurotransmitter are being formulated. Deficiencies of other neurotransmitters are constantly being discovered. Heredity seems to play some part, since a family history of the disease makes some individuals more likely than others to develop the condition. It is generally agreed that hardening of the arteries is not a cause. Alzheimer disease does not appear to be contagious, nor is it caused by emotional upsets.

Symptoms

Symptoms vary considerably from one person to another and may occur days or months apart. They begin with small memory lapses, almost always first involving loss of recall for recent events. Such lapses can happen to anyone, but in Alzheimer disease they grow more serious with time. A person may forget a close relative's name, get lost coming home from the office, forget to turn off the oven, misplace articles, recheck to see if a task was done, or repeatedly ask questions that have already been answered. Eventually, the gaps in memory and the failure to recognize friends and family members will interfere with normal life.

As the disease progresses, the victim of Alzheimer disease becomes confused, frustrated, and irritable. Although at first the person seems physically unaffected by the disease, as the condition advances, the patient becomes restless, always moving about, and must be watched so that he or she does not wander away or into danger. Endless repetition of unnecessary actions, such as the opening and closing of drawers, is another characteristic of the disease. Some victims of Alzheimer disease may even become extremely agitated with little or no provocation.

The course of the disease may range from 1 year to as many as 20 years. The disease may eventually result in deterioration of the rest of the nervous system and other parts of the body and in loss of control over bladder and bowels. It may cut life expectancy by contributing to death from another cause, such as pneumonia or heart or kidney failure.

Diagnosis

Other conditions can cause many of the symptoms of Alzheimer disease, and many of these conditions are treatable. Therefore, it is very important for the patient to undergo a thorough medical evaluation, which sometimes includes extensive neurologic and psychological examinations and other diagnostic studies, such as computed tomography (a special X-ray technique for obtaining cross-sectional images), electro-encephalography (a study of brain waves), blood tests, and sampling of cerebrospinal fluid.

These procedures can rule out or identify possible causes of nervous system malfunctioning, such as a series of "little strokes," brain tumors or infections, pernicious anemia (can be cured by taking vitamin B_{12}), overmedication with barbiturates or bromides, alcoholism, the side effects of certain medications, abnormal functioning of the thyroid, or hydrocephalus (blockage of cerebrospinal fluid in the head).

Problems with memory can also be linked to depression. Depression can be brought on by major life changes, including death of a loved one or moving to a nursing home. Its symptoms, which include apathy, irritation, and poor concentration, are treatable.

Treatment

Medical science does not yet know how to prevent or treat Alzheimer disease. However, it is important to find a physician who is able to help the patient and the patient's family handle the many problems that are bound to arise. At times, tranquilizers can lessen agitation and anxiety and reduce the incidence of undesirable behavior. Medication may also help to improve sleeping patterns and treat depression caused by the disease.

It is important that a patient continue the daily routine, exercise as usual, and keep in touch with friends. Memory aids, such as lists of daily chores, reminders about safety, and a large calendar, can help in day-to-day living. As care of the patient becomes more difficult, it may be best to move the patient to a health facility where a professional staff can provide around-the-clock care.

Recently, a drug called *tacrine* was released for the treatment of Alzheimer disease. This medication appears to improve function in some patients. However, careful monitoring of liver function with frequent blood tests is required, and the drug can have unpleasant side effects. This medication is not a cure, but it does seem to have some beneficial effects.

Amnesia

Amnesia is the loss of memory and the inability to form new memories. It can be a temporary or permanent condition. The causes of amnesia range from brain damage to severe anxiety.

Retrograde amnesia

This type of amnesia usually follows any severe head injury that produces unconsciousness. The patient is not able to recall what happened immediately before the accident, the accident itself, or some of the events of the recovery period. In most cases, this type of amnesia is not significant because no other memory is affected and no treatment is needed.

Korsakoff syndrome

An inability to record new memory along with a defect in recent memory, usually accompanied by confabulation (storytelling of fabricated events), is known as *Korsakoff syndrome*. It can be caused by head injury, stroke, encephalitis (inflammation of the lining of the brain), deficiency of vitamin B_{12}, cancer of the brain, or poor blood supply to memory tissue or pathways in the brain. However, heavy drinking of alcohol, with resultant brain damage, is commonly the cause.

Although there may be little or no loss of memory or skills that were acquired before the disease began, the person with Korsakoff syndrome cannot effectively learn new skills or remember recent events. To hide this loss, from themselves as well as from others, patients may create experiences to take the place of the missing experiences. Sometimes the stories are so convincing that Korsakoff patients appear normal.

Treatment of Korsakoff syndrome is limited to treating the condition that caused it. Permanent brain damage may make it incurable. Frequently, however, the condition will disappear with time, especially if it was caused by a concussion (a swelling in the head that puts pressure on the brain).

Psychological amnesia

Amnesia of psychological origin is less common than other forms of amnesia. A man disappears from home, job, and family; he travels to a new place and assumes a new identity—all without being aware that anything has changed. After days or weeks, he "awakens," becomes his old self, and wonders what happened. There is no memory of the period of amnesia.

Anxiety is the cause of this type of amnesia. The person is faced with an intolerable situation of high emotional stress or pain. To protect itself, the mind forgets the anxieties and everything related to them.

Treatment may not be necessary, since most affected persons recover without help. However, if the problem that caused the amnesia still remains, it must be faced and solved. Family therapy and change of work or activities may help. Hypnosis may be used to bring back the memory of the "lost days" and unlock the ideas and feelings that caused the original flight from home and self.

Ataxia

Ataxia is a condition characterized by muscular incoordination, producing irregular and inaccurate movements of the body. The result may be a clumsy manner of walking, with feet wide apart, a lack of balance, tremor (shakiness) of the arms, or slurring of speech.

Causes

Ataxia can be caused by anything that affects the motor control centers of the brain or the nerve pathways leading from them. One of the most common causes of ataxia is a stroke in the brainstem (the portion of the brain that controls the most basic body functions, such as breathing and circulation) or cerebellum (the portion of the brain responsible for fine control of muscle movements). Drunkenness can produce a temporary staggering ataxia. Permanent ataxia is caused by damage to the brain, spinal cord, or spinal nerves.

Locomotor ataxia may be a late result of untreated syphilis. Its symptoms include sharp, stabbing pains, usually in the legs; an unsteady walk; and a feeling of walking on foam rubber. There also may be an increased sensitivity of the skin, sometimes with sensations of burning, prickling, creeping, or crawling.

Ataxia occurs in one case in ten of cerebral palsy, which is a movement disorder caused by damage to the brain or nerve pathways before or around the time of birth. Weakness, unsteadiness, clumsy walking, and difficulty with fine or rapid movements are typical. Physical and occupational therapies help patients handle daily life despite their condition.

Ataxia may also be caused by any one of a group of hereditary diseases that attack the central nervous system. They cause degeneration of the spinal cord and cerebellum and also frequently damage the brain stem and various nerves. Inherited disorders of body chemistry and body chemicals are believed to be involved, but little is known about them. Only one of these disorders—Refsum syndrome—can be treated, by reducing the excessive level of a body chemical known as *phytanic acid*.

Symptoms

Symptoms of the hereditary ataxias include unsteadiness in walking, tremor of the arms, muscle weakness, and wasting away of muscles. Various other abnormalities may be present, depending on the disease. For example, Friedreich ataxia causes scoliosis (curvature of the spine) and damages heart tissue.

Treatment

All of these diseases continue throughout life. With the exception of Refsum syndrome, none can be treated effectively.

Bell palsy

Bell palsy is total or partial paralysis (loss of function or movement) of one side of the face. It is believed to be caused by an inflammation of the nerve that controls the facial muscles. The inflammation causes the nerve to swell and to be compressed inside its bony passage in the skull. This compression reduces the blood supply to the nerve and thus its ability to function.

Symptoms

This disorder can occur in someone of any age but is most common from ages 20 to 50. The first sign may be an aching pain behind or below the ear. Paralysis may develop in a few hours or more slowly, causing the entire side of the face to be flat and without expression (this is different from the facial paralysis caused by stroke or brain tumor, in which the weakness is mostly below the forehead). The mouth droops on the weak side and the sense of taste may be impaired. The eyebrow cannot be raised. In most cases, the eye cannot be shut. When the patient tries to close the affected eye, it can be seen to roll upward (which also happens in a healthy person but is not seen because the eyelid normally closes). Unprovoked tears may come from the affected eye.

Diagnosis

In making a diagnosis, the doctor must determine if the paralysis might be caused by other disorders affecting the facial nerve, including ear infections, cancer, or a skull fracture. In such disorders, there is usually involvement of other nerves as well, and distinctive signs and symptoms are frequently present. X-ray studies of the head may be performed.

Treatment

Primary treatment is aimed at reducing the inflammation of the nerve before any permanent damage is done to it. An oral corticosteroid, such as prednisone, may be given for this purpose. However, in many (if not most) uncomplicated cases, treatment with medication is unnecessary. After two weeks, if there has been no improvement in the ability of the muscles to move, the muscles of the weak side of the face may be stimulated electrically to maintain muscle tone.

The affected eye should be covered with an eye patch, especially when the patient is outdoors, and protected from dirt and wind. Application of moist, moderate heat on the affected side of the face can reduce pain. Brief periods of upward facial massage help maintain muscle tone, as do specific facial exercises.

Fortunately, most Bell palsy patients recover in one to eight weeks. Elderly patients may take much longer—up to two years. Complete recovery usually follows within several months if the paralysis is partial.

Carpal tunnel syndrome

Carpal tunnel syndrome is characterized by weakness, pain, tingling, numbness, or burning in the palm, the thumb, the index finger, the middle finger, and the ring finger caused by entrapment of the median nerve in the wrist. (This condition, like any syndrome, is not a disease in itself but rather a collection of symptoms.) The condition most often affects women in their 30s, 40s, and 50s. It may develop or become worse because of work that requires repeated grasping, twisting, or turning of the hand and wrist, especially against resistance or while using vibrating tools.

The carpal tunnel is formed by the bones of the wrist (*carpal* means wrist) and the tough band of connective tissue known as the *transverse carpal ligament*. Among the structures inside the tunnel are the median nerve and the tendons that flex the fingers and thumb. Any swelling or thickening of tissue within the tunnel can cause the median nerve to be compressed between the transverse carpal ligament and the tendons and other contents of the tunnel. The squeezed nerve, which controls the thumb, index finger, and third finger, cannot work as it should, and the symptoms of carpal tunnel syndrome result.

Causes

The most common causes of carpal tunnel syndrome are repeated and forceful grasping with the hands or repeated bending of the wrists (such as while typing or playing the piano). Pregnancy and other conditions that produce generalized swelling of body tissues may also be a cause of carpal tunnel syndrome, as can localized swelling caused by a dislocation, sprain, or fracture of the wrist. Rheumatoid arthritis can cause inflammation of the sheaths (coverings) of the tendons, causing compression. Other possible causes include an inflamed wrist joint, a benign (noncancerous) tumor, myxedema (tissue swelling due to lack of thyroid hormone), tuberculosis, amyloidosis (a disease characterized by abnormal deposits of the protein amyloid), acromegaly (overgrowth of connective tissue), and diabetes mellitus.

Symptoms

Aching pain may travel up the forearm and even into the shoulder joint, neck, and chest. (This type of pain can usually be relieved by shaking the hand vigorously or dangling the arm loosely from its socket; occasionally, however, such pains are caused by compression of the median nerve in the forearm or upper arm.) Other signs include an inability to make a fist, deterioration of the nails, and dryness and shininess of the skin over the involved surfaces. The pains may occur in both hands at the same time. They may be constant or intermittent and are increased by manual work or movement that flexes the wrist or palm. Weakness of

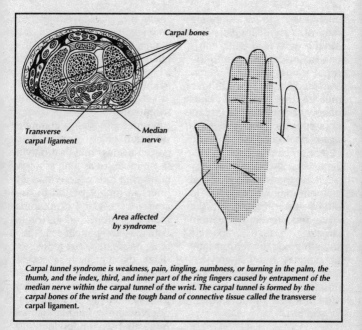

Carpal tunnel syndrome is weakness, pain, tingling, numbness, or burning in the palm, the thumb, and the index, third, and inner part of the ring fingers caused by entrapment of the median nerve within the carpal tunnel of the wrist. The carpal tunnel is formed by the carpal bones of the wrist and the tough band of connective tissue called the transverse carpal ligament.

the fingers occurs later than other symptoms and accompanies atrophy (wasting away) of the muscles. Symptoms are usually worse at night and in the morning.

Diagnosis

Preliminary diagnostic tests include tapping the wrist, which causes tingling in the area of pain if carpal tunnel syndrome is present, and forced flexion of the wrist, which may also reproduce the pain. Though rarely

necessary, an X-ray examination may reveal abnormalities of the wrist bones. Testing of the conduction of nerve impulses is the most specific means of diagnosing the condition.

Treatment

Treatment is aimed first at relieving pressure on the median nerve. If soft-tissue swelling is a cause, elevating the hand may eliminate the symptoms. It may help to place the forearm in a splint at night, which keeps the hand turned upward, extending the wrist. If an inflammation inside the wrist is at fault, cortisone may be injected into the carpal tunnel. Anti-inflammatory medication can relieve some of the pressure. Other causes or aggravating factors associated with the disorder are treated appropriately.

If conservative forms of treatment prove ineffective, surgery to release the transverse carpal ligament may be necessary to relieve the pressure on the nerve and prevent permanent damage. Usually, muscle strength gradually returns after such surgery, but if surgery has been delayed too long and muscles have severely deteriorated, full strength does not always return.

Concussion

Concussion is an injury to the brain, caused by a violent jar or shock, such as a blow to the head. The force of the shock causes the brain to strike against the inside of the skull, producing temporary brain swelling and malfunctioning and often loss of consciousness. The shock may even be strong enough to cause cerebral contusion (bruising of brain tissue),

cerebral hemorrhage (bleeding between the covering of the brain and the skull or inside the brain covering), or formation of a hematoma (collection of clotted blood).

Symptoms

Unconsciousness is a common symptom of concussion. Unconsciousness may last only a few minutes or as long as a few hours, but rarely more than 24 hours (a longer period of unconsciousness or a deep coma indicates more serious brain damage). The patient may then feel nauseated, irritable, or dizzy or may have a severe headache; these symptoms may continue for days or weeks (or longer) after the accident. Frequently, the individual cannot remember what happened just before the injury and later may not be able to recall anything that happened in the first few hours or on the day following the concussion.

A person who suffers an accident serious enough to cause a cerebral contusion; laceration of nerve tissue, blood vessels, and brain covering; or edema (fluid buildup) within or around the brain often shows symptoms other than those accompanying a simple concussion. Some signs of serious damage to the brain include partial paralysis of the body, posture with the arms and legs extended and with the jaws clenched, and unequal or pinpoint pupils.

Diagnosis

A simple concussion usually requires no special care. The purpose of the doctor's examination is to determine if a more serious injury may have occurred. The patient is observed for level of consciousness, mental sharpness (if awake), and proper nerve and muscle functions and reflexes. If the patient acts out of character or does not respond correctly to the tests, hospitalization and evaluation by a neurologist or neurosurgeon may be necessary. An X-ray study of the head may be performed to rule out a skull fracture (although most simple undepressed skull fractures are usually allowed to heal without treatment). A computed tomographic (CT) scan, which provides a cross sectional picture of the brain, can be used to detect bleeding in the brain.

Treatment

Once a doctor has determined that a patient has only a simple

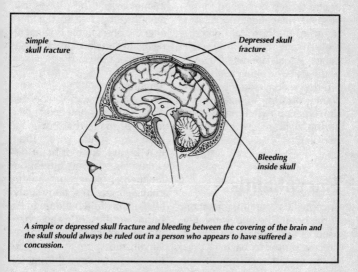

A simple or depressed skull fracture and bleeding between the covering of the brain and the skull should always be ruled out in a person who appears to have suffered a concussion.

concussion, the patient may be allowed to return home without hospitalization. For the next 24 hours, the person is advised to relax and to take no medication stronger than an aspirin substitute (acetaminophen). The individual should also avoid eating solid foods; vomiting is common after concussion.

A parent, roommate, or spouse is usually asked to wake the patient every two hours during the night and ask three questions: What is your name? Where are you? What is my name? If the patient cannot answer these questions, will not awaken, or has convulsions, he or she should be rushed to the hospital. The patient should also return to the hospital immediately if any of the following danger signals are noted: a continuing or worsening headache, blurring vision, extreme or constant vomiting, unusual eye movements, twitching, a staggering walk, or any change in personality.

Encephalitis

Encephalitis is an inflammation of the brain. The term is usually used to describe an infectious process caused by bacteria, parasites, vaccines, or, most often, viruses. Noninfectious agents such as poisons, metabolic abnormalities due to liver or kidney failure, and tumors can cause conditions that closely resemble encephalitis.

Causes

Viruses can cause encephalitis either as a primary disease or as a complication of an infection. Some of these viruses are mosquito-borne and afflict humans only in warm weather, when mosquitoes are in season. Many cases of encephalitis occur as complications of viral infections, such as measles, mumps, chicken pox, and rubella (German measles). These cases usually develop five to ten days after the onset of the original illness, but can develop as long as six weeks afterward.

Symptoms

Encephalitis may be associated with meningitis (infection of the layers of tissue that cover the brain and spinal cord). There may be evidence of brain disturbances, such as alterations in mental state, personality changes, seizures, and paralysis. Edema (fluid buildup) in the brain is present, and there may be petechial hemorrhages (small, red spots that indicate bleeding) scattered throughout parts of the brain and spinal cord. Fever, headache, vomiting, a general feeling of illness, and a stiff neck may be among the first symptoms of encephalitis to appear.

Diagnosis
Prompt diagnosis and supportive treatment are essential in any case of encephalitis or suspected encephalitis. Even patients who have been seriously or critically ill with encephalitis often recover. One diagnostic problem is differentiating encephalitis from bacterial meningitis and other similar ailments. Even with ideal circumstances for diagnosis, the encephalitis virus is often not identified. Viruses can sometimes be isolated directly from cerebrospinal fluid or from the tissues.

Since many forms of encephalitis, such as the mosquito-borne forms, have important public health implications, blood is often drawn whenever encephalitis is suspected; the blood sample is sent to the local department of health, which can provide a more precise diagnosis.

Treatment
With a form of encephalitis called *herpes simplex* encephalitis, early recognition and treatment with a medication that inhibits the reproduction of viruses significantly reduce the chances of death and neurologic impairment. However, for maximal effectiveness, the drug should be given before coma or paralysis occurs. Supportive therapy involves bed rest and maintaining fluid balance to avoid dehydration (loss of body fluids).

Epilepsy

Epilepsy is a disorder characterized by sudden surges of disorganized electrical impulses in the brain, which lead to seizures.

There are several categories of seizures; they can be so mild as to go almost unnoticed or so severe that, if untreated, they can cause serious harm.

Causes
Epilepsy is usually divided into two categories: idiopathic (of unknown cause) and acquired (caused by some known factor, such as a brain tumor or an injury). Idiopathic epilepsy is a very common cause of seizures in people under 25. Seizures beginning after the age of 25 are more often a sign of acquired epilepsy due to injury, tumors, or other brain disorders

93

(such as cerebral palsy, infection, or malformations of blood vessels).

Although its cause is unknown, idiopathic epilepsy has several consistent attributes. It appears with highest frequency between the ages of two and five years and again at puberty and has a tendency to run in families.

Symptoms
The symptoms of epilepsy vary according to the type of seizure experienced. Not all seizures are convulsions. A convulsion involves the nerves that control movement and is characterized by jerking, spastic muscle movements. It is also marked by alterations in sensation and consciousness; loss of consciousness is common.

Seizures are classified according to the symptoms present. In the past, classifications were *grand mal* (French for "big sickness"), *petit mal* (French for "little sickness"), *psychomotor,* and *focal.* The current classification separates seizures into partial and generalized types, depending on the extent of brain involvement.

One classification is as follows:
• Simple partial seizures, confined to small areas of the brain, may be accompanied by a tingling sensation in the arm, finger, or foot; perceiving a bad odor; seeing flashing lights; or speaking unintelligibly. The patient remains conscious.
• Complex partial seizures include episodes of "automatic behavior," in which the patient remains conscious but sits motionless or moves or behaves in a strange, repetitive, or somehow inappropriate way.
• Generalized convulsive seizures have a number of symptoms: The patient may cry out, stiffen and fall to the ground unconscious, lose urinary and bowel control, and have muscle spasms or thrashing movements that cause the limbs to jerk. Spasm of the jaw muscles can cause the victim to bite his or her tongue. After the convulsion, the patient falls into a deep sleep and then awakens dazed, often with a headache and no recollection of the seizure. A warning sensation, called an *aura,* may precede the seizure in the form of headache, sleepiness, yawning, or tingling in the arms or legs.
• Generalized nonconvulsive, or absence, seizures are characterized by periods of staring into space, rhythmic blinking,

and what appears to be day-dreaming. The patient remains conscious but is totally unaware of the seizure. This type of seizure, which is most common in children, may be mistaken for a short attention span or a learning disability.

Diagnosis

Epilepsy is diagnosed by observing the symptoms and by obtaining an electroencephalogram (EEG), which is a visual record of the electrical activity of the brain. Abnormal electrical discharges can be detected if they are present in the brain. However, an abnormal EEG in the absence of symptoms is by no means proof of epilepsy, nor does a normal EEG rule it out.

Treatment

Nonmedical treatment of an epileptic seizure should be limited to preventing injury and keeping the patient as comfortable as posssible by loosening clothing or placing a pillow under the head. The patient should not be left in any position in which vomit can be swallowed or inhaled or in any position in which he or she might suffocate. *Never* attempt to pry open the mouth or insert any object into the mouth of an individual who is having a convulsion.

Epilepsy cannot be cured, but it can usually be controlled with a program of anticonvulsant drug therapy. Patients who tend to have seizures following emotional or physical stress may also benefit from tranquilizers. After two to five years of drug control of idiopathic epilepsy, the dosage is sometimes decreased and, occasionally, when enough time has elapsed during which no seizures have occurred, medication can be discontinued.

Headaches

A headache is a symptom, not a disease. A headache is rarely the symptom of a serious illness, but severe or frequent headaches can be exhausting and can affect daily life.

There are three basic types of headaches. The vascular headache occurs when blood vessels in the head enlarge and press on nerves, causing pain. The most common vascular headache is the migraine.

The second type of headache is the muscle contraction headache, which results when the muscles of the face, neck, or scalp contract and tighten. A tension headache is an example of a muscle contraction headache.

The third kind of headache is the inflammatory headache. Such a headache is the result of pressure within the head. The causes range from relatively minor conditions, such as sinusitis, to more serious conditions, such as brain tumors.

MIGRAINE HEADACHE

One theory about migraine headaches is that they occur when the blood vessels in the head expand and press on the nerves, causing pain. However, another theory is that they result from the blood vessels constricting and thus blocking blood flow to parts of the brain; this may cause the visual impairment and numbness that often accompany or precede a migraine headache. The blood vessels then become full of blood and press on surrounding nerves, causing pain.

Women are more prone to migraines than are men, and a certain personality type—compulsive, perfectionist, and very success-oriented—seems to be more susceptible to migraine headaches.

Causes

A number of physical and emotional factors may contribute to migraine headaches. Migraines may be triggered by a sharp reduction in caffeine intake or by allergies to certain foods or food additives (among them chocolate, coffee, fatty foods, alcohol, citrus fruits, monosodium glutamate, and nitrates).

Emotional stress can also cause migraine headaches, as can drinking alcohol, smoking, or an interruption in routine eating and sleeping habits (all of which may be responsible for "weekend" headaches suffered by some patients). Cyclical, seasonal, or emotional factors may also be associated with the tendency to develop migraine headaches. A tendency to develop this type of headache may be inherited.

Symptoms

The predominant symptom of a migraine headache is a sharp, pulsating pain on one or both sides of the head. Paleness, sweating, nausea, and sensitivity to light may accompany the pain.

A warning sensation, or aura, may indicate an approaching migraine headache. Before the pain begins, some individuals may see flashing lights or "shooting stars," hear noises, smell fragrances or odors, or feel a tingling sensation in the arms or legs.

Cluster headaches are a form of migraine most commonly experienced by men. Cluster headaches have an abrupt onset and can happen at any time. The headaches can occur daily for days, weeks, or months. Their chief symptom is intense pain on one side of the head, accompanied by tearing of the eye and a runny nose on the same side. Drinking and smoking may aggravate these headaches.

Diagnosis

Vascular headaches are diagnosed by a careful review of the circumstances surrounding the headaches as well as by a physical examination to rule out any other disorder that might be causing the symptoms. Elimination tests may be done to identify the exact cause of migraines suffered by people who seem to react to certain foods or changes in eating and sleeping habits. In an elimination test, all the substances that are suspected of causing the trouble are eliminated and then reintroduced one at a time to identify the specific cause of the migraine headaches.

Treatment

Treatment of a migraine already in progress usually consists of a drug therapy program chosen from a variety of painkillers, sedatives, and special prescribed medications.

Prevention

Prevention of migraines is possible with several types of medication. A commonly prescribed drug called ergotamine (and its close relative dihydroergotamine) constricts the blood vessels and thus prevents the swelling that causes pressure on the surrounding nerves. This drug is usually taken to stop an approaching migraine; it may have no effect on the aura symptoms some patients experience. Antidepressant drugs have been shown to prevent migraines in some patients.

A mainstay in migraine treatment is the use of beta-blocking drugs. These drugs work in the body to block what are called the *beta effects,* one of which is dilation of the blood vessels. Drugs known as *calcium-channel blockers,* such as verapamil, nifedipine, and diltiazem, are also effective in the prevention of migraines. While it is not yet known exactly how these drugs provide relief, research suggests that they act by preventing the initial constriction of blood vessels that causes migraine.

Sumatriptan succinate, a relatively new drug, is available in pill form or via injection. This drug has offered dramatic relief to many migraine sufferers who fail to respond adequately to other medications. Individuals with a history of heart disease or other vascular conditions are advised to use extra caution, however. If used inappropriately, this drug can have serious side effects.

MUSCLE CONTRACTION HEADACHE

A muscle contraction headache occurs when muscles of the face, neck, or scalp remain tightened for long periods of time. These muscles are then said to be in spasm.

Causes

A muscle contraction headache usually occurs after a specific event that has caused the muscles to tense. The tension is then translated into physical discomfort in the form of a clenched jaw, aching neck, and tightened muscles of the face and head.

Muscle contraction headaches can also be brought about by abnormalities in the eyes, neck, teeth, or jaws or by poor posture—especially by holding the head at an awkward angle while reading, driving, or watching television.

Symptoms

The major symptom of these headaches is a tight, squeezing pain in the forehead or jaws or around the back of the head or neck. This constant, dull pain usually occurs on both sides of the head.

Diagnosis

Diagnostic evaluation involves a review of the events that usually precede the headaches, as well as a physical examination to rule out any other disorder that might be causing them. A psychological examination may also be conducted to detect any emotional problems that may be contributing to the headaches.

Treatment

Treatment usually begins with eliminating the tension or correcting the physical problem that is causing the headaches. Painkillers, muscle relaxants, and tranquilizers may be used occasionally to treat muscle contraction headaches. Also, antidepressant drugs may be effective in preventing these headaches in those individuals who suffer from them regularly.

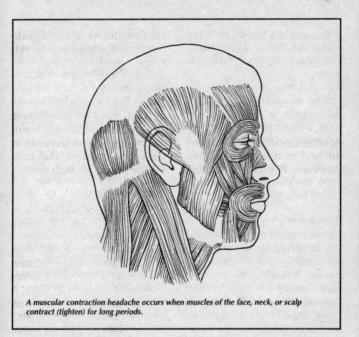

A muscular contraction headache occurs when muscles of the face, neck, or scalp contract (tighten) for long periods.

INFLAMMATORY HEADACHE

An inflammatory, or traction, headache is caused by pressure within the head, due to any of a variety of disorders.

Causes

Clogged sinuses and sinus infections are probably the chief cause of this type of headache. The sinuses are the cavities within the facial bones. When mucus, which normally flows freely through the sinuses and drains down the nasopharynx or out the nose, cannot drain properly, it collects in the sinuses and causes excess pressure on the surrounding tissues, leading to headache.

Other causes of inflammatory headaches include an aneurysm (a bulge in a blood vessel) in the head and a brain tumor. Aneurysms may not cause pain until they rupture or enlarge rapidly. Brain tumors are usually associated with swelling in the surrounding tissues, which

99

may cause increased pressure within the skull and, as a result, a dull, constant painful headache.

High blood pressure, which causes blood to rush through the vessels with too great a force; infections, which inflame sensitive tissue; and fever, which may enlarge the blood vessels, can also cause headache due to excess pressure within the skull.

Symptoms

The symptoms of an inflammatory headache are a dull, aching pain, often occurring early in the day, accompanied by a feeling of pressure in the head. The pain is heightened by sneezing, coughing, bending over, or doing anything that increases the amount of blood in the head.

Diagnosis

This type of headache is diagnosed by determining first whether sinus problems are causing it. If not, the doctor may order an electroencephalogram (EEG), which is a visual record of electrical activity in the brain; X-ray studies; a computed tomographic (CT) scan, which provides a cross-sectional picture of the brain; or a magnetic resonance (MR) imaging study, which yields images comparable to those obtained with CT but without the use of X rays. These tests can detect the presence of a tumor, an aneurysm, or another abnormality in the brain that may be responsible for causing the headache.

Treatment

Inflammatory headaches are treated according to their causes. Those triggered by a sinus infection can be treated with painkillers, antibiotics to fight the infection, or antihistamines and decongestants to dry out and help drain the sinuses. Headaches resulting from more serious disorders, such as a brain tumor, will almost certainly require surgery.

Prevention

Prevention of these headaches is sometimes possible if the cause is as simple as a sinus infection. For example, if you suffer from frequent sinus headaches, you should stop smoking. Smokers seem particularly prone to sinus infections.

Meningitis

Meningitis occurs when bacteria or viruses enter the spinal

fluid and infect the meninges, the three layers of membrane that surround the brain and spinal cord. Meningitis can prove to be fatal, although this is becoming less common because of the increased use of effective medications.

Meningitis seems to strike males more often than females and is most commonly seen in children up to the age of four years and in adults over the age of 60. Swelling of the brain, as well as epilepsy, blindness, amnesia, and deafness, can result when meningitis is not properly and promptly treated.

The three layers of meninges are the dura mater (the outermost layer), the arachnoid (the middle layer), and the pia mater (the innermost layer). The space between the inner two layers, called the subarachnoid space, is filled with clear cerebrospinal fluid, which is produced in the brain. When bacteria or viruses invade this fluid and form pus, the surrounding membranes soon become infected, resulting in meningitis.

Causes

Meningitis is caused by an infection that enters the system through a serious head wound or through the bloodstream from a source of infection in another part of the body. The bacteria may also reach the meninges from an abscess (localized infection) of the brain itself, but this is quite rare.

A deficiency in the immune system, which can be either inherited or acquired over time, may lead to a greater chance of contracting this disease as well.

Also, newborns may be at a greater risk of contracting meningitis if the mother had a genital infection, such as herpes, during the last week of pregnancy, if the membranes of the uterus ruptured prematurely, or if labor was prolonged.

Symptoms

The symptoms of meningitis are a "bursting" headache, high fever, rising pulse rate, irregular breathing, vomiting, and sensitivity to light.

Pain extends down the neck, into the back and lower limbs; the neck may be stiff, and it will be difficult for the patient to bend forward. As the disease progresses, the patient may suffer convulsions, or coma may occur.

Diagnosis

Unless increased pressure in the brain is suspected, meningitis is

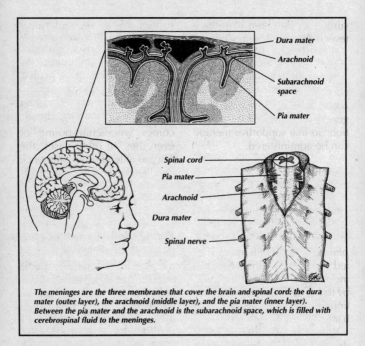

Dura mater

Arachnoid

Subarachnoid space

Pia mater

Spinal cord

Pia mater

Arachnoid

Dura mater

Spinal nerve

The meninges are the three membranes that cover the brain and spinal cord: the dura mater (outer layer), the arachnoid (middle layer), and the pia mater (inner layer). Between the pia mater and the arachnoid is the subarachnoid space, which is filled with cerebrospinal fluid to the meninges.

diagnosed with a test called a *lumbar puncture,* or *spinal tap,* in which a sample of the cerebrospinal fluid is withdrawn and examined to see if it is clear (healthy) or cloudy (pus-filled) and to identify the bacteria causing the infection. A physical examination, blood cultures, and cultures from the secretions of the respiratory tract may also be useful in determining the type of bacteria present. A viral infection is much harder to diagnose; it may not show up on any tests.

Treatment
Because meningitis must be treated immediately, medication may be prescribed before the specific infecting agent has been identified. Once the cause has been determined, a more appropriate medication can then be administered. The patient will be admitted to the hospital, where necessary mea-

sures can be taken to reduce fever and control brain swelling.

Viral infections are much more difficult to treat. Fortunately, most cases run their course without causing serious consequences. Treatment is generally limited to hospitalization, so that supportive therapy can be administered.

Prevention

Prevention of meningitis caused by certain strains of bacteria may be possible with some vaccines that are now available. Immunization against *Hemophilus influenzae* in infants has led to dramatic decreases in the incidence of meningitis caused by this organism. Research continues on vaccines against other bacterial strains.

Rifampin, an antituberculosis drug, is used for prevention of meningococcal meningitis, which is caused by the bacteria *Neisseria meningitidis*. The drug is given orally to individuals who have been in close contact with a person who has a documented case of meningococcal meningitis.

Multiple sclerosis

Multiple sclerosis is a chronic disease of the central nervous system (the brain and spinal cord) in which the protective myelin sheath (the insulating covering) of the nerve fibers degenerates. When this protection disappears, body functions may become impaired. In some cases, the patient ultimately becomes wheelchair-bound or even dies. In other cases, the disease may flare up only once in a lifetime and leave the individual with no or only minimal disabilities.

Causes

Researchers have not yet determined the exact cause of multiple sclerosis. Some studies indicate that the disease follows exposure to a virus that may lie dormant until some factor, such as stress or a second exposure to the virus, triggers the disease.

Another theory suggests that multiple sclerosis affects people who have some defect in their immune system. It is thought that after viral exposure, the immune system mistakenly identifies the myelin covering of the nerves as foreign tissue and tries to destroy it.

Symptoms

Initial attacks of multiple sclerosis are most common in people in their late 20s and early 30s. The disease often begins with one or more of the following symptoms: tingling and numbness in the arms and legs, muscle spasms, partial loss of vision, difficulty in walking, and impaired bladder control. After the first attack, there is usually a period of remission (a time without symptoms) for as long as two to three years.

Subsequent attacks may occur at irregular intervals and cause gradually increasing disability. Frequent episodes cause weakness, general incoordination, impaired speech, and burning sensations. Sexual function deteriorates, and mood swings are common.

More extensive nerve damage may result in loss of muscle control and may necessitate the use of a wheelchair. Usually, the earlier the onset of disease, the more slowly it progresses. Ten years after onset, fewer than half of patients with multiple sclerosis can continue regular daily activity. After 20 years, fewer than one fourth are able to function normally. (An individual may suffer one attack, however, and never have further symptoms.)

Diagnosis
Physicians diagnose multiple sclerosis through physical examination and observation of

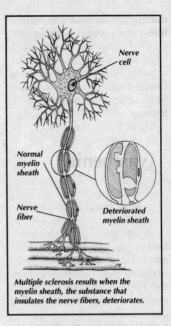

Multiple sclerosis results when the myelin sheath, the substance that insulates the nerve fibers, deteriorates.

symptoms. Often, diagnosis remains unconfirmed until a second attack occurs. Analysis of the spinal fluid in conjunction with magnetic resonance (MR) imaging studies is very useful in establishing the diagnosis.

Treatment
Since there is no cure for multiple sclerosis, treatment concentrates on relieving the symptoms. Muscle relaxants may ease muscle spasms and corticosteroid drugs may shorten attacks by re-

ducing nerve tissue inflammation. Many patients are more comfortable if they are well rested; afternoon naps and adequate sleep at night are advised. Cold temperatures sometimes relieve symptoms, whereas heat tends to make them worse.

Myasthenia gravis

Myasthenia gravis is an uncommon disease of the nerves and muscles, characterized by great fatigue and weakness in the muscular system, most notably in the face and throat. Although the muscles do not wither or waste away, there is slow and progressive paralysis. The disease is most likely to strike adults, especially women between the ages of 18 and 25 and men older than 40, but it can affect people of any age.

Causes
Myasthenia gravis is sometimes associated with thyroid disease, excessive growth of the thymus (a gland in the chest that is an essential part of the immune system), or tumors in the thymus.

The condition is a neuromuscular disorder; the muscles fail to receive messages from the nerves because of a lack of the important neurotransmitting chemical acetylcholine. Experts believe that the disorder originates in the immune system and causes the body to destroy or block the sites responsible for receiving acetylcholine.

Symptoms
The muscular weakness first shows up in the face: The eyelids droop, often causing squinting and double vision; there is an inability to move the mouth and lips, with subsequent difficulty in talking, chewing, and swallowing; and the cheeks generally droop or sag. Sometimes the arms and legs are afflicted, affecting basic motor movements, like walking and standing, and the performance of simple tasks, like lifting a cup. The progressive muscular weakness can also impair breathing. The degree of paralysis or weakness varies from hour to hour and day to day, although it tends to be least severe in the morning and worst at night. Blood tests and chest X rays aid in the diagnosis.

Treatment
Myasthenia gravis is usually not curable, but drugs are available that restore nerve transmission to the muscles. The drugs

neostigmine and pyridostigmine have been used to reestablish muscle strength and enable the patient with myasthenia gravis to live a more normal life. If a disorder of the thymus gland is found to be the underlying problem, the gland can be surgically removed. Corticosteroids are often used to help regulate the immune system.

Narcolepsy

Narcolepsy is a disorder in which an individual is recurrently subject to an irresistible, uncontrollable desire to sleep.

Causes
Narcolepsy is not necessarily related to any other abnormal condition, although it may be the result of an abnormality in the hypothalamus that causes a disorder in the body's endocrine system.

Symptoms
The most obvious symptom is the pattern of uncontrollable lapses into deep sleep during waking hours, often at inopportune times. These episodes of sleep last only a few minutes; the person wakes up feeling refreshed but is likely to fall asleep again a few hours later.

The condition may be associated with cataplexy, a disorder in which stress or an unexpected emotional reaction causes collapse due to a sudden attack of muscle weakness.

Diagnosis
The diagnosis is confirmed by observation of the patient in a sleep laboratory or by special electroencephalographic (EEG) studies.

Treatment
Central nervous system stimulants are often prescribed.

Neuralgia

Neuralgia is pain that runs along the course of a damaged nerve. The condition ranges from mild and temporary to severe and chronic. The pain is sharp and extreme, lasting only a few seconds but tending to recur. There are many types of neuralgia.

Peripheral neuropathy
In peripheral neuropathy, impairment of the peripheral nerves (those outside the brain and spinal cord) occurs as a complication of another disorder, such as diabetes mellitus, alcoholism, certain vitamin de-

ficiencies, anemia, or a tumor, or as a result of overexposure to particular chemicals or drugs. The first symptom of peripheral neuropathy is frequently a tingling sensation in the hands and feet, which slowly spreads up the limbs to the trunk; numbness follows in the same pattern, the skin becomes sensitive, and neuralgic pain ensues. Numbness in the hands leads to a loss of dexterity and susceptibility to accidents. A special risk is that a numbed part of the body can sustain an injury without the patient's awareness until it becomes infected or ulcerated. The muscles gradually atrophy (wither away), and paralysis may set in.

Shingles

Shingles, or herpes zoster, is a viral infection characterized by intense pain and skin rash along the course of a nerve. Red blisters appear in a band, usually along one side of the chest, trunk, or abdomen.

Shingles occurs almost exclusively in people who have already had chicken pox (which is caused by the same virus) and appears during times of stress or after a subsequent exposure to the chicken pox virus. Shingles can often be diagnosed by sight. (For additional information on shingles, see pages 56.)

Trigeminal neuralgia

Trigeminal neuralgia, or tic douloureux, primarily affects elderly people (most commonly, those over age 70), although it may also occur in younger people with multiple sclerosis. The pain arises from the trigeminal nerve, which controls sensation in the face, teeth, mouth, and nasal cavity and movement of the jaw. The pain, usually excruciating, covers one side of the face and can be set off by eating, by washing, or even by being exposed to a gust of air. With time, the stabbing pains occur more and more frequently, until they become constant. The cause is unknown. Although the condition is not life-threatening, it can become very disabling.

Treatment

Treatment for the various types of neuralgia depends on the location of the damaged nerves, the severity of the pain, and the reason behind the impairment. Therapy may vary from cold or hot packs and aspirin to stronger prescription painkillers. For shingles, ointments may soothe and dry up blisters, and an antiviral drug such as acyclovir or famciclovir, may shorten the course of the illness. A physician may refer a patient with neuralgia to a neurologist (a specialist in problems of the nervous system). In rare instances, neurosurgery to sever a damaged nerve is necessary to eliminate the pain.

Prevention
There is virtually no way to prevent neuralgia, except to treat underlying diseases that may precipitate nerve damage and to avoid overexposure to certain chemicals and drugs.

Paralysis

Paralysis is the loss of the ability to move a part of the body, usually brought on by damage either to the muscles or to the nervous system. The condition can vary in severity—from paralysis of one small muscle to paralysis of almost the entire body.

Irreversible and permanent paralysis results when a nerve is completely severed and destroyed, whereas paralysis caused by some diseases that cause inflammation without actual destruction of nerve tissue may diminish as the condition is treated and the body begins to recuperate.

Causes
There are numerous causes of paralysis. Brain damage resulting from disease or a stroke can lead to partial or total paralysis of various parts of the body. Such damage interferes with the transmission of nerve impulses from the brain to the muscles. Certain other diseases (for example, myasthenia gravis, a severe muscular disorder of the neurochemical transmission system) and poisons (such as nerve gas and the toxin that causes botulism) also prevent nerve impulses from making contact with muscles but do not necessarily cause complete loss of movement.

Damage to the spinal cord at the level of the middle or lower back can cause paralysis of the legs and the structures located in the lower part of the body; this condition is called *paraplegia*. Injury to the spinal cord at the level of the neck affects both arms and both legs; this condition is known as *quadriplegia*.

Diabetes, cancer, alcoholism, vitamin deficiency, and reactions to certain drugs, among other conditions, can injure peripheral nerves (those outside the brain and spinal cord), occasionally weakening or totally immobilizing the muscles they control, as well as causing loss of sensation in the areas they serve.

Treatment
Well-being and survival depend on the cause and extent of the paralysis. Obviously, paralysis that affects the muscles involved in breathing is life-threatening, and the job of breathing must be taken over by machines (called *ventilators* or *respirators*) until the paralysis improves or disappears.

Patients whose paralysis does not require artificial measures for survival may benefit from physical or occupational therapy. These patients can learn to reuse a muscle or to develop other muscles to compensate for a disabled muscle. All patients with disabled muscles require special attention to prevent muscle atrophy (withering away) and ulcers (pressure sores or bed sores).

Parkinson disease

Parkinson disease is a progressive disorder characterized primarily by uncontrollable tremors in the limbs, a shuffling gait, and generalized muscular rigidity. It most often strikes people over the age of 60.

Parkinson disease is usually not fatal, but it leads to changes in the entire body, making the patient more susceptible to other diseases. It can be present in a mild form for 20 or 30 years, but a severe form can lead to serious disability within 5 to 10 years.

Cause
The cause of Parkinson disease is unknown. No inherited, physiologic, or environmental factors have been identified as causes of the disease. It is known, however, that Parkinson disease is a reflection of a chemical imbalance in the brain. Those with the disease have been shown to have low levels of a neurotransmitter called *dopamine*. (Neurotransmitters are chemicals in the brain that transmit impulses across junctions between neurons; the delicate balance of neurotransmitters in the brain is responsible for brain function and muscular control.) To date, no cause for this chemical deficiency has been found.

Symptoms
The symptoms of Parkinson disease are uncontrollable shaking of the limbs, stiff muscles, drooling, reduced blinking, an

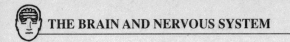

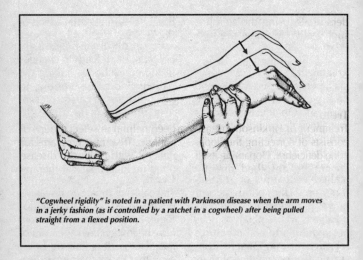

"Cogwheel rigidity" is noted in a patient with Parkinson disease when the arm moves in a jerky fashion (as if controlled by a ratchet in a cogwheel) after being pulled straight from a flexed position.

expressionless face, stooping posture, and a shuffling walk. Tremors may worsen during rest periods and times of increased anxiety. Interestingly, the tremors may decrease when the patient makes a conscious effort to perform some action.

As the disease progresses, speech may slur and sentences may trail off. Small muscle movements become increasingly difficult—reducing the ability to write, eat, chew, and swallow—and all movements seem overly stiff and slow. The term "cogwheel rigidity" is often used to describe the typical arm motion these patients display: When the arm is pulled straight from a flexed position, it seems to jerk up and down as if controlled by a ratchet in a cogwheel.

Excitement and tension can cause these symptoms to worsen, as can depression. Depression is common among Parkinson disease victims, who are understandably upset by their loss of muscle control.

Diagnosis

Diagnostic evaluation involves a medical history, physical examination, and observation of the symptoms. If tremors are the only symptom displayed, tests may be done to rule out the possibility that other disorders are causing the tremors, such as liver disease, multiple sclerosis (a debilitating nervous disorder), chronic alcoholism, or overactivity of the thyroid gland.

Treatment

Treatment of Parkinson disease consists of correcting the dopamine deficiency. Dopamine itself cannot be absorbed directly into the brain from the bloodstream, so a substance called *levodopa* is prescribed to help the brain manufacture more of its own dopamine.

Levodopa has several undesirable side effects, such as nausea (which is decreased if the drug is taken with meals), an uneven "on-off" effect (causing symptoms to disappear and then reappear), and a loss of effectiveness over time. Levodopa preparations are often given in combination with anticholinergic drugs, which decrease nerve-to-muscle transmission, thereby reducing tremor and rigidity, and also decrease drooling. Levodopa is most often prescribed in combination with carbidopa, a substance that prevents destruction of levodopa in the body before it reaches the brain, thus allowing the use of smaller amounts of levodopa. Bromocriptine, a

drug that enhances the effects of dopamine, has also been successful. Selegiline, a newer anti-Parkinson drug given in addition to existing drug regimens, appears to be quite helpful in many patients as well.

Surgery to halt tremors has been helpful in select groups of patients. Treatment programs for patients with Parkinson disease often include physical therapy and exercise regimes. In addition, emotional support and understanding are critical to the patient's well being.

Rabies

Rabies (formerly known as *hydrophobia*) is an acute infectious viral disease of mammals, especially carnivores (meat eaters), which is characterized by central nervous system irritation followed by paralysis and, in some cases, death. Human infection is usually caused by the bite of a rabid animal (dogs, skunks, cats, bats, foxes, and coyotes are among those that may be affected).

The disease is marked by paralysis of the swallowing muscles and by throat spasms, which are set off by drinking or even the sight of liquids (hence the name *hydrophobia*, meaning fear of water). In late stages of the disease, convulsions, tetanus (a condition characterized by severe muscular contractions), and paralysis of the respiratory (breathing) muscles may occur. Fortunately, because of animal immunization programs, only a handful of cases of rabies are reported in the United States each year.

Cause

Rabies is caused by a virus that is present in the saliva and respiratory secretions of rabid animals. Rabid animals transmit the infection by biting other animals or human beings. Rabies can be acquired by exposure of a mucous membrane or an open skin wound to infected animal saliva or by inhalation of the virus.

The rabies virus travels from the site of entry to the spinal cord and brain, where it multiplies. It then spreads to the salivary glands and into the saliva itself.

In human beings, the incubation period (the time between exposure to the virus and development of symptoms) may extend from ten days to one year, but the average incubation period is 30 to 50 days. The incubation period is shortest in people who have been bitten on the head or trunk and in those who have multiple bites.

Symptoms

The first symptom is a short period of mental depression, restlessness, and fever. In the next stage of the disease, the restlessness increases to uncontrollable excitement and hyperactivity. There is excessive salivation ("foaming at the mouth") and painful spasms of the throat muscles. The spasms can be easily initiated—by a breath of air, a slight breeze, an attempt to drink water. Generally, the patient experiences overwhelming thirst but cannot drink. In untreated cases, death occurs within three to ten days. However, patients often survive the disease if diagnosis and treatment are prompt.

Diagnosis

In human patients, rabies is usually suspected if there has been a report of an animal bite or exposure to the saliva of a rabid animal. The diagnosis is confirmed by testing for the virus once the symptoms appear. A domestic animal with no symptoms that suddenly bites a human should be confined and observed by a veterinarian for ten days. If the animal still shows no symptoms, it was most likely not infectious at the time of the bite and is usually released. However, if the animal is apparently rabid or is a wild animal, it should be captured. The police or local health department should be notified so that they can capture and examine the animal for rabies. Only an experienced professional should attempt to capture an animal suspected of being rabid.

Treatment
As soon as possible after the bite or exposure of an open wound to animal saliva occurs, the contaminated area should be cleaned thoroughly with soap and water or an antiseptic solution.

The next step is administration of antirabies serum or human rabies immune globulin for passive immunization. This is followed immediately by vaccine for active immunization. A new active immunization, called *HDCV,* is said to have only mild side effects for most people. Subsequent HDCV injections are given on days 3, 7, 14, and 28 after exposure. The World Health Organization recommends that a sixth injection be given routinely 90 days after the first injection.

Prevention
The best preventive measure for rabies is to minimize contact with animals that may be rabid. In many cases, people with a high occupational risk of animal bites receive preexposure injections. This is especially helpful for zoo personnel and people whose work or hobbies take them into areas where they might encounter rabid animals.

As for domestic animals, restraining dogs and cats from contact with wild animals and impounding stray animals are important preventive measures. Immunizing 70 percent or more of the dog population of major cities has helped to restrict transmission of rabies, even in areas where wild animals have the disease.

Controlling rabies in wildlife areas is more difficult, although rabies as a disease is self-limiting because it tends to kill off susceptible hosts in an area. Expensive control efforts are generally limited to areas where humans are apt to be exposed to wildlife—in campgrounds, parks, and wildlife preserves.

Sciatica

Sciatica is a condition characterized by pain that extends

along the entire length of the sciatic nerve (which runs down the lower back and outer side of the thigh, leg, and foot), radiating across the back of the pelvis through the buttocks and into the leg.

Cause

Sciatica is commonly associated with injury to or rupture of a lumbar disk, one of the cartilaginous disks located between the lumbar (lower back) vertebrae. When the injured disk exerts pressure against the sciatic nerve, pain radiates down the nerve. There may be numbness and tingling in the afflicted area.

Symptoms

The symptoms of sciatica vary in intensity, depending on the extent to which the injured disk presses on the sciatic nerve and according to the individual's susceptibility to pain. In mild cases, the pain may be a slight discomfort in the lower back and along the leg. In severe cases, the pain is excruciating and often completely immobilizes the victim. Since the cause is frequently a ruptured ("slipped") disk, it is difficult to know when an attack will begin. A sudden cough may cause the disk to move and

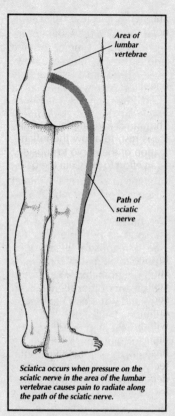

Area of lumbar vertebrae

Path of sciatic nerve

Sciatica occurs when pressure on the sciatic nerve in the area of the lumbar vertebrae causes pain to radiate along the path of the sciatic nerve.

press on the sciatic nerve, resulting in pain. (It is commonplace for sciatica patients to be free from pain one moment and in agony the next.)

Repeated problems with a ruptured lumbar disk can cause general inflammation of the sciatic nerve. In these cases, it is not a matter of pain that comes and goes. Depending on the inflammation, it may be a matter of having somewhat less pain at one time than at another.

Treatment

The primary treatment of sciatica is rest, to allow the inflammation of the nerve to subside. In an effort to alleviate the pain, various medications, such as analgesics and muscle relaxants, may be prescribed or anesthetic agents may be injected into the area around the spinal cord.

In cases that do not respond to such conservative measures, surgery may be necessary. Recently, new surgical techniques, such as microsurgery and percutaneous (through the skin without cutting, as with a needle) removal of disk fragments, have been developed. These techniques have considerably decreased hospital stays and loss of work time. So far, success at relieving pain and neurologic symptoms has been good. Not all individuals with disk problems, however, are suitable for this surgery.

Physical therapy is often used to relieve the pain of sciatica. This treatment includes hydrotherapy, in which a stream of water is directed at the affected area. Many therapists advise their patients to overcome the effects of a ruptured disk by developing the core muscles (the four muscle groups that form the waist) in order to provide a supportive column of muscle that will help keep the disk in place.

THE SKIN

The skin is the largest organ of the body, covering 18 square feet and weighing about seven pounds in an average adult. The skin acts as a waterproof barrier that affords protection from invasion by dirt, bacteria, and other harmful substances and helps to regulate body temperature.

The skin is composed of three layers—the epidermis, the dermis, and the subcutaneous layer.

Epidermis

The outermost layer of skin is the epidermis. The epidermis contains pigment cells that determine skin color and shield the skin against damaging sun rays. Specialized cells within this layer manufacture keratin, a tough substance also found in hair and nails.

Epidermal cells are continuously being worn away and replaced. This reconstruction process is usually invisible. Since the outer skin layer repairs itself quickly, any injury to the epidermis rarely causes injury to the body as a whole.

Dermis

The dermis contains blood vessels, nerve endings, hair follicles, sweat glands, and sebaceous (oil) glands. Damage occurring at this level can send infection into the bloodstream and throughout the body.

Within the dermis, blood vessels and sweat glands help the body regulate heat. If the temperature of blood rises, the brain stimulates secretion by the sweat glands. Sweat then flows to the surface of the skin through ducts and cools the skin by evaporating. The sebaceous glands prevent excessive evaporation by coating the surface of the skin with an oily substance called *sebum*.

Subcutaneous layer

Beneath the dermis is the subcutaneous layer, in which the sweat glands originate and fat is stored. This layer also supports the blood vessels and nerves that supply the outer layers of the skin.

Because the dermis and the subcutaneous layer are rich

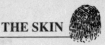

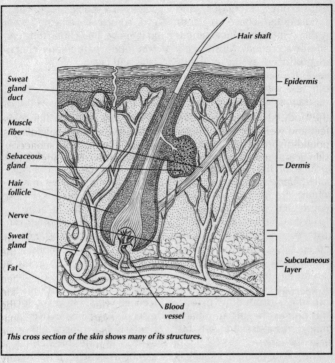

This cross section of the skin shows many of its structures.

with nerve endings, the skin is also a sensory organ. Nerves throughout these layers transmit tactile perceptions to the brain.

Acne

Acne is a condition of the skin that ranges in appearance from small raised bumps to pimples and large cysts. Acne is so common that 80 percent of the population will have some form of it at some time in their lives.

Causes

Although there are several theories about what causes acne, authorities generally believe that acne is a by-product of hormonal changes during puberty. Production of hormones (particularly the male hormone testosterone) increases and stimulates the sebaceous glands in the skin to produce sebum (an oily secretion). Most excess oil produced by these glands leaves the skin through the hair follicles. Sometimes, oil clogs these tubes and creates comedones (blocked hair follicles). Comedones are what form the initial lumps in acne.

If comedones are open to the surface of the skin, they are called *blackheads*. They contain sebum from the sebaceous glands, bacteria, and any skin tissue that accumulates near the surface. Comedones that are closed at the surface are called *whiteheads*. Plugged follicles can rupture internally, resulting in a discharge of their contents into the surrounding tissues. This process begins an inflammatory response that sets the stage for acne.

The role of bacteria in acne is unclear. Bacteria may act by causing chemical reactions in the sebaceous fluid, leading to the release of very irritating compounds called *fatty acids*. These in turn may cause inflammation that increases susceptibility to infection.

Authorities disagree about the role of diet in acne. Diet alone does not cure acne, nor does acne stem from an allergic re-

action to a specific food. However, some cases of acne appear to improve after eliminating certain foods, particularly chocolates and fats.

Symptoms

Acne causes raised swellings, most frequently on the face, neck, back, chest, and shoulders. In severe cases, there may be pus-filled sacs that break open and discharge fluid. Soreness, pain, and itching may accompany the bumps. These symptoms could be acne, or they could indicate other skin reactions to such substances as cosmetics or medications.

Since puberty plays a role in the onset of acne, the condition usually appears during the teenage years. However, it can extend to age 25 and over, particularly in women. Although acne is not life-threatening, it can be a problem. If untreated, acne lesions can leave permanent scars.

Treatment

Acne has no prevention or cure, but there are several treatments. The simplest home remedy is to wash the affected areas thoroughly at least twice a day with warm water and mild soap. Washing gently will not dry or irritate sensitive skin.

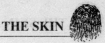

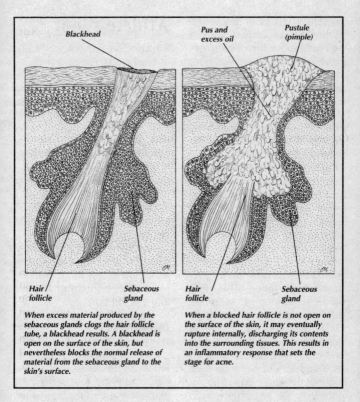

Blackhead

Pus and
excess oil

Pustule
(pimple)

Hair
follicle

Sebaceous
gland

Hair
follicle

Sebaceous
gland

When excess material produced by the sebaceous glands clogs the hair follicle tube, a blackhead results. A blackhead is open on the surface of the skin, but nevertheless blocks the normal release of material from the sebaceous gland to the skin's surface.

When a blocked hair follicle is not open on the surface of the skin, it may eventually rupture internally, discharging its contents into the surrounding tissues. This results in an inflammatory response that sets the stage for acne.

Use of makeup should be limited. In addition, skin may heal with exposure to the sun. However, sunlamps and ultraviolet lamps should be used only under a doctor's supervision.

Do not pick or squeeze pimples, since more inflammation and scarring may result. Also, the risk of infection is increased.

Some over-the-counter acne medications, particularly lotions or creams containing benzoyl peroxide, can help troubled skin. However, most of these preparations tend to dry the skin if the manufacturer's directions are not followed carefully.

For persistent acne, a doctor may prescribe an antibiotic

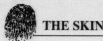

preparation that can be applied to the surface of the skin or an oral antibiotic, such as tetracycline or erythromycin. These antibiotics act to suppress bacterial growth, which may be a factor in worsening acne.

Another drug, tretinoin (vitamin A acid), has reduced acne in more than 50 percent of the people who have tried it. This drug can be taken independently or in combination with an antibiotic, and must be used under a doctor's supervision. A newer drug, isotretinoin, is related to tretinoin and is used to treat severe cystic acne. It is usually not prescribed, however, unless all other acne treatments have failed. This drug works by temporarily suppressing the production of secretions by the sebaceous glands. It is important to note that this drug can have very serious side effects and should never be used without the knowledge and supervision of an experienced doctor. In addition, isotretinoin should not be used by any woman who is, who thinks she may be, or who intends to become pregnant. Use of this drug in any amount for even short periods during pregnancy is associated with an extremely high risk of fetal abnormalities and spontaneous abortion.

Athlete's foot

Athlete's foot (known medically as *tinea pedis*) is a fungal infection of the foot. It is also known as ringworm of the foot, although it is not caused by a worm.

Symptoms
Athlete's foot causes itching, burning, and stinging sensations. The skin between the toes may redden, peel, and crack. In extremely long-lasting cases of athlete's foot, the toenails may become infected, discolored, and overgrown. The fungus may spread to the underside of the foot, beneath the arch, producing groups of itching blisters and peeling skin.

Diagnosis
It is important to rule out other causes of similar symptoms. For example, hot, tight shoes may make the feet sweaty in warm weather; the moisture and friction may cause softening and peeling of the skin on the soles. Dyes, adhesive cements, and other substances inside the shoes may cause irritation, as may some powders and nail polishes. Eczema, psoriasis, and scabies are other possible causes of similar symptoms.

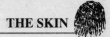

Treatment

Most people can treat athlete's foot at home using one of several good salves, powders, or liquids obtainable without a prescription from the drugstore. These include undecylenic acid ointment, tolnaftate, and miconazole. Clotrimazole is another effective medication, but it must be prescribed by a physician. Directions usually call for application morning and night, until one week after all symptoms have vanished. If skin is peeling, soak feet and remove loose skin before applying ointment.

If sweaty feet are the cause of your athlete's foot, ointments should not be used. Instead, you should ask your doctor for suggestions about controlling the excessive sweating. Changing shoes may eliminate the problem if the feet are sensitive to chemicals inside the shoes.

Severe cases of athlete's foot call for treatment by a physician. To relieve symptoms, the doctor may prescribe soaking the feet in a solution of aluminum sulfate and calcium acetate (often called *Burow's solution*). An antiseptic solution may be added to the Burow's solution if a secondary infection is present.

Prevention

Athlete's foot can recur despite any treatment, especially during hot weather. The organisms that cause athlete's foot thrive in a hot, moist setting. However, there are several things you can do to help prevent the disease. You can keep your feet clean, dry between your toes after bathing, and change socks frequently. Use dusting and drying powders to keep the feet dry. Separate your toes with small wads of cotton when you are sleeping. Wear wooden or rubber clogs in motel and community showers and wear sandals, open-toed shoes, or no shoes at all (when safe and practical) during hot weather.

Baldness

Baldness (known medically as *alopecia*) is partial or complete loss of hair on the head. This may be caused by an inherited tendency or by aging, fever, drugs, radiation, or disease.

Male-pattern baldness

Male-pattern baldness is the most common form of hair loss. There seems to be an inherited tendency toward it; androgen (a male hormone) contributes to it as well. However, the exact

121

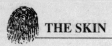

mechanism by which it occurs is not known. Hair loss is gradual, occurring at the forehead, at the temples, and on top of the head. It can begin as early as age 15 or 16, in which case it may indicate that considerable baldness is likely in the future. However, male-pattern baldness does not usually advance at a steady or predictable rate.

Female-pattern baldness
Female-pattern baldness is fairly common in menopausal women

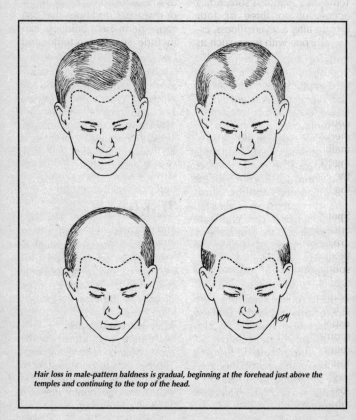

Hair loss in male-pattern baldness is gradual, beginning at the forehead just above the temples and continuing to the top of the head.

and usually involves only the area around the crown of the head. Female-pattern baldness, like male-pattern baldness, is believed to have hormonal causes.

Temporary baldness

Temporary baldness sometimes occurs up to three or four months after a severe illness, especially one with fever, such as scarlet fever. Temporary baldness can also result from decreased activity of the pituitary or thyroid gland, early stages of syphilis, pregnancy, use of birth control pills and certain other medications, crash dieting or malnutrition, or a diet containing too much vitamin A. When the cause is removed, the missing hair usually returns.

Spotty baldness

Spotty baldness, or *alopecia areata*, may affect areas of the head and beard. The cause of spotty baldness is unknown. If the condition first occurs in adulthood and there are just a few bald spots, hair growth usually resumes after a few months. The condition may recur, however. The outlook is less favorable if the condition begins in childhood or if hair loss is widespread. Occasionally, all body hair is lost. If there

is no apparent cause for widespread hair loss, such as fever or severe illness, hair growth is not likely to resume.

Permanent baldness

Permanent baldness occurs when the scalp becomes scarred as a result of burns, other injury, or disease. Conditions that can cause permanent baldness can include severe bacterial and fungal infections, tuberculosis, ulcers, lupus erythematosus, and certain slow-growing tumors.

Treatment

There is no totally satisfactory medical treatment at this time to cure or prevent baldness. However, hair transplants can be effective. Scalp plugs containing active hair follicles are taken from the back of the head and transplanted to areas affected by hair loss. In the new location, the transplanted follicles continue to produce hair just as before.

A topical form of the antihypertensive drug minoxidil has been shown to stimulate hair growth in some individuals. This over-the-counter preparation must be applied on a continuous basis, however, and only seems effective in treating male pattern baldness.

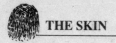

Boils

A boil, or furuncle, is caused by a bacterial infection and irritation of the skin and its underlying structures. It is a painful swelling in the skin that is easily detected by touch. When a group of boils interconnects below the surface of the skin, a growth called a *carbuncle* forms.

Causes

Boils develop when *Staphylococcus* bacteria enter the skin through a hair follicle and multiply in its warm, moist environment. Bacteria continue to grow while producing substances that invade surrounding cells. White blood cells (which attack and kill invading organisms) travel to the infected hair follicle and enclose bacteria. As more white blood cells gather, they eventually consume the bacteria and eliminate the infection. This buildup by the white blood cells is what produces the pustule (large cyst) in the center of the boil. When the pustule ruptures, pus and dead skin cells killed by the bacteria drain out, and the boil heals.

Staphylococcus bacteria are often found in the nose and throat. From there—or from other parts of the body—the bacteria can spread to a hair follicle. The bacteria can also be transmitted via contact with an infected person or an infected article, such as a washcloth or towel. In most cases, however, people who come in contact with the bacteria do not get boils.

Those at risk

People who are run-down or who suffer diseases such as anemia (deficiency of red blood cells), diabetes, or infections that weaken their natural defenses against bacteria seem more susceptible to boils. Those who work with greasy or oily substances are more likely to develop boils because these materials trap bacteria against the skin. Poor bathing habits also invite infection, especially in the summer months, when sweaty skin provides the moist climate conducive to bacterial growth.

Symptoms

Boils can develop anywhere on the skin. They appear most frequently on the neck, face, and back, and they can erupt in several places during an infection. Although boils vary in size, they characteristically form white or yellow pustules. As the infection progresses, the pustule becomes red and hot. Excess fluid in the boil produces pressure on the nerves underneath, which can result in considerable pain. When boils contain little pus, they are called *blind boils;* the inflammation recedes slowly without rupturing, but sometimes it leaves a scar.

If boils are large or extensive, the person may also experience fever and a general feeling of weakness. Sometimes, the infection gets into the bloodstream and spreads throughout the body. The same bacteria that cause the boil may also produce a toxin (poison) that causes blood clots, usually in the blood vessels that are around the boil.

Treatment

Boils and carbuncles should *never* be squeezed, particularly if they are on the face. Squeezing may force the infection deeper into the skin and possibly into the bloodstream. Only a physician is qualified to lance a boil to encourage drainage. Afterward, the doctor may prescribe an oral antibiotic, such as penicillin or erythromycin, to fight further infection.

Many boils will rupture and heal on their own. However, holding a soft cloth soaked with warm water against the boil for 15 to 20 minutes at least four times a day will speed the process. These warm compresses increase blood flow to the area and encourage pustule formation. Since bacteria from the boil are contagious, the cloth should be disinfected in boiling water or in the hot cycle of a washing machine.

When a boil bursts, the infected area should be washed thoroughly and covered with an antibiotic cream and sterile gauze. If the boil does not heal within a few days, or if the boil is located on or near the face, a physician should be consulted.

Prevention

To prevent new eruptions, the skin needs to be kept cool and dry. Sometimes, physicians advise their patients to wash the entire body with an antiseptic (germ-fighting) soap twice a day. If boils frequently recur, underclothing and bed linen should be changed on a daily basis.

Calluses

Calluses are thickened areas of the skin. They develop most often on the balls and heels of the feet and on the hands.

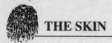

Causes

Skin buildup is the result of excessive friction or pressure against the surface of the skin. As pressure mounts, dead skin cells accumulate, and the skin thickens. After a blister heals, calluses may form at the site—perhaps the body's way of protecting the area against further injury.

Shoes that fit improperly are often the cause of calluses on the feet. Calluses on the hands also result from pressure or friction; even holding a pencil too tightly can result in callused fingers. Those who wear high heels are also prone to calluses because of the increased pressure the shoes exert on the balls of the feet.

Flat-footed people have a greater incidence of calluses. The small bones in the front of the foot are forced downward against the skin when the individual walks, resulting in calluses.

Symptoms

Calluses vary in size and shape depending on where they grow and how much skin is affected. Sometimes, calluses grow so thick that the skin becomes inflexible and cracks.

When pressure is relieved, calluses usually produce no pain. However, continued irritation, especially involving areas where the skin is split, can cause discomfort that interferes with physical activities.

Treatment

Immediate treatment involves removal of the pressure that caused the callus in the first place. Extremely persistent or painful calluses should be examined by a doctor. In rare instances, surgery may be necessary to alleviate intense pressure. In milder cases, calluses can often be eased by padding the exposed area to reduce further friction.

There are over-the-counter remedies that soften the callused tissue, making it easier to remove. Salicylic acid plasters, which are sold in medicated sheets, can be placed over the callus after bathing and secured with tape. (The pad should be removed just before the next bath so that the softened skin can be gently removed with a pumice stone.)

These home remedies should not be used by people who have diabetes, atherosclerosis, or other disorders affecting circulation. They should consult their doctor before attempting to remove calluses because of the high risk of infection.

Canker sores

Canker sores (medically known as *aphthous ulcers*) are inflamed tissue cavities, usually found in the mouth. They can be quite painful, often inhibiting eating ability. Even though up to one out of every four people develops canker sores, they are not contagious.

Causes

Researchers disagree about the cause of canker sores. One unconfirmed theory suggests that the sores are the result of an autoimmune response, whereby the body develops antibodies to its own tissue.

Other factors that have been thought to trigger canker sores include fever, menstruation, fatigue, tension, and allergies. Some people get canker sores after eating certain foods. Poor dental hygiene, ill-fitting dentures, and stiff toothbrushes may also contribute to the development of the sores.

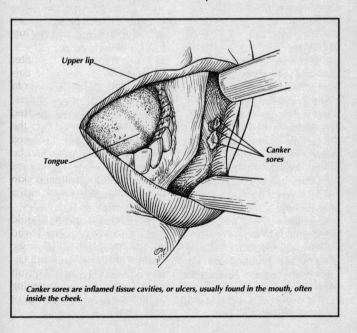

Upper lip

Tongue

Canker sores

Canker sores are inflamed tissue cavities, or ulcers, usually found in the mouth, often inside the cheek.

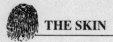

Symptoms

Canker sores can occur singly or in groups. They can be found almost anywhere in the mouth—inside the cheek and on the tongue, lips, or gums.

A canker sore begins as a small blister. After the blister breaks, a small ulcer develops and enlarges until there is a bright red sore surrounding the whitish-yellow cavity. This sore can last about 10 to 14 days before healing. Canker sores leave no scars. However, they often recur, sometimes every few weeks or months.

Treatment

Canker sores have no cure, but there are several treatments that may relieve pain. Some physicians prescribe the antibiotic tetracycline for canker sores. Treatment involves dissolving the capsule in an ounce of warm water and swishing the mixture in the mouth for five to ten minutes, three or four times a day for five to seven days. Therapy may also include soaking a cotton wad in the solution and applying it directly to the sores.

There are also various over-the-counter preparations designed to reduce discomfort from canker sores. Ask your doctor to recommend one that might work well for you.

Prevention

People who have repeated attacks of canker sores should see a physician or dentist. Recurrence may be lessened by improving oral hygiene or by avoiding certain foods or other substances.

Corns

Corns are small, round mounds of firm, dead skin that form on or between the toes. Their hard, waxy core, which bores down into the skin and presses on the underlying tissue and nerves, can cause extreme pain.

Causes

Corns, like calluses, are caused by a great deal of pressure or friction on the toes, usually from ill-fitting shoes or high heels. Since the skin acts as the body's protector from the outside environment, corns form when the body attempts to protect the troubled area from more pressure by building up a mass of dead skin cells and secreting a hard substance called *keratin*. People who have abnormal bone structure in their feet or certain types of arthritis tend to develop corns. Generally, however, if you don't wear high heeled or tight-fitting

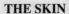

shoes, you should be able to avoid the development of corns.

Symptoms
Corns are usually regular in shape, and can be white, gray, or yellow. They most often form on the outside of the first or fifth toes, where pressure most often occurs.

Corns that form between the toes are called *soft corns;* they are not as firm as other corns because of the moistness between the toes.

Treatment
Corns are best treated by first eliminating the cause of the pressure. Over-the-counter preparations are available. These include padding to reduce the friction on the area, ointments, and medicated pads. Severe or persistent corns must be treated by a doctor, but only rarely do they necessitate surgery. Because of the risk of infection, people with diabetes, atherosclerosis, or other circulatory diseases should *never* treat a corn themselves.

Cysts

A cyst is an abnormal sac or membrane containing a fluid or semisolid material.

Cysts can develop virtually anywhere in the body. They can form around a foreign body, such as a particle in the lung or beneath the skin, or around a parasite. They may entrap an escaping body liquid, such as blood hemorrhaging into tissue or fluid leaking from a bursa (a sac containing lubricant for a joint).

Types and treatment
Perhaps the most common cysts are those of the skin and mucous membranes.

A *sebaceous cyst* occurs when a sebaceous gland (the tiny oil gland at the base of each hair root) becomes plugged. Ordinarily, this plugging results in a blackhead or, if the blackhead becomes infected, a pus-filled pimple. Occasionally, however, the pimple does not break, and the swelling becomes entrapped beneath the surface of the skin. Sebum (oil from the sebaceous gland) continues to flow into the sac that forms in the cavity, and the cyst grows to the size of a marble or larger.

Sebaceous cysts—which can occur in any part of the body where there is hair, including the neck, scalp, and back—can easily be removed surgically if bothersome; if they become infected, they must be drained be-

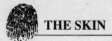

fore removal. A type of tiny cyst known as *milium,* which usually occurs on the face and scrotum, can simply be opened and drained. Larger cysts must be removed completely, or they will recur.

Mucous cysts that occur in the mouth, on the tongue, or on the lower lip are caused by plugged mucous glands and can grow to the size of a pea or larger. They can be removed surgically as well.

Traumatic epithelial cysts usually result from the trapping of a piece of skin, a blood clot, or foreign material beneath the skin because of some injury. These cysts may or may not need to be removed.

Dermatitis

Dermatitis is an inflammation of the skin. There are many different kinds of dermatitis.

Chronic dermatitis

Chronic dermatitis often occurs on the hands or feet, and may simply be the result of continued irritation, especially by contact dermatitis. It is marked by thickened skin, inflammation, and scaling. It is sometimes caused by excessive hand washing or by accumulation of

soaps or detergents under rings. Occasionally, a fungal infection is the cause.

Contact dermatitis

This skin inflammation is caused by a substance that has touched the skin. It may be a harsh chemical or a detergent or soap that irritates skin directly, or it may be a substance that produces an allergic reaction that does not appear until five or six days after the initial contact. Less commonly, the reaction appears only after years of repeated use.

Common causes of allergic contact dermatitis are poison ivy, chemicals in shoes and clothing, metal rings, antibiotic salves, and cosmetics. There are also cases in which a substance, such as a shaving lotion or cosmetic, produces a "photoallergic" reaction—that is, a skin rash develops from exposure to sunlight.

Eczema

This inflammation of the skin is marked by small blisters (when severe), redness, fluid in the tissue, oozing, scales, crusts or scabs, burning or itching, and sometimes dryness. The skin of flexor surfaces (those subject to bending movements, such as the back of the knee and the top of the elbow) is most commonly affected.

There are several different forms of eczema. One of the more common types is atopic dermatitis, which is caused by an allergy. Susceptible people often have a family history of allergic diseases, such as asthma or hay fever. Typically, atopic dermatitis begins in infancy, subsides by age 3, and may reappear by age 10 or 12. Certain foods (such as wheat, milk, and eggs) and other substances (such as pollen and fur) may also bring on symptoms of eczema.

Exfoliative dermatitis

This condition produces shedding of skin all over the body, together with hair loss. The entire skin surface is red, scaly, and thickened. The cause is unknown in most cases, but it sometimes occurs after a less severe case of dermatitis or as a side effect of a drug. (Consult a doctor about any medication you are currently taking.) Hospitalization is frequently necessary because the condition can be life-threatening.

Localized neurodermatitis

This condition is characterized by thick, sharp-bordered, scaly breaks in the skin, occasionally with little blisters. Localized neurodermatitis is caused by habitual scratching of an insect bite or other real or imagined irritation of the skin. It is corrected by covering the area to prevent scratching. In the case of an itch in the area around the vagina and anus, however, warts, pinworms, hemorrhoids, infections, or certain diseases may be the cause.

Nummular dermatitis

Coin-shaped patches of blisters that later ooze and crust over mark this condition, which is usually accompanied by dry skin and itching. Most often, nummular dermatitis appears on the legs, buttocks, and trunk.

Seborrheic dermatitis

This is a scaling and inflammation of the scalp. This condition sometimes affects the face and other parts of the body as well. Seborrheic dermatitis is the cause of dandruff in adults and cradle cap in infants.

Stasis dermatitis

This stubborn skin inflammation of the lower legs is usually the result of poor blood return from the area. There is redness, mild scaling, and a brown discoloration of the skin. If the condition is neglected, the skin may swell and become infected, or ulcers may develop.

Treatment

Because there is such a variety of skin diseases—and because some can be dangerous if neglected—it is important to seek medical care for any dermatitis. In general, this care usually begins with very simple measures. Dry skin needs lubricating agents, while moist or oily skin may require powders or other drying substances. Inflamed skin is commonly treated with cortisone-type creams, cool wet dressings, or baths.

Hardened, dried skin may be peeled off with strong substances available only by prescription. If possible, the cause of the dermatitis is sought and eliminated. Cortisone ointments are often used to make the patient more comfortable by reducing inflammation, although continuous use is not usually recommended. Antibiotics are employed promptly to eliminate any infection that may spread to other parts of the body. Patients must resist the temptation to scratch itchy areas or remove scabs; this simply prolongs and even worsens the problem. In addition, while cleanliness is desirable, some patients need to reduce hand washing and the number of baths they take, because they may be washing away the natural oils that protect the skin. Patients should not use any medication that has not been recommended by a doctor, and medications should not be used more frequently than directed: In some cases, overmedication of skin diseases may be worse than undermedication.

Fever blisters

Fever blisters, also called *cold sores*, are fluid-filled blisters that appear on the border of the lips and on or around the nose. They are the result of a very contagious virus that affects most of the population at one time or another.

Causes

Fever blisters are caused by a type of herpes simplex virus. It enters the body most often through the mouth or nose areas, where the skin is easier to penetrate.

At first, characteristic blisters may not result. Antibodies (protective substances) in the body defend against the invading virus. The inactivated virus withdraws to a nearby nerve, where it remains until stress to the body or a diminished capacity to fight off infection triggers a recurrence. When the virus is reactivated, it overruns the body's protective system and progresses back along the nerve to the general area of original infection. Factors that seem to bring on the appearance of blisters include fever, colds, menstruation, skin injury from dental work, excessive sun and wind exposure, and emotional stress.

Symptoms

Initially, the virus may present no symptoms, so some people are unaware of infection. For others, the infection begins with numbness or tenderness in the affected area. Then small, fluid-filled blisters appear. These blisters break, encrust, and heal within one to two weeks.

Complications

Occasionally, excessive pain or swelling of lymph nodes develops. These symptoms may indicate a secondary bacterial infection that needs medical attention.

Other complications can be more serious. Herpes simplex keratitis is a painful viral infection of the cornea (transparent covering of the eye) that can result in blindness if not treated.

Herpes virus has been shown to cause serious complications in infants and extremely ill patients who contract the disease.

Treatment

Treatment involves relieving symptoms, since there is no known cure for fever blisters. Some over-the-counter remedies may relieve pain and help dry blisters. Topical corticosteroid creams, however, should not be applied unless prescribed by a physician; the possibility of spreading infection increases because the corticosteroid can depress the immune response.

Frostbite

Frostbite is damage to skin tissue resulting from exposure to low temperatures. The condition can affect any part of the body, but the areas most often involved are the face, hands, and feet—areas with poor circulation that are often the most exposed.

Causes

When exposed to cold, the body tries to protect its vital organs. Blood vessels near the surface of the skin constrict to preserve internal body heat.

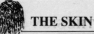

This tightening causes blood to be diverted from the outside of the body, thereby reducing the supply of blood to skin tissues. The skin and underlying tissue may freeze as a result of the lack of a warm blood supply. Frostbite develops after prolonged exposure to cold. Extremely low temperatures or forceful winds can also cause the condition.

Wearing insufficient or improper clothing increases susceptibility to frostbite. Skin can also freeze to the surface of a metal object and block circulation to the area. In addition, any health problem that weakens the body or reduces circulation increases the likelihood of frostbite.

Stages of frostbite

Frostbite develops in three stages, and each stage can produce varying degrees of pain. First-degree frostbite appears as whiteness or slight yellowness of the skin accompanied by burning or itching sensations. In this stage, symptoms can be reversed if the affected area is gradually rewarmed.

Should exposure to cold continue, sensation in the affected area ceases. Disappearance of pain and reddening and swelling of the tissue signals second-degree frostbite. At this stage, warming the area may produce blisters.

Skin with third-degree frostbite becomes waxy and hard. At this stage, skin tissue dies and edema (excess fluid retention in the tissues) may occur. Severe frostbite can damage muscles, tendons, and nerves. Blood clots may form in small blood vessels and inhibit or block circulation, which can lead to gangrene.

Treatment

Initial treatment focuses on what *not* to do, since there are many misconceptions about the proper course of action. Frostbitten tissue should not be rubbed with snow. In fact, the affected part should not be rubbed at all, because further damage to tissue can result. Exercising the frostbitten area will aggravate the condition as well.

To reduce tissue loss and avoid complications, frostbitten tissue should be immersed in lukewarm water rather than exposed to the extreme heat of a radiator, stove, or fire. Ideally, water temperature should be between 100°F and 110°F. Any temperature above 110°F can burn skin that lacks sensation, and thawing that is too rapid may produce pain, redness, and blisters. Gently patting (but not rubbing) the skin dry helps prevent additional injury to the area.

If the patient must remain outdoors, affected areas can be warmed by placing them in contact with warm portions of the body, such as under the armpits or between the thighs. Frostbitten areas can also be wrapped in a warm, dry blanket. They should be kept clean to prevent infection. Drinking warm, nonalcoholic drinks can help aid circulation. Smoking should be avoided because it causes constriction of blood vessels.

Once frozen tissue has been rewarmed, the affected area should be elevated to promote increased blood circulation and to maintain the skin at room temperature. All cases of frostbite should be examined by a physician, who may prescribe medication to prevent infection and formation of clots in blood vessels.

Prevention

The best prevention is to wear adequate clothing to protect the skin from frostbite. Feet, hands, and the nose and ears need to be covered because these areas are likely to have the poorest blood circulation and are the most exposed. When weather is unusually cold or windy, try to remain indoors as much as possible and keep outside trips to a minimum.

Head lice

Infestation with head lice (known medically as *pediculosis capitis*) has become a relatively common occurrence among school-age children; however, people in all age groups are susceptible. Sometimes erroneously thought to be an indication of an unsanitary lifestyle, lice infestation can actually afflict anyone, without regard for social status or personal hygiene.

Cause

Head lice are tiny parasites, less than one eighth of an inch long. They are grayish-white, almost transparent, six-legged creatures that live exclusively on humans. Lice can be passed easily from one person to another (for example, by using the comb of an infested person). Head lice live on or close to the scalp, where they bite and suck blood. Their eggs, which are called nits, are milk-white and about the size of a flake of dandruff.

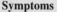

Symptoms

Head lice cause itching of the scalp and sometimes a red, scaly rash on the back of the neck at the hairline. Scratching may cause sores. The lymph nodes at the base of the skull may be enlarged.

Diagnosis

Unless hundreds are present, it is difficult to see lice in the hair. However, the nits attached to the shafts of the hairs are usually clearly visible. Although nits are about the same color and size as flakes of dandruff, they can be easily distinguished from dandruff: Flakes of dandruff can be blown or brushed away; nits are somewhat difficult to remove.

Treatment

Both prescription and nonprescription medicated shampoos (called pediculicides) are used to combat lice infestations. It is important to remember that these substances can be poisonous if swallowed or absorbed through the skin or if they come in contact with the eyes. Care must be taken to use them exactly as directed and neither more nor less often than recommended, especially in pregnant women and young children. Sometimes a vinegar rinse is

recommended to loosen the nits after using the medicated shampoo. The nits can then be removed with a fine-tooth comb.

If infected sores on the scalp or enlarged lymph nodes at the base of the skull accompany a lice infestation, consult a physician.

Prevention

The best measure for preventing head lice is to avoid sharing combs, brushes, towels, and hats.

If one member of the family has head lice, it is usually necessary to treat the rest of the family as well. (A physician may have special recommendations for infants and pregnant women.) Lice cannot be transmitted by pets, however. Combs and hairbrushes should be discarded or thoroughly cleaned in boiling water. Pillowcases, hats, and clothing that may have been in contact with an infested person should be cleaned by washing in very hot water.

Heat rash

Heat rash, or prickly heat, is a mild skin condition that produces an itchy, burning sensation. It is found most often in

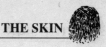

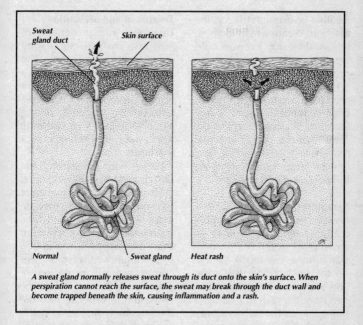

Sweat gland duct   Skin surface

Normal   Sweat gland   Heat rash

A sweat gland normally releases sweat through its duct onto the skin's surface. When perspiration cannot reach the surface, the sweat may break through the duct wall and become trapped beneath the skin, causing inflammation and a rash.

infants and in overweight people who have overlapping folds of fat.

Causes

The sweat glands in the skin normally work with blood vessels to regulate the body's heat. When the blood temperature rises, the brain triggers a reflex in the sweat glands to encourage secretion of sweat. Sweating reduces body temperature by releasing sweat to the surface of the skin, where it evapo-

rates and cools the skin. However, when skin surfaces press together, the sweat ducts, which carry secretions from the sweat glands to the skin's surface, become temporarily blocked. If sweat cannot reach the skin's surface, it may break through the duct wall and remain trapped in an inner layer of the skin, where it can cause inflammation and a rash.

Heat rash can result any time the body is unable to perspire adequately. Most often, hot

137

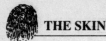

weather or exertion triggers the reaction. Wearing tight clothing or overdressing, even in cold weather, may compound the problem.

Heat rash in infants occurs primarily because their sweat ducts cannot transport large amounts of perspiration to the surface of the skin. The sweat remains trapped within the skin, which causes the characteristic inflammation and irritation.

Symptoms

Usually, heat rash (known medically as *miliaria*) appears on moist parts of the body where skin surfaces can touch, such as on the neck, under the arms, and between the legs. An infant can have the rash from a tight-fitting diaper. The rash looks like tiny, pinhead-sized red pimples, and it can cause itching and a prickling or burning sensation. Under extreme conditions, the warm, moist areas where heat rash develops can become breeding grounds for microorganisms that cause a secondary fungus infection.

Heat rash is sometimes confused with chafing because the symptoms are similar. However, chafing is caused by friction between two skin surfaces rubbing together and not by obstructed sweat ducts.

Treatment and prevention

Treatment and prevention of heat rash involve eliminating the stimulus for sweating. The affected person should stay in a cool environment and refrain from exertion. Cool showers followed by thorough drying can also help. Once sweating stops, the rash disappears in a few hours.

Babies who suffer from heat rash should be bathed and dried thoroughly. Cloth diapers are recommended because they are more likely to allow the natural evaporation process to occur than are disposable diapers. If an infant's discomfort becomes unusually prolonged or extreme, a doctor should be consulted in order to rule out the possibility that some disorder other than heat rash is causing the symptoms.

Leukoplakia

Leukoplakia is a tough, fibrous lesion that occurs on a mucous membrane. When it occurs in the mouth, it is often referred to as a *smoker's patch* or *smoker's tongue*. Although these oral lesions are generally not painful, they may cause some discomfort when the person talks or swallows.

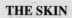
Causes

This oral condition may be caused by badly fitted dentures, excessive smoking, overconsumption of alcohol, or a diet containing spicey foods. Leukoplakia is also a symptom of syphilis and can develop into a cancerous growth.

Symptoms

Leukoplakia most often appears in the form of a white patch on the lips, tongue, or gums or in other areas that are lined by mucous membranes, such as the female genital organs.

Diagnosis

If a person notices these persistent white patches, a physician should be consulted immediately. A biopsy specimen is often obtained to determine the presence of cancer.

Treatment

One should never attempt to treat leukoplakia without first consulting their doctor. After a physician has examined the lesion, he or she may advise having dentures refitted or cutting down on smoking and the consumption of alcohol or spicy foods. These patches should be examined by a physician frequently, since cancer may develop in the future. In most cases, however, the physician will probably advise that the lesion be surgically removed.

Mole

A mole is a cluster of cells, usually pigmented (colored), that appears on the skin. Moles are sometimes present at birth, but more often they appear during childhood, adolescence, or pregnancy. Although moles can become cancerous, the occurrence is quite rare.

Symptoms

Moles vary in size, shape, and color. They can be large or small, flat or raised, smooth or warty. They can be the same color as the skin, or their color may vary from yellow-brown to black. Some moles have one or more hairs in them.

The most common type of mole is the intradermal nevus, which forms in the lower layer of skin. It is a raised cluster of cells that ranges in color from pink to black. Other types of moles include the lentigo nevus (a flat, uniformly pigmented brown or black spot), the junctional nevus (a flat or slightly raised blemish that ranges in color from light brown to nearly black), the compound nevus (a raised mole that is usually dark in color), and the halo nevus (a pigmented mole in the middle of a ring of skin from which the pigment has been lost).

Treatment
Moles are often removed solely for cosmetic reasons. However, any mole that enlarges suddenly, becomes darker, begins to bleed, or changes in any other unexplained way should be removed by a physician and examined microscopically.

Onychomycosis

The most common of inflammatory nail disorders, onychomycosis is a fungal infection of the nails that is prevalent among people with a low resistance to infection (people with diabetes and patients taking corticosteroid or other hormonal drugs), those who work with their hands in water and who are prone to paronychia (inflammation of the skin around the nail), and those with ingrown toenails.

Symptoms
The condition is chronic but painless. The affected nails look dull, opaque, flaky, and brittle and are marked with grooves or

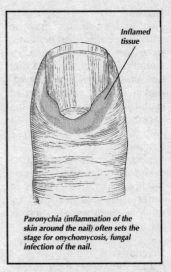

Paronychia (inflammation of the skin around the nail) often sets the stage for onychomycosis, fungal infection of the nail.

ridges. The surrounding cuticle may become red, tender, and swollen and may ooze pus if a bacterial infection accompanies the disorder. The fungi can be identified by examining nail scrapings in the laboratory.

Treatment
The condition is sometimes treated with griseofulvin, an antifungal drug that can be taken orally or applied topically to the affected area. The condition, however, may take months to cure or may never clear up at all, especially if the toenails are affected. Cutting the nails short or having the entire nail re-

moved by a physician can help the healing process.

Prevention
To prevent onychomycosis, fingernails and toenails should be dried thoroughly after bathing, because fungi thrive in a moist environment. Footwear should be changed often if the feet tend to perspire.

Photosensitivity

Photosensitivity is an abnormally increased sensitivity of the skin to the rays of the sun.

Causes
The causes of this condition are not fully understood, although it is known that certain substances, when combined with ultraviolet light, produce the reaction. Among those substances are contraceptive pills, hexachlorophene (a skin antiseptic), sandalwood oil, coal tar, certain perfumes and soaps, certain sunscreen agents, and a variety of orally administered drugs, including chlorothiazides, phenothiazines, sulfonamides, and tetracyclines.

Symptoms
The symptoms of photosensitivity include immediate burning reactions similar to those ordinarily suffered after prolonged exposure to the sun, rashes, scaling, welts (raised areas), dizziness, nausea, and vomiting. The most common symptom of photosensitivity is a rash.

Treatment
Treatment of photosensitivity symptoms is similar to that used for sunburn: ointments, topical anesthetics, and creams. Though these treatments are standard topical therapy for the skin, they do not eliminate the underlying causes of photosensitivity. The most effective treatment is to discover the basic cause of the heightened sensitivity and to eliminate it. If, for example, photosensitivity is a reaction to a contraceptive pill, a different kind contraception should be considered.

If it is impossible to isolate the cause of photosensitivity, the next best step is to avoid exposure to sunlight by wearing light-colored clothing, white gloves, and broad-brimmed hats. Commercial sunscreen products are also helpful.

Psoriasis

Psoriasis is a persistent skin disease characterized by thick, red

141

eruptions, often covered by silvery scales, either in small patches or over large areas of the body. Psoriasis is fairly common, affecting 1 to 2 percent of the population. The condition often first appears between the ages of 15 and 30 years and usually requires lifelong treatment.

Cause

Psoriasis is not contagious. The cause of psoriasis is unknown, but researchers believe that the condition is related to a malfunction in the process of skin growth and regeneration. With normal skin, old cells are continuously being shed from the epidermis and replaced by new cells formed in the deeper layers. Cells live for about one month before they die and flake off. With psoriasis, the rate of cell growth accelerates. Skin cells move to the surface and die in as short a time as four or five days. Increased cell growth causes buildup that can be extremely dry and irritating. The normal shedding process is usually unnoticeable, but psoriasis can produce very obvious blemishes.

Psoriasis seems to involve a strong hereditary factor, although only one third of its victims can recall having a relative with the disease. There also seems to be some relationship between the condition and a certain type of arthritis.

Once psoriasis develops, outbreaks of the disorder can be triggered in several ways. Injury to the skin, such as a cut, may provoke a flare-up, usually 8 to 18 days after the trauma. Seasonal changes also affect psoriasis, with the disease usually worsening during the winter months. Many patients also have greater problems during periods of physical and emotional stress. Infections, particularly upper respiratory tract infections, can also aggravate psoriasis.

Symptoms

Psoriasis is characterized by reddened, raised patches of skin with silvery scales called *plaques.* These clearly defined plaques appear most commonly on the elbows, knees, trunk, and scalp, although the underarm and genital areas may also be involved. Patches on the scalp shed large, silverwhite scales at the hairline that resemble severe dandruff. Those patches found in moist areas, such as the underarms, are usually not as scaly. All patches may itch. If fingernails are involved, they may be pit-

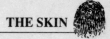

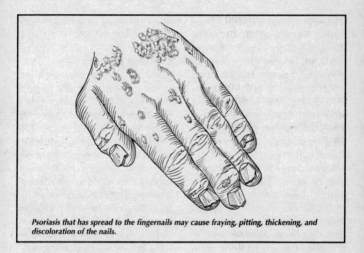

Psoriasis that has spread to the fingernails may cause fraying, pitting, thickening, and discoloration of the nails.

ted, frayed, thickened, or discolored; in more advanced cases, the nails separate from the nail beds.

Usually, psoriasis produces no general health problems. Sometimes, however, the disease becomes so severe that chills, painful reddening of the skin, cracking of the skin around the joints, and shedding of large areas of scaled skin result. This condition, called *exfoliative psoriasis,* may require hospitalization for intensive therapy.

Treatment
As yet, there is no known cure for psoriasis, and treatment offers only temporary relief from symptoms. Normal cleaning of the skin around the affected areas is important to prevent infection. Over-the-counter lotions and creams can cleanse irritated skin and reduce itching as well. These preparations often contain small amounts of coal tar and other ingredients designed to remove scales. If the skin becomes sensitive after application, use of these preparations should be discontinued. Many patients find exposure to sunlight helpful as well. Where sunlight is scarce, a special sunlamp may be used, but only under a doctor's supervision.

Various drugs have recently been shown to be effective in

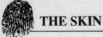

relieving the symptoms of psoriasis. Cortisone and newer steroids (hormonally based medications) can clear plaques in about 50 percent of the cases when applied directly to the affected skin. Many physicians recommend covering the treated areas with a thin plastic wrapping in addition to the cream. This is called *occlusive therapy*.

Some drugs slow the growth rate of cells. The most commonly used of these drugs, methotrexate, reduces symptoms in severe cases. Because its side effects may be severe, however, the drug is prescribed for use only under the close supervision of a physician.

Another form of treatment is called *PUVA therapy*, which combines medication and ultraviolet light treatments. The benefits of this form of therapy should be carefully weighed against the premature skin aging and skin cancer that may result.

Purpura

The term purpura refers to a group of bleeding disorders that are characterized by purplish or brownish-red discolorations, easily visible through the skin's outer layer, that are caused by hemorrhaging (internal bleeding) into the tissues.

Common purpura

Common purpura (also called *simple purpura* or *senile purpura*) is the most widespread of the disorders and is marked by easy bruising and increased blood vessel fragility. Common purpura is an inherited condition that occurs most commonly in post-menopausal women. The condition often affects thigh tissue and produces large bruises rather than hemorrhages. The bleeding may be intensified by surgery or injury.

Henoch-Schönlein purpura

Henoch-Schönlein purpura (also known as *allergic purpura* and *anaphylactoid purpura*) most often affects children. Henoch-Schönlein purpura may be associated with some forms of arthritis, gastrointestinal disorders, kidney failure, and erythema (redness of the skin).

Purpura fulminans

Purpura fulminans is most often seen in children, occurring mainly after an infectious disease. The condition is marked by fever, shock, anemia, rapidly spreading symmetrical skin hemorrhages in the lower limbs, intravascular thrombosis (block-

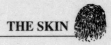
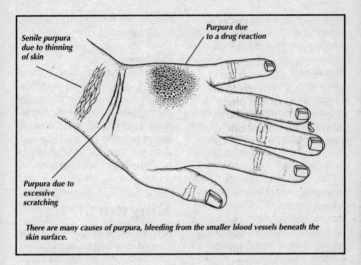

Senile purpura due to thinning of skin

Purpura due to a drug reaction

Purpura due to excessive scratching

There are many causes of purpura, bleeding from the smaller blood vessels beneath the skin surface.

age of a blood vessel by a solid mass), and gangrene.

Thrombocytopenic purpura

Thrombocytopenic purpura is a disorder in which the number of platelets (the tiny elements in the blood that are vital to clotting) is decreased, whether because of a primary disease or as a consequence of another blood disorder. This form of purpura is characterized by anemia, side effects in the nervous system, and blood clots in tiny blood vessels.

Causes

Causes vary with the type of purpura. Common purpura in postmenopausal women appears to result from decreased estrogen (female hormone) levels and thinning of the deep layers of the skin. Henoch-Schönlein purpura may result from sensitivities developed after an infection or allergic reaction. Purpura in the elderly is often due to the fragility of their skin. There are also temporary forms of purpura in which vascular bleeding occurs as a result of fever, hypothyroidism (low output of thyroid hormone), generalized illness, defects in the small blood vessels, or a drug reaction to certain medications, such as aspirin. Purpura can sometimes stem from wearing overly tight clothing or from sustaining an injury, such as a black eye.

Diagnosis

Laboratory testing is essential in all cases of possible purpura in order to exclude other causes. Perhaps the most difficult of the forms of purpura to diagnose is Henoch-Schönlein purpura. Joint pain and bouts of abdominal pain in this disorder may mimic acute abdominal conditions or forms of arthritis. Later, kidney involvement during the course of this form of purpura may cause a misdiagnosis of kidney disease.

Treatment

In the case of Henoch-Schönlein purpura, it is advisable to eliminate the possible allergic cause. Corticosteroid medications (artificial hormones) are often prescribed, but may produce disappointing results. Immunosuppressive therapy (suppression of the immune system by means of drugs) is sometimes useful in treating the various forms of purpura.

If the purpura is thrombocytopenic, the spleen (an abdominal organ that is a component of the circulatory system) may be removed if it is hoarding too many platelets. Milder cases of the condition often improve spontaneously.

Prevention

Estrogen therapy has proved helpful in preventing or relieving common purpura in postmenopausal women. Other than preventive measures to avoid infections or allergic reactions, there is little that can be done to prevent purpura.

Ringworm

Ringworm is a skin infection caused by a fungus, not a worm. The name originated because the infection is often characterized by round patches that enlarge as healing proceeds from the center, leaving red rings that persist on the skin for a few months.

Types

There are several different types of ringworm, each caused by a different type of fungus. Ringworm of the scalp, or *tinea capitis*, appears as scaly patches with stubs of broken-off hairs or as bald areas. Ringworm of the body, or *tinea corporis*, appears as round or oval, scaly, red patches on the torso. Ringworm of the groin, or *tinea cruris* (popularly referred to as "jock itch"), is characterized by a scaly, red or brown rash in the crotch and genital area. Ringworm of the feet, or *tinea pedis*, is more commonly called *athlete's foot*.

Cause
Ringworm spreads by direct contact with an infected person or pet or by contact with contaminated objects, such as combs, pillows, towels, and clothing. Tight-fitting clothing, obesity, and heavy perspiration may be contributing factors in the development of ringworm of the body and the groin.

Diagnosis
Though ringworm infections are generally unsightly, they are not threatening to general health. However, several other skin infections resemble ringworm, so it is important that a physician makes the diagnosis. The doctor may want to examine the rash under ultraviolet light and obtain a skin scraping to be examined microscopically.

Treatment
An antifungal ointment to be applied to the skin may be prescribed for ringworm of the body or the groin. Special medicated shampoos are available to treat ringworm of the scalp.

In some especially resistant cases, an oral medication called griseofulvin may be necessary as well.

Prevention
To prevent spread of the infection, personal articles that have been in contact with infected areas should be discarded or laundered in very hot water.

Sunburn

Sunburn is an inflammation of the cells of the skin caused by overexposure to the ultraviolet radiation of the sun or a sunlamp. Damage to the skin can be either insignificant or serious, depending on the intensity of the light source, the length of exposure, and the sensitivity of the individual to ultraviolet radiation.

Causes
Sunburn is caused by overexposure to ultraviolet radiation. Substances (such as deodorants, soaps, perfumes, cosmetics, and certain medications) may produce heightened sensitivity to ultraviolet radiation, with a corresponding increase in the severity of the burn. While light-skinned people usually burn more easily than dark-

147

skinned people, skin color is not always a dependable guide to individual susceptibility.

Symptoms

Irritation of the skin and a prickling sensation mark the onset of sunburn; the skin also feels hot to the touch. Capillaries (tiny blood vessels) in the skin become congested because of the release of certain inflammatory agents, thus producing the characteristic redness. Oral contraceptive users may develop irregularly shaped dark splotches, and some sensitive individuals may have allergic reactions in the form of rashes or welts.

As the burn progresses in severity, the skin will feel tight, swollen, and dry or brittle and may become hypersensitive to touch. Overheating and loss of fluids through the damaged skin may also produce dizziness, nausea, vomiting, hyperventilation (rapid breathing, which causes excessive loss of carbon dioxide from the blood), impaired vision and hearing, irregular heartbeat, and loss of consciousness.

The aftermath of severe sunburn often includes blistering and peeling, as well as permanent freckling, splotching, or scarring of the skin. Long-term effects may include premature skin aging, which is marked by chronic dryness, wrinkling, leathery texture, and loss of elasticity. In some cases, melanoma (a form of skin cancer) may be induced by chronic overexposure to sunlight.

Treatment

Minor sunburn can be effectively treated by a wide variety of nonprescription ointments, oils, powders, creams, and sprays that restore fluids and prevent further drying, relieve discomfort, and promote healing. Many over-the-counter medications contain mild anesthetics to relieve stinging and suppress the desire to scratch itching areas. Infection of blistered and peeling areas of the skin is a common complication. This condition should be treated by a physician.

In the case of severe sunburn, overheating and dehydration (loss of too much fluid) must be avoided. The victim should be taken out of the sun immediately and placed in a cool, shaded area until medical attention can be obtained. Cool (but not cold), wet cloths can be applied to the arms, the head, and the legs. If the victim is perspiring profusely, a fan may help evaporate the water on the skin's surface, thus aiding a natural cooling process.

Prevention

The best prevention of sunburn is simply to avoid prolonged exposure to the direct rays of the sun or a sunlamp. When this is not possible, the first line of defense is to cover exposed areas of the skin completely, preferably with loose-fitting, light-colored clothes made of loose-weave fabrics. Wearing a widebrimmed hat will also help block the sun's harmful rays.

The second line of defense is a sunscreen with an SPF of at least 15, available as an oil, cream, paste, or liquid. Most sunscreens are intended to block ultraviolet rays. Many contain paraaminobenzoic acid (PABA). This compound may affect some individuals adversely, particularly those with photosensitivity. For these people, many opaque (light-blocking) creams, pastes, and lotions are available, as well as sunscreens known as benzophenones.

Warts

Warts are infectious growths in the outer layers of the skin. Because they are contagious, they can spread from person to person or from one site to another on the same person. Most frequently, warts appear on the hands and fingers and on the soles of the feet. However, they can emerge anywhere on the skin, including the genital and anal areas.

Causes

Common warts are caused by exposure to a virus called the *human papilloma virus*. The virus can remain inactive for up to six months after contact before causing the eruption of abnormal skin masses.

The virus is transmitted to another person or another site on the body by direct contact. For example, brushing or combing the hair can spread the virus from a wart on the scalp. Shaving or scratching a given area on the body and then touching another area will also transmit the virus. In addition, moist parts of the body, such as the soles of the feet, provide a breeding ground for growth of the virus.

As people become older, they seem to develop an immunity or resistance to the wart virus. For this reason, children tend to acquire warts more frequently than adults. Nevertheless, warts can occur at any age.

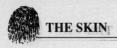
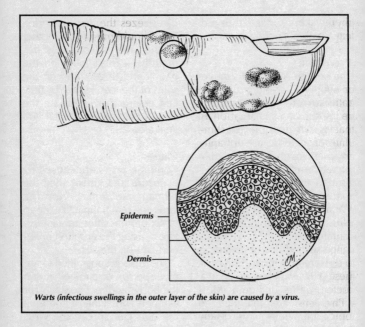

Epidermis ——

Dermis——

Warts (infectious swellings in the outer layer of the skin) are caused by a virus.

Symptoms

Usually, warts appear as firm gray masses that feel tender or itchy. Their size and shape vary depending on the location and severity of the viral infection. Children are most likely to have flat warts, particularly on the face. This variety looks smooth, flat, and yellowish brown.

Plantar warts grow on the soles of the feet, where they can become as large as two inches in diameter. These warts cause considerable pain because the tissue swelling pushes inward. (The discomfort from plantar warts feels like walking with a pebble in your shoe.)

Most warts are not health-threatening. However, when they are extensive in number, they can cause extreme sensitivity or pain.

Treatment

Studies have shown that two out of every three warts disappear on their own, usually within two years. Consequently,

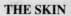

physicians usually recommend leaving warts alone unless they are causing discomfort or obstruction.

Doctors sometimes treat one or two warts and find that the patient's other warts also clear up. A possible explanation is that the original treatment stimulates the manufacture of antibodies (protective substances) that fight the virus in other warts.

There are over-the-counter preparations to aid removal of warts. Most of these remedies contain a form of acid, which is dangerous if not used according to directions. Although some of these drugs are effective, only a doctor should remove a wart.

Physicians may try a variety of topical preparations to loosen the warts. A solution containing cantharidin, a substance that causes blistering, may be applied directly to the wart. About one week after application, the doctor should be able to remove the wart with a surgical knife or scissors. Corn plasters containing salicylic acid soften the wart so that it can be scraped away.

When a wart persists, physicians may advise surgery to remove affected tissue. Electrosurgery dissolves wart tissue with electric current. Cryotherapy freezes the area with dry ice or liquid nitrogen; freezing allows the wart to be lifted off easily.

BONES AND MUSCLES

The musculoskeletal system is an intricate structure of interconnecting parts. Every movement of the body is the result of the coordination of bones, muscles, tendons, and ligaments.

Bones

Bones are hardened masses of living tissue. They collect calcium for the entire body, storing 99 percent of the body's supply of this mineral. Within some bones is a substance called *marrow,* which produces red and white blood cells and platelets.

There are 206 bones in the human skeleton. The skeleton maintains the body's shape and protects internal organs. For example, the bones in the skull shield the brain, and the bones in the rib cage encircle and protect the lungs.

The place where two or more bones meet is called a *joint.* This juncture usually allows movement of the bones that are involved. However, movement is governed by *ligaments* (bands of fibrous tissue) attached to the bones and by *cartilage* (elastic tissue) covering the ends of the bones. Ligaments connect one bone with another. Cartilage cushions and protects bones with the aid of various joint fluids and bursae (small sacs containing lubricating fluid that encompass the joints). Other bands of connective tissue called *tendons* attach bones to muscles. Muscles are specific kinds of tissues that have the ability to contract. It is this contraction that pulls on the tendons and makes movement possible.

Muscles

There are three types of muscle: striated, smooth, and cardiac. Striated, or striped, muscle consists of layers of tissue divided into bundles of interwoven fibers that run parallel to one another. These layers are attached to the skeleton, and they aid the body in voluntary movement.

Smooth, or organic, muscle is present in several of the internal organs, including the intestines and the bladder, and in

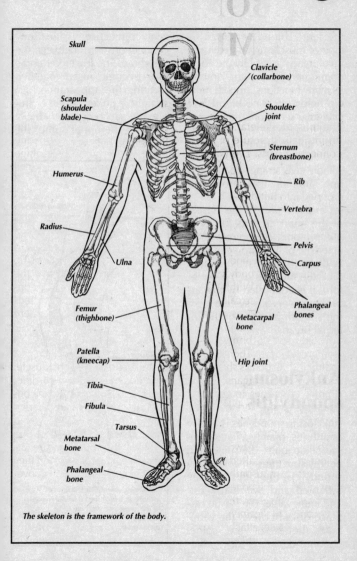

Skull

Clavicle (collarbone)

Scapula (shoulder blade)

Shoulder joint

Sternum (breastbone)

Humerus

Rib

Vertebra

Radius

Pelvis

Carpus

Ulna

Phalangeal bones

Femur (thighbone)

Metacarpal bone

Patella (kneecap)

Hip joint

Tibia

Fibula

Tarsus

Metatarsal bone

Phalangeal bone

The skeleton is the framework of the body.

the larger blood vessels. This type of muscle functions under involuntary control by the autonomic nervous system. Among its many functions, smooth muscle helps circulate blood and glandular secretions, moves material through the digestive tract, and regulates breathing. Smooth muscle contains elongated, spindly cells arranged parallel to one another that are often grouped into bundles.

Cardiac muscle is the muscle of the heart, and its job is to pump blood. The unique characteristic of the cardiac muscle is that although it is striated (like the muscles of the skeleton), it is controlled by the autonomic nervous system (like the smooth muscles of the internal organs).

Ankylosing spondylitis

Ankylosing spondylitis is a form of arthritis, mainly affecting the sacroiliac joints, the spine, and nearby structures. In ankylosing spondylitis, the joints become inflamed and eventually stiff and immovable. The elastic cartilage disks between the vertebrae (bones of the spine) become dense, as does adja-

cent connective tissue. Bony connections form between the vertebrae. The lower vertebrae may become fused together, creating the appearance of a straight "poker spine," frequently accompanied by a curve in the upper spine (see illustration below).

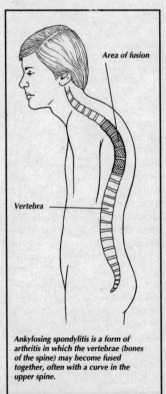

Area of fusion

Vertebra

Ankylosing spondylitis is a form of arthritis in which the vertebrae (bones of the spine) may become fused together, often with a curve in the upper spine.

Causes

The cause of ankylosing spondylitis is unknown, but there appears to be an inherited tendency toward the disease. The disease affects men ten times more often than women. People born with a certain trait in their blood, called HLA-B27, are more likely to suffer the disease.

Ankylosing spondylitis is predominantly a disease of young men, occurring most commonly between the ages of 15 and 40. The disease may progress slowly for 10 to 20 years and then stop or slow down.

Symptoms

Chronic low-back pain and stiffness is a chief sign of the disease; hip pain is also quite common, as is an inflammation of the eye known as *anterior uveitis*. Symptoms, such as low backaches, begin gradually. There may be morning stiffness and pain extending down the leg along the sciatic nerve, commonly alternating from one side to the other. The back pain and stiffness eventually affect the upper spine and sometimes the neck. In up to a third of the cases, large joints (such as those of the hips and shoulders) are affected. Knees and other smaller joints may be affected by symptoms matching those of

rheumatoid arthritis. The heart is affected in approximately 3 percent of cases (after many years of disease), and inflammation of the lining of the eye occurs in about 25 percent of cases. As the disease progresses, it is more difficult for the patient to flex the back and expand the chest.

X rays of the back-related joints—especially those between the upper portion of the hip bone and the sacrum (the bony structure at the base of the spine)—reveal changes typical of ankylosing spondylitis. A sign of advanced disease is "bamboo spine," in which bony bands around the disks cement the vertebrae together.

Treatment

Although there is no cure for ankylosing spondylitis, certain measures can lessen the effects of the disease. These include rest; breathing exercises; and exercises designed to help maintain posture and keep the back as flexible as possible. To prevent curvature of the upper spine, sleeping on the back on a firm mattress with a small pillow or no pillow is advised. Locking the fingers behind the head and pushing the elbows back as far as possible is a good way to straighten the upper back and stretch the chest muscles. Painkillers and anti-inflammatory drugs may be given. Corticosteroid drugs are generally not prescribed because of side effects. Surgery is rarely needed.

Arthritis

Arthritis is an inflammation of the joints (the junctures where the ends of two or more bones meet).

Types

Inflammation develops in various ways. With *osteoarthritis*, there is gradual wearing away of cartilage in the joints. Healthy cartilage is the elastic tissue that lines and cushions the joints and allows bones to move smoothly against one another. When this cartilage deteriorates, the bones rub together, causing pain and swelling.

Osteoarthritis can cause permanent damage, stiffness, and deformity of the joints. Although osteoarthritis can result from direct injury to the joint, it commonly occurs in adults over age 55 because of long-term wear and tear.

Rheumatoid arthritis can attack individuals of any age. This form of arthritis affects all the connective tissues, as well as other organs. The precise cause of rheumatoid arthritis is unknown. Some researchers believe that a virus triggers the disease, causing an autoimmune response whereby the body attacks its own tissues. (Evidence for this theory is inconclusive, however.)

In rheumatoid arthritis, the synovium (the thin membrane lining and lubricating the joint) becomes inflamed. The inflammation eventually destroys the cartilage. As scar tissue gradually replaces the damaged cartilage, the joint becomes misshapen and rigid.

Rheumatoid arthritis may damage the heart, lungs, nerves, and eyes.

Those at risk

Arthritis is not an inherited disease. Nonetheless, people who have a family history of arthritis are more likely to develop the disease. Women are at greater risk than men, although the reason for this is unclear.

Excess body weight may promote osteoarthritis because of the increased pressure on the joints. While inactivity can also aggravate the problem, constant sports- or job-related abuse to joints may also encourage arthritis.

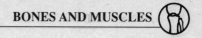
Symptoms

Symptoms of osteoarthritis include swelling, tenderness, pain, stiffness, and redness in one or more joints. For many patients, pain is greatest in the morning and subsides as the day progresses. Damp weather and emotional stress can make symptoms worse.

With rheumatoid arthritis, these symptoms may be accom-

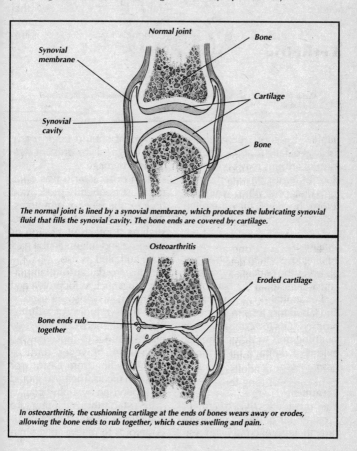

Normal joint

Synovial membrane

Synovial cavity

Bone

Cartilage

Bone

The normal joint is lined by a synovial membrane, which produces the lubricating synovial fluid that fills the synovial cavity. The bone ends are covered by cartilage.

Osteoarthritis

Bone ends rub together

Eroded cartilage

In osteoarthritis, the cushioning cartilage at the ends of bones wears away or erodes, allowing the bone ends to rub together, which causes swelling and pain.

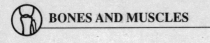

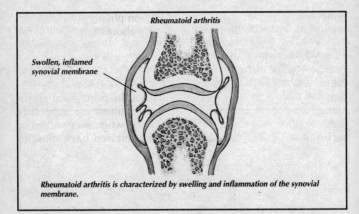

Rheumatoid arthritis

Swollen, inflamed synovial membrane

Rheumatoid arthritis is characterized by swelling and inflammation of the synovial membrane.

panied by more generalized feelings of fatigue and fever. This form of arthritis may go into periods of remission, when symptoms disappear. When symptoms return, however, they are often more severe.

Diagnosis

To diagnose arthritis, a physician observes the patient's symptoms and administers a standard physical examination. X-ray studies and laboratory tests may be recommended to confirm joint swelling and to determine the extent of damage the arthritis has caused.

Treatment

The most effective treatment program for arthritis consists of drug therapy, exercise, and rest.

Treatment should begin early after diagnosis to prevent permanent damage.

High-dose aspirin was once the most frequently prescribed drug for the relief of symptoms. Although effective, side effects such as stomach ulceration or bleeding and ringing in the ears have curtailed its use.

Nonsteroidal anti-inflammatory drugs such as ibuprofen and naproxen may also be used to treat the symptoms of arthritis. These medications can cause side effects similar to those caused by aspirin, however, particularly bleeding from gastritis or stomach ulcers. Their use should be supervised by a physician.

In osteoarthritis, joints are sometimes injected with corticosteroids to relieve inflammation and pain. Though these drugs are quite effective, they do have side effects. They should be used only under close and continuous medical supervision.

Oral or injectable gold may prove helpful in treating rheumatoid arthritis. Drugs usually used for cancer chemotherapy, such as methotrexate, may also be helpful.

Moderate daily exercise, such as swimming, walking, or physical therapy, is critical to maintaining mobility in arthritic joints. A supervised exercise program interspersed with rest periods helps to reduce joint inflammation. To lessen pain while increasing movement, moist heat often helps. In addition, maintaining correct posture and body weight reduces extra burden on sore joints.

Severe cases of rheumatoid arthritis may require surgery to remove inflamed synovial tissue. With either form of arthritis, artificial joints may be implanted to replace those damaged beyond repair.

Backache

A backache is generally a gripping pain near the inward curve of the back above the base of the spine. It is one of the most common physical ailments, affecting about 80 percent of the population at some time in their lives.

Causes

Pain results from a variety of causes. Strains are especially common when overworked or underexercised back muscles perform beyond their normal capacity. The muscles will then contract or go into spasm and become a tight mass of tissue. Meanwhile, the body transmits a sharp pain signal as nearby muscles tighten in an effort to protect strained muscles and prevent further damage. A strain can be caused by exercise, sudden jerking motions, or a reflex action, such as sneezing.

Overweight is a leading factor in backache, because it increases the stress on back muscles. Similarly, pregnancy can produce back pain because of the weight or position of the fetus. For some women, menstruation is also associated with back discomfort.

Many people experience back pain as they age and their joint tissues deteriorate or shift. Psychological tension, stress, or anxiety about everyday problems can also lead to backache. In addition, back pain can result from diseases of the kidneys, heart, lungs, intestinal tract, or reproductive organs.

Backache occasionally stems from a congenital (present from birth) malformation. In such cases, pain generally results from the unusual stresses that the deformity imposes on surrounding muscular structures rather than from the abnormality itself. For example, if one leg is shorter than the other, the muscles in the lower part of the body are forced out of alignment, causing back pain.

Symptoms

Backaches can appear abruptly after physical activity or may develop slowly. The pain may feel like a sharp jab or a dull ache. The pain sometimes becomes so piercing that a person who is bending over may not be able to straighten up. Severe back pain may also be accompanied by pain or numbness radiating down one or both legs. Though most muscular back pains disappear within a week or two of their onset, some can last one to two months. Pain may recur unless preventive measures are taken.

Diagnosis

Prolonged back pain (lasting for more than one or two weeks) should be brought to the

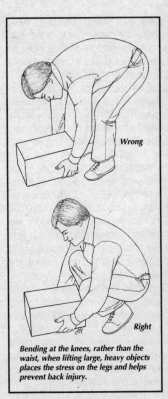

Wrong

Right

Bending at the knees, rather than the waist, when lifting large, heavy objects places the stress on the legs and helps prevent back injury.

attention of a physician, who will check for underlying disorders, such as kidney, bone, or lung problems, that may be causing the backache. Once other medical causes have been ruled out, an orthopedic surgeon (a physician who specializes in bone and muscle conditions) may be able to determine the cause of the discomfort.

During the examination, the physician may ask questions about the type of pain and its location, general health, previous illnesses, and physical activity routines. The patient walks, sits, stands, and performs exercises while being observed. An X-ray study may be used to reveal adverse changes in the spine.

Treatment

If there are no apparent physical causes for the backache, physicians usually recommend an exercise program to strengthen weak back muscles. Losing weight can also relieve pressure on the back.

For immediate treatment of symptoms, using a heating pad or ice at the site of the pain will usually reduce soreness. Nonprescription analgesic creams containing methyl salicylate (oil of wintergreen) or a similar ingredient produce a soothing warm sensation when applied to the pain site. Muscle relaxants and/or anti-inflammatory drugs may also be prescribed.

When backache is the result of some deformity or damage to a disk (the soft material that lies between the bones of the spine), surgery may be necessary to correct the problem.

Braces, corsets, or shoe lifts can sometimes improve the condition. Physical therapy may be useful because it strengthens back muscles, which helps to prevent the recurrence of back strain. Your doctor may prescribe at-home exercises to strengthen affected muscles as well.

Almost all types of musculoskeletal backaches respond well to rest, which allows muscles to relax and inflammation to subside. Time is often the best healer of back pain.

Prevention

To prevent back pain, stress to the spine should be avoided. Good posture, when awake and asleep, relieves tension on the spinal column. Wearing properly fitted shoes encourages good posture, as does sleeping on a semifirm bed. Contrary to popular belief, a hard mattress is no better for your back than a soft one: It can distort the alignment of the spine and cause back pain. A semifirm mattress conforms to the arch of the back and helps maintain spinal alignment.

Good posture is also important when performing daily activities. Bending at the knees, rather than from the waist, when lifting large, heavy objects places the stress on the legs, not on the lower back. One should also avoid looking down for long periods of time while seated at a desk.

Bunion

A bunion is a swelling on the foot, usually located at the joint of the big toe. Often, a bony protuberance is present at the joint of the big toe, which gives the bunion its bulging appearance.

Causes

Bunions are most commonly caused by wearing poorly fitting footwear, but they can also be the result of inherited deformities in bone structure of the foot. In a normal foot, the two main bones of the big toe must align to fit together. However, some people have loose joints in the foot that allow their big toes to point toward the other toes. This inherited condition causes problems when footwear forces the big toe inward and the big-toe joint outward. Friction from the joint rubbing against the inner surface of the shoe can produce a bunion. The same action results when a tight or pointed-toe shoe puts pressure on the joint—regardless of whether or not the person has loose joints in the foot.

Symptoms

A bunion is characterized by swelling at the big-toe joint, which may be accompanied by pain and tenderness. Bunion formations can be acute or chronic. Acute bunions are a type of bursitis, which is an inflammation of a bursa (a fluid-filled sac that cushions joints). With an acute bunion, the bursa covering the big-toe joint becomes inflamed from friction, often producing considerable pain. Chronic (long-term) bunions develop into inflexible bony protrusions.

Complications

Complications can occur if the bunion grows and increases the pressure on the big toe. This pressure may force the other toes to overlap, encouraging the development of corns (mounds of dead skin) or other problems that result from friction among the distorted toes.

Diagnosis

A physician diagnoses a bunion by general physical examination. To identify bone problems, an X-ray examination may be necessary.

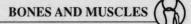

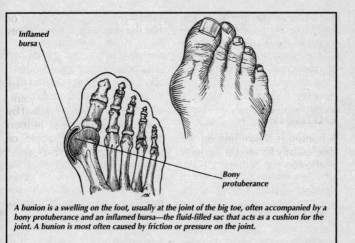

A bunion is a swelling on the foot, usually at the joint of the big toe, often accompanied by a bony protuberance and an inflamed bursa—the fluid-filled sac that acts as a cushion for the joint. A bunion is most often caused by friction or pressure on the joint.

Inflamed bursa

Bony protuberance

Treatment

Surgery is the only permanent cure for bunions. The procedure may entail the simple removal of the excess bone. Local anesthetic is often used and pain from surgery is minimal. With this treatment, the patient has full use of the foot again in about six weeks.

More extensive surgery requires a complex realignment of the affected bones, muscles, and tendons. The patient is admitted to the hospital, and the recuperation time is longer. Usually, an orthopedic surgeon performs this type of surgery.

Nonsurgical devices can often relieve the pain and discomfort of bunions. Padding can be used to shift the weight of the foot in the shoe, lessening friction. Protective shields can also prevent contact between the bunion and the inside of the shoe.

Prevention

Wearing properly fitting footwear is the best preventive measure. A child's first shoes should be wide enough to accommodate all the toes without cramping, since early childhood is when many foot problems begin.

When buying shoes, the width and length of each foot needs to be measured separately. If

163

one foot is larger than the other, the shoe size should correspond to the size of the larger foot. A one-inch gap between the big toe and the tip of the shoe allows enough space for movement. Even more room is needed with pointed-toe shoes. Shoes should be comfortable from the first wearing—no breaking-in period should be necessary.

People who wear high heels are also at risk of developing bunions. Heels about one inch in height are best. However, if higher heels are preferred, open-toe styles seem to cause fewer problems than closed-toe styles.

Bursitis

Bursitis is an inflammation of a bursa (a fluid-filled sac that cushions joints). Bursae (the plural of bursa) contain lubricating fluid that normally eliminates friction in the area and maintains smooth muscle movement over the bones.

Continual stress on a particular joint increases the probability of injury and inflammation. In advanced cases of bursitis, swelling and calcium deposits within a joint may render it immobile.

Causes

The inflammation can result from either sudden extreme pressure or from continual strain. Some occupations and sports that require constant use of certain joints contribute to acute or chronic bursitis. For example, "typist's shoulder" and "tennis elbow" are forms of chronic bursitis. Acute bursitis can develop suddenly and may be triggered by physical stress or injury. Bursitis seems to be more common in men than in women.

Symptoms

Inflamed bursae produce tenderness and swelling near the affected joint. Pain from bursitis can be so severe that movement of the joint becomes impossible. Any joint in the body can be the site of bursitis, but shoulders, knees, and elbows are the most commonly affected areas.

Diagnosis

To diagnose bursitis, an X-ray examination may be ordered to determine whether there are calcium deposits in the bursa or if other problems, such as a fracture, exist. In the case of stress-related bursitis, however, an X-ray study will show only swelling of the bursa.

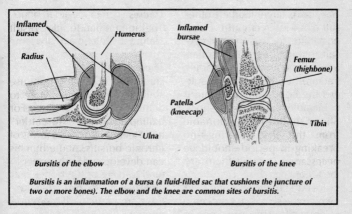

Bursitis of the elbow

Bursitis of the knee

Bursitis is an inflammation of a bursa (a fluid-filled sac that cushions the juncture of two or more bones). The elbow and the knee are common sites of bursitis.

Treatment

Acute bursitis may heal with time if the joint is immobilized. Complete bed rest or use of a sling or crutches may be recommended to relieve pressure on the affected area.

Applying moist heat to the area of the inflamed joint frequently reduces the discomfort of bursitis, although some patients find cold compresses more effective. Aspirin and other over-the-counter pain relievers may also help. In some cases, anti-inflammatory corticosteroid drugs may be injected directly into the inflamed area. But, because they have been known to cause serious side effects, corticosteroid drugs must be used judiciously and only under the supervision of a physician.

For severe cases of bursitis, a doctor may recommend surgery by an orthopedic surgeon to remove calcium deposits or free the area from chronic inflammation by removing all or part of the bursa.

Fracture

A fracture is a break in a bone or cartilage. Among the possible consequences of a fracture are infection and damage to nearby nerves, blood vessels, and internal organs.

Causes

Most often, fractures are caused by direct stress, such as a blow from a heavy object, or a severe strain, such as a violent twist.

They can, however, be the result of an indirect cause. A fall on a hand, for example, may result in a fracture of the collarbone. There are also pathologic fractures, in which disease softens the bone, making it more vulnerable to a break.

Types

There are many different types of fractures, among them are the following:

- Closed fracture—one in which the skin is not broken
- Comminuted fracture—one in which the bone is splintered into several pieces
- Complicated fracture—one in which significant injury has been done to internal organs, blood vessels, or nerves
- Greenstick fracture—one in which only one side of the bone is broken and the bone is not severed
- Impacted fracture—one in which the ends or fragments of bone are jammed together
- Open fracture—one in which one or more of the broken ends of the bone pierce the skin
- Stress fracture—one in which there is a tiny crack (or cracks) in a bone; the crack causes severe pain but may be undetectable by conventional X ray. This type of fracture is commonly seen in the small bones of the foot due to injuries relating to athletic activity.

Those at risk

Fractures are common among children and the elderly. Children have relatively soft, elastic bones. Because of this elasticity, however, breaks are often incomplete, affecting only one side of the bone. Elderly people tend to have brittle bones that break easily; for them, hip fractures are particularly common injuries.

Symptoms

The symptoms of a fracture include pain, swelling, loss of strength, abnormal movement, and a grating sound that results from pieces of broken bone rubbing together. An individual who has suffered a severe fracture may go into shock, especially if large amounts of blood have been lost.

Treatment

Bone fractures are treated by closed (nonsurgical) or open (surgical) reduction. Reduction is a procedure in which the broken bone is manipulated (for example, by pulling or bending) so that its ends will be in the best position for healing. Most fractures are treated

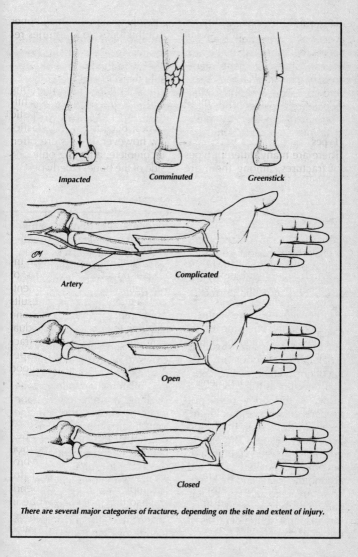

Impacted   *Comminuted*   *Greenstick*

Artery

Complicated

Open

Closed

There are several major categories of fractures, depending on the site and extent of injury.

through closed reduction. However, open reduction may be necessary when damage to bones, joints, ligaments, tendons, or other internal parts is severe or extensive. In open reduction, the pieces of bone are often held together by pins, metal plates, or rods; some are left in the body permanently, and others are removed after healing has taken place.

Gout

Gout is a form of recurrent acute arthritis. Most gout victims are middle-aged men. If gout appears in women, it usually occurs after the period of menopause.

Cause
The underlying cause of gout is a defect in the body's processing of uric acid, a chemical normally found in the blood and urine. If the body does not properly process uric acid, the level of uric acid in the blood becomes elevated. The excess uric acid may crystallize and become deposited in and around the joints and their tendons. An acute attack of gout is caused by the body's inflammatory response to the deposits of uric acid crystals.

The high levels of uric acid can also lead to deposition of crystals in areas of the body other than the joints, most notably the skin and the kidneys. Uric acid deposits in the kidneys may form kidney stones. About 20 percent of patients with chronic gout also have kidney stones. If the kidneys become blocked by stones, the kidneys can fail.

Symptoms
Gout usually first appears as a sudden and extremely painful attack in a single joint, usually the big toe. Later attacks can involve several joints, such as the ankle, knee, wrist, and elbow. The pain, which commonly begins at night during sleep, may occur without warning or may be preceded by excessive alcohol consumption. The pain grows in intensity and is often described as throbbing or crushing. Inflammation follows, with swelling, warmth, redness, and tenderness over the affected joint. The pain is sometimes so severe that the individual cannot tolerate the weight of a bed sheet over the joint.

Other symptoms that may accompany the joint pain and swelling include fever, rapid heartbeat, chills, and an overall feeling of being unwell. Uric acid deposits in the skin, called *tophi*, may be noted as white lumps under the skin, most often appearing in the hands, the feet, the elbows, and the rims of the outer ears.

The first attacks usually last only a few days, but if the disorder goes untreated, later attacks may last for weeks. Symptoms eventually disappear, and joint function returns to normal between attacks. As the disease progresses, the periods of remission become shorter and shorter, and more and more attacks occur each year.

Treatment

The drug colchicine has traditionally been used to relieve a gout attack, but nonsteroidal anti-inflammatory drugs are now more often prescribed to relieve the inflammation and pain. Though these drugs are quite effective, they do have side effects. They should be used only under close and continuous medical supervision.

Once the acute attack is under control, prevention of future attacks becomes the main goal. This can be done with the drug allopurinol, which interferes with the production of uric acid and thus prevents the deposition of uric acid crystals. Allopurinol usually has to be taken for long periods of time in order to maintain normal blood levels of uric acid. There are also other drugs called *uricosurics* that speed up the excretion of uric acid by the kidneys. These drugs, however, should not be used if there is known kidney damage.

Hernia

A hernia is an abnormal protrusion of part of an organ through the tissues that normally contain it. In this condition, a weak spot or opening in a body wall, often due to laxity of the muscles, allows part of the organ to protrude. A hernia may develop in almost any part of the body; however, the muscles of the abdominal wall are most commonly affected.

Types

A hernia can be congenital (present at birth) or acquired (often the result of some physical stress or strain). Although there are various types of hernias, the following are some of the most common:

- Umbilical hernia—protrusion of part of the intestine at the umbilicus (navel). This type is seen mostly in infants.
- Inguinal hernia—protrusion of

a loop of intestine into the groin (where the folds of abdominal flesh meet the thighs). This type of hernia, which accounts for about 75 percent of all abdominal hernias, is often the result of increased pressure in the abdomen because of lifting, coughing, or straining. This type of hernia is more common in men than women.

• Scrotal hernia—an inguinal hernia that has passed into the scrotum (the sac containing the testes).

• Femoral hernia—protrusion of a loop of tissue into the femoral canal, which carries nerves and blood vessels from the abdomen into the upper thigh and groin area. This type of hernia is more common in women than in men.

• Incisional hernia—a hernia that occurs at the site of a surgical incision. This type of hernia is often due to strain on healing tissues by excessive muscular effort, lifting, coughing, or extreme pressure.

• Hiatal hernia—protrusion of part of the stomach through the diaphragm and into the chest (for more information, see page 351).

Symptoms

The symptoms vary slightly, depending on the cause and the structures involved. Most hernias begin as small breakthroughs that are hardly noticeable. At first, they may be soft lumps under the skin, a little larger than a marble, and there is usually no pain. As time goes by, the pressure of the internal contents against the weak wall increases, and the size of the lump increases.

In the early stages, the hernia may be reducible, that is, the protruding structures can be pushed gently back into their normal locations. If those structures cannot be returned to their normal positions by manipulation, the hernia is said to be irreducible, or incarcerated.

If an incarcerated hernia progresses, bulging out farther through the weakest points in its containing wall, the opening in the wall will close behind it, forming a narrow neck. If the neck is pinched tightly enough to cut off the blood supply to the protruding tissue, the hernia will swell quickly and become strangulated—that is, the blood supply will be totally cut off. Unless treated, a strangulated hernia can cause tissue death.

Fortunately, the symptoms of strangulation of a hernia are usually detectable. When a hernia suddenly grows larger, becomes tense, will not go back into place, and is accompanied by pain and nausea, the hernia is most likely strangulated. Sometimes, however, there is no pain or tenderness when this happens. This type of condition is more likely to occur in elderly patients.

Diagnosis

A physician can usually diagnose a hernia by performing a thorough physical examination and by studying the patient's medical history and physical symptoms.

Treatment

For small nonstrangulated and nonincarcerated hernias, various supports and trusses may offer temporary, symptomatic relief. However, the best treatment is herniorrhaphy (surgical closure or repair of the muscle wall through which the hernia protrudes). When the weakened area is very large, some strong synthetic material may be sewn over the defect to reinforce the weak area.

Postoperative care involves protecting the patient from respiratory infections that might cause coughing or sneezing, which would strain the suture line. Recovery is usually quick and complete.

Prevention

Avoiding strain or pressure on any body wall, especially the abdominal wall in men, is the only real preventive measure against hernias.

Lupus erythematosus

Lupus erythematosus is a disorder that frequently affects the skin and the connective tissues (particularly the joints and muscles) but it can affect every tissue and organ in the body. The disorder occurs in two different forms—discoid lupus erythematosus and systemic lupus erythematosus.

Discoid lupus erythematosus

Discoid lupus erythematosus is a chronic disease of the skin that is characterized by a red rash that most commonly appears on the cheeks and nose, but may appear on other parts of the body as well. It often appears for the first time after the skin has been exposed to sunlight. Discoid lupus erythematosus is usually treated with drugs commonly used in the treatment of malaria. (The two conditions are not at all related, however).

Systemic lupus erythematosus

Systemic lupus erythematosus is a widespread autoimmune inflammatory disease of the blood vessels and connective tissues. The condition affects the joints, skin, and numerous other organs in the body, including the heart, lungs, liver, intestines, and kidneys. A red patch that resembles an open-winged butterfly may appear on the cheeks and nose. Symptoms may include severe pain in the joints, intermittent fever, and unusual fatigue. The inflammation can cause severe and irreversible damage to the blood vessels and to the kidneys.

Cortisone and other steroids are used to control the inflammation in the joints and in other parts of the body; aspirin and other analgesics are used to control the pain. As with discoid lupus erythematosus, antimalarial drugs are used in the treatment of the rash.

Systemic lupus erythematosus may be mild, or it may progress rapidly to seriously affect many organs. Death may result in severe cases.

Osteoporosis

Osteoporosis is a relatively common disorder characterized by a decrease in the calcium content of the bones, which leaves them thin and susceptible to fracture.

Causes

The causes of osteoporosis are largely unknown. However, chances of acquiring the condition seem to increase dramatically with age, especially for women. One prevailing theory maintains that osteoporosis results from a loss of the female hormone estrogen, which affects the calcium content of the bones. Menopause (cessation of menstruation) may lead to osteoporosis because the body's production of estrogen is greatly reduced at that time. Almost one third of all women over 60 years of age have osteoporosis to some extent.

For reasons not entirely known, osteoporosis is more likely to affect white and Asian women than black women. In addition, slender women, especially those with fair skin, run a higher risk than stouter, darker-skinned women.

Osteoporosis can also occur as a result of other conditions. Surgical removal of both ovaries (the female sex glands, which produce estrogen) and chronic arthritis (inflammation of the joints) may lead to osteoporo-

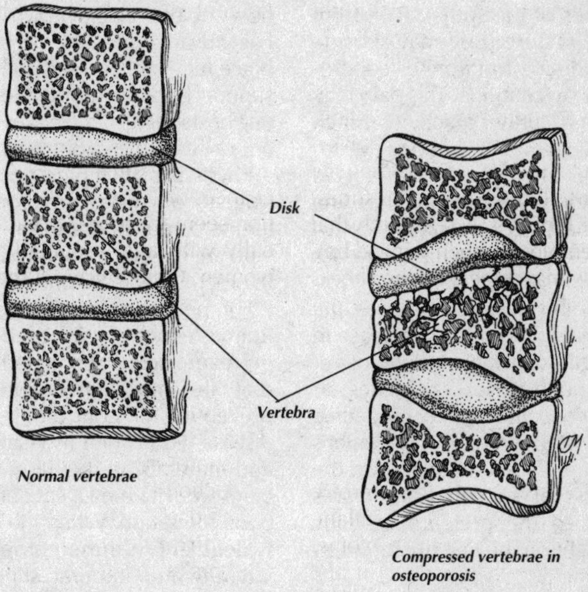

Normal vertebrae

Disk

Vertebra

Compressed vertebrae in osteoporosis

Osteoporosis, a condition in which the bones weaken and break easily, may lead to compression of the vertebrae (bones of the spine).

sis. People who are inactive, either by choice or due to confinement because of illness, seem more susceptible to the disorder. A diet deficient in nutrients, especially calcium (which promotes bone development), may also contribute to osteoporosis. Additional risk factors include smoking, early menopause, and a family history of osteoporosis.

Symptoms

Depending on the strength of the bones, osteoporosis may initially cause either no symptoms or extreme pain. If there is pain, it is most commonly in the lower back. The disease is not life-threatening, but it may lead to fractures, which, for the elderly, can result in serious complications. Initially, sudden back pain could be caused by fracture of the vertebrae (the bones of the spine). Pain from the fracture itself may subside but discomfort from osteoporosis may continue. This pain may lead to further inactivity, which may weaken additional vertebrae. Hence, a vicious cycle develops whereby pain leading to inactivity encourages osteoporosis, which in turn increases bone fragility.

As the disease progresses, the spinal column may decrease in length, causing a height loss of as much as several inches, or may become curved, producing the characteristic "dowager's hump." These changes are the result of successive fractures due to the pressure of body weight on the deteriorating vertebrae.

Diagnosis
Often, osteoporosis progresses undetected until a bone is fractured and an X ray is taken. At that time, a physician may notice that bone thinning has become a generalized condition throughout the body.

Treatment
Physicians urge patients with osteoporosis to follow an exercise program that will strengthen the muscles supporting weakened bones. To protect bones in the spinal column, however, lifting heavy objects should be avoided. For advanced cases, a back brace may be necessary to help support body weight while sitting or standing. Crutches, walkers, or canes may assist walking.

Physicians often prescribe estrogen or estrogen–progesterone combinations to women who are no longer menstruating in order to decrease bone loss.

For people prone to injury from osteoporosis, weight-bearing exercises and a balanced diet are important factors in preventing or controlling the disease. Foods rich in vitamins and minerals, particularly calcium and vitamin D, encourage bone formation. When the diet is deficient in these nutrients, vitamin and mineral supplements may be prescribed by a doctor.

Paget disease

Paget disease (known medically as *osteitis deformans*) is a disorder in which the normal process of breakdown and replacement of bone tissue is greatly accelerated. The disease develops in three stages. In the first, or destructive, stage, bone tissue breaks down and is replaced with blood vessels and dense fibrous tissue, making the bones very vascular (having a greater-than-normal number of blood vessels). During the second, or mixed, stage, new bone formation takes place at a rate geared to the breakdown process. In the third, or sclerotic, stage, the breakdown process slows, allowing the hardening of new bone, which becomes quite dense.

Although any bone can be affected, Paget disease most commonly invades the pelvis, skull, thighbones, shinbones, vertebrae (the bones of the spine), collarbones, and ribs.

The condition affects 1 to 3 percent of the adult population. Men are more commonly afflicted than women. The incidence of the condition is higher in some European countries than in others; it is rare in Asia, Africa, and South America. The cause of Paget disease is unknown.

Symptoms and complications

Bone pain is one of the most prevalent symptoms. Complications sometimes develop. The thickened, enlarged bones are susceptible to fracture, particularly during the destructive phase of the disease. When the disease attacks the skull bones, the auditory nerve, which relays signals from the ear to the brain, is often compressed, causing deafness. Heart failure can result from the stress of the increased blood flow through the bones. Malignant bone tumors are another complication, but they are uncommon. The disease can affect appearance if it enlarges the head, bends the back, or bows the legs. In some severe cases, particularly if the person is immobile, calcium levels in the blood and urine increase and may lead to formation of kidney stones.

Diagnosis

An individual's medical history, a physical examination, blood tests, and X-ray studies are used to confirm the diagnosis of Paget disease.

Treatment

Although there is no cure for Paget disease, some analgesics (painkillers) such as aspirin offer relief. Severe pain and other complications are sometimes managed with drug therapy. Injections of calcitonin (a hormone normally produced in the thyroid gland, which promotes the calcification of bone) may help block excessive breakdown of bone. Oral drug therapy is now also available.

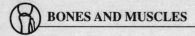

Slipped disk

A slipped disk is a back problem involving the disks of soft elastic tissue located between the vertebrae (bones of the spinal column). The vertebrae are loosely strung together by bands of tissue called ligaments, which allow body movement and flexibility. The main function of each disk is to prevent friction and trauma between adjacent vertebrae as the body moves.

When this intricate spinal structure experiences strain and overexertion, the rim of a disk may weaken and tear, causing part of the gelatinous center of the disk to be forced out of position ("slip" or "herniate"). In its new location, the protruding material often presses against an adjacent spinal nerve, which causes pain along the path of the affected nerve.

Causes

Often, a slipped disk occurs when there is strain or injury to the spinal structure caused by bending and straightening of the back to lift heavy objects. Damage to the disk may not be realized for many months. More often, low-back pain radiating into the buttocks and thighs occurs soon after the injury.

Disks also seem to deteriorate with age. They lose some fluidity and become more compressed. This form of degeneration usually results in only mild pain and intermittent backache and stiffness.

Symptoms

Symptoms may vary with the location of the disk. The most common site for a slipped disk is the lowest movable disk in the small of the back. Injury to this disk causes pain along the sciatic nerve, a condition called *sciatica.* Mild or disabling pain and tenderness may result. Any straining, such as coughing or moving, can aggravate the discomfort. Weakness, tingling, or numbness in parts of the arms, legs, or feet may also result from damage to a particular disk in the neck or back.

Diagnosis

To determine the source of back pain, a physician obtains a medical history; observes the patient sitting, walking, and bending; and explores for sensitive areas by maneuvering the patient's legs in different positions, checking reflexes, and testing muscle strength. Structural changes in bones, joints, or disk spaces (but not the disks themselves) can be determined on an X-ray study.

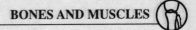
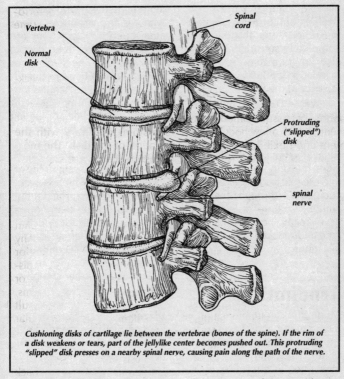

Cushioning disks of cartilage lie between the vertebrae (bones of the spine). If the rim of a disk weakens or tears, part of the jellylike center becomes pushed out. This protruding "slipped" disk presses on a nearby spinal nerve, causing pain along the path of the nerve.

Magnetic resonance imaging (MRI) is also used in the diagnosis of disk problems.

Treatment

The first course of treatment for a slipped disk involves bed rest on a firm mattress. Rest relieves pressure exerted by the disk on the nerve. Some form of back support may improve comfort when moving about. Under no circumstances should a patient lift heavy objects.

For severe pain, a physician may prescribe an analgesic or anti-inflammatory drug. Frequently, direct injection of a steroid (cortisone) drug and local anesthetic into the area around the spinal cord (epidural space) will break the cycle of pain and nerve-root swelling and provide long-lasting relief. After the pain has completely subsided, an exercise program may be recommended to gradually strengthen muscles in the region.

Partial or complete relief from the pain of a slipped disk can usually be obtained without surgery. However, in some cases, surgical removal of the disk provides the only remedy. Newer microscopic techniques and percutaneous (through the skin without cutting) disk removal have greatly shortened recovery time and reduced surgical complications.

Tendinitis

Tendinitis is an inflammation of a tendon (a band of fibrous tissue connecting muscle to bone). The condition appears most often as a result of physical activity. It also can be a symptom of a more generalized inflammatory disease, such as rheumatoid arthritis.

Causes
Improper activity, lack of conditioning, and poor athletic equipment encourage the development of tendinitis. Nonathletes who suddenly begin athletic activity and athletes who resume strenuous sports after a period of inactivity are especially susceptible. People who wear high heels or shoes with run-down heels put needless tension on the Achilles tendon, which joins the calf muscles on the back of the leg to the back of the heel bone.

Symptoms
Tendinitis causes pain in the affected tendon, which is worsened by activity. The tendon may grow thicker than normal and be tender to the touch or very painful. When an already inflamed tendon is continually placed under stress, it can rupture, causing further complications.

Diagnosis
Physicians diagnose tendinitis problems by first acquiring the patient's exercise history. Muscle lengths in the area of inflammation are also evaluated. (Short or inflexible muscles are often the cause of tendinitis.)

Treatment
Treatment for tendinitis begins with resting the affected area. Pain relievers and anti-inflammatory drugs are used to ease immediate symptoms, but they will not cure the condition or

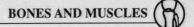

keep it from recurring. Injecting cortisone and a local anesthetic into the area surrounding the tendon usually provides substantial relief within 24 to 72 hours.

In rare cases, surgery is necessary to repair damaged tendons. In the past, tendons were replaced with artificial tissues that never achieved the strength and flexibility of natural tissues.

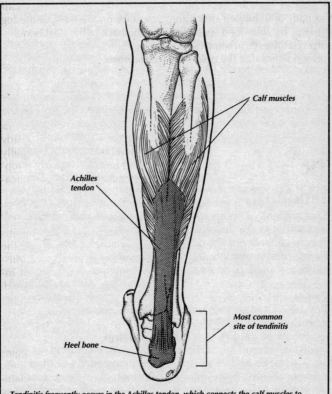

Calf muscles

Achilles tendon

Most common site of tendinitis

Heel bone

Tendinitis frequently occurs in the Achilles tendon, which connects the calf muscles to the heel bone.

More effective techniques and materials have since been developed.

Prevention
People participating in sports can prevent tendinitis by taking time to warm-up before exercising. For example, stretching the leg and calf muscles before and after running may help prevent inflammation of the Achilles tendon. When tendinitis does occur, wearing supports in shoes during physical activity can correct instability of the foot and lessen the level of pain.

Tic

A tic is a spasmodic movement or twitching that is generally a brief, repetitive, purposeless, semivoluntary or involuntary muscle contraction. The movement is most commonly seen in the face, shoulders, or arms.

Causes
Tics are caused by involuntary muscle contractions. With the exception of the tics that develop as a result of nerve or brain damage and other specific conditions, however, the physiologic basis of most tics is largely unknown. They often accompany emotional upset or psychological problems. Tics in children may be a sign of Gilles de la Tourette syndrome, a disorder marked by multiple tics and compulsive use of profane language (see page 534).

Symptoms
A typical "nervous tic" is a twitching of the corner of the eye or the mouth, grimacing, blinking, or making repetitive motions involving the hands, arms, or shoulders.

Tics in children often first occur between the ages of five and ten years and may gradually disappear as the child grows older; however, the tics can persist into adulthood. When nervous tics first arise, they can usually be voluntarily controlled, but persistent tics often become automatic after a period of time.

Diagnosis
Certain types of tics are, at the beginning, hard to distinguish from many neurologically based illnesses.

Treatment
For mild childhood or adult tics, tranquilizers or muscle relaxants may be prescribed. Gilles de la Tourette syndrome responds to medication. Psychotherapy may help to relieve

the emotional stress that precipitates attacks or intensifies the symptoms of some tics.

Trichinosis

Trichinosis is a condition caused by the infestation of the body by *Trichinella spiralis*, a parasitic worm sometimes found in meat.

Cause
Trichinosis is most commonly caused by ingestion of bear meat that has not been cooked for a sufficient length of time or at a sufficiently high temperature to kill the *Trichinella spiralis* worms.

The worms are encapsulated in the meat itself. When the meat is eaten, the worms emerge from it and begin their life cycle in the human host. This begins in the small intestine, where the larvae mature within two days after they emerge from the meat. The adult *Trichinella spiralis* worms breed, the males die, and the females produce more larvae, which invade the tissues of the bowel and are then dispersed to muscles throughout the body, where they lodge.

The muscles around the eyes, the tongue, and the diaphragm (the muscle separating the chest cavity from the abdomen) and the muscles between the ribs are the areas of the body most commonly affected by the condition.

Symptoms
Quite often, the infested patient is entirely unaware of the presence of trichinosis. When large infestations do occur, however, they are accompanied by a variety of symptoms.

One to two days after consumption of the contaminated meat, a severe flulike illness consisting of fever, nausea, vomiting, diarrhea, and abdominal pain occurs. Tenderness and swelling around the infested muscles are common.

After about a week, a rash, swelling of the eyelids, and neurologic disorders may develop. Eventually, the larvae in the muscles die and become calcified. Symptoms of the condition gradually disappear within a few months.

Treatment
Since there is no way to get the larvae out of the muscles, treatment is aimed at relief of the patient's discomfort.

Analgesics, such as aspirin, are administered for pain, and anti-inflammatory steroids (cor-

181

tisone drugs, such as prednisone) are administered for allergic symptoms, myocarditis, and central nervous system involvement. Thiabendazole (which tends to kill worms such as the *Trichinella*) is often given with good results. The patient is watched closely for fever, abdominal pain, vomiting, and dermatitis (skin inflammation).

Prevention
The only way to avoid contracting trichinosis is to make sure that meat is sufficiently cooked (an internal temperature of 170°F) to kill the larvae.

THE EYES AND VISION

The eye is the organ of sight. This complex structure works by capturing light and transforming it into impulses that the brain can interpret as images.

To understand visual perception, it is important to know the functions of the parts of the eye. The eye includes the eyeball and all structures within and surrounding its almost spherical mass. This delicate organ is nestled within the bony socket of the skull. A layer of fat cushions the socket; the eyebrow, eyelashes, and eyelid provide a barrier against incoming irritants. Lining the inside of the

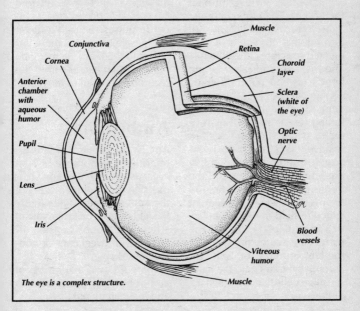

The eye is a complex structure.

eyelid and continuing over the exposed surface of the eyeball is the conjunctiva, a thin protective membrane. Tears released from the lacrimal glands in the upper eyelid moisten the conjunctiva and keep the eye clean. The sclera is the tough, white, outer layer of the eyeball. The sclera covers the entire eyeball, except for the circular area in front that admits light, which is covered by the transparent cornea. The choroid layer contains blood vessels that nourish the eye.

Light enters the eye through the cornea. The curved cornea helps to focus the light inward. Behind the cornea is a pigmented structure called the iris. The iris surrounds an opening known as the pupil. The iris changes the size of the pupil, depending on the amount of light present in the environment: If the surroundings are relatively dark, the pupil is enlarged to admit more light; if the environment is bright, the pupil is made smaller. Behind the iris is the lens, a transparent structure held in place by elastic, muscular-type tissue. The tissue can change the shape of the lens to finely focus the incoming light rays onto the light-sensitive cells that line the back of the eye.

Between the cornea and the lens is a space, the anterior chamber, which is filled with a fluid called aqueous humor. Aqueous humor contains nutrients that nourish the cornea and the lens. The fluid also allows light rays to pass through easily.

The chamber of the eyeball behind the lens holds a clear jelly called vitreous humor. In the retina (the layer of light-sensitive cells that lines the back of the eyeball) are the specialized cells, called rods and cones, that convert light focused from the cornea and lens into electrical impulses. Sensitive nerve endings then transmit these impulses to the brain via the optic nerve, which extends from the rear of the eyeball to the brain.

Amblyopia

Amblyopia is the name for diminished vision in one or both eyes, usually without any obvious defect. (Amblyopia is not the same as nearsightedness, farsightedness, or astigmatism. (These conditions can be corrected with eyeglasses or contact lenses.)

There are two main types of amblyopia: lazy-eye amblyopia and toxic amblyopia.

LAZY-EYE AMBLYOPIA

Lazy-eye amblyopia occurs frequently in young children whose eyes do not line up correctly (a condition known as strabismus). To prevent double vision (in which the patient sees two images instead of one), the brain suppresses the sight of one eye; the other eye does all the work. Without treatment, the brain structures dependent on the eye that is not working may atrophy (waste away) or fail to develop.

Symptoms

There are usually no obvious symptoms of this form of amblyopia. By the time the condition is recognized, the eye may be permanently damaged. Usually, the child appears to see as well as the next child. Sometimes, however, the condition that causes the amblyopia is very noticeable: The eyes may turn either inward or outward, or one eye may be looking up while the other is looking down.

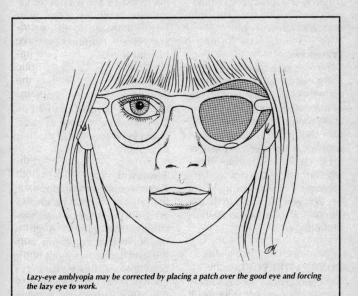

Lazy-eye amblyopia may be corrected by placing a patch over the good eye and forcing the lazy eye to work.

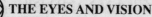

Treatment

To restore sight in the lazy eye fully, treatment must begin before the child is four to six years of age. If the eyes are out of focus because some of the muscles of the lazy eye are weaker than others, the condition may be corrected by wearing special glasses or contact lenses, by doing eye exercises, by patching the good eye and prescribing corrective lenses for the amblyopic eye (thereby forcing the lazy eye to work), or by surgery. Periodic reexaminations are needed until the child is at least ten years old.

Prevention

If the eyes of a baby are continually out of alignment in the first weeks of life or are still out of alignment from time to time at six months of age, the condition should be investigated. A simple eye test given in the doctor's office should show whether one eye is not working properly. Evaluation should not be delayed. A child will not "grow out" of either strabismus or amblyopia.

TOXIC AMBLYOPIA

Toxic amblyopia, which usually occurs in both eyes, can result from excessive drinking of alcoholic beverages over a long period of time. (This may be due mainly to the poor nutrition of heavy drinkers, who get most of their calories from alcohol.) It may also be found in heavy cigarette smokers and in people exposed to various chemicals and drugs, including lead, methanol (wood alcohol), digitalis, chloramphenicol, and arsenic. The toxic substance causes swelling and irritation of the optic nerve around the site at the rear of the eye where the nerve leaves the eyeball. If the irritation continues, it can cause lasting damage to the nerve, sometimes resulting in total blindness.

Symptoms

Symptoms include pain on moving the eyeball and an increasing area of poor eyesight in or near the center of the field of vision.

Treatment

Treatment is to stop exposure to the poison, if it can be discovered. In the case of lead poisoning, the patient is given medicine that combines with the lead and draws it out of the body tissues (this treatment is known as *chelation therapy*). If the cause is removed at once, vision may improve—unless there has been permanent damage to the optic nerve.

Astigmatism

Astigmatism is a type of distorted vision caused by a defect in the curvature of the cornea or lens of the eye. This prevents the rays of light entering the eye from being properly focused onto the retina at the back of the eyeball. Some rays are misplaced, causing the image to be partially out of focus.

Types

There are several types of astigmatism. Most people with astigmatism can see clearly those objects directly in front of them, but their peripheral vision is defective. Others have vertical astigmatism, in which the areas above and below their direct

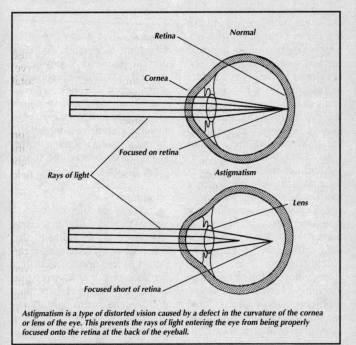

Astigmatism is a type of distorted vision caused by a defect in the curvature of the cornea or lens of the eye. This prevents the rays of light entering the eye from being properly focused onto the retina at the back of the eyeball.

gaze are imperfectly visualized. Some may have horizontal astigmatism, in which the right and left sides of their field of vision are defective. The astigmatism may be diagonal as well.

Treatment

Fortunately, a defect in the curvature of the cornea or lens is usually uniform and can be easily corrected by eyeglasses or contact lenses. The fault is usually in the shape of the cornea (the clear "window" in front of the iris and pupil of the eye), which may be slightly flattened vertically or horizontally. The eyeglass lenses or contact lenses are curved to adjust the angle of rays entering regions of the eye that are defective; the glasses or lenses do not bend the rays entering the areas of clear vision.

Although most people with astigmatism were born with a tendency toward the condition, a few cases are caused by eye disease or injury. In these situations, the condition causing the astigmatism may be more difficult to correct.

Regardless of the cause, astigmatism—as with any vision problem—should be corrected as early as possible. If astigmatism goes uncorrected, children, in particular, are at risk for

development of permanently defective vision.

Blepharitis

Blepharitis is an inflammation of the edges of the eyelids. Redness, scales and crusts, or shallow ulcers may also appear. The disease is common, especially in children, and often affects the upper and lower eyelids of both eyes.

Causes

Infection of eyelash follicles and oil glands by *Staphylococcus* bacteria causes blepharitis with ulcers. The nonulcerous variety may be due to an allergic reaction or lice, or it may be linked to seborrheic dermatitis, an inflammatory scaling of the scalp, the eyebrows, and sometimes the ears.

Symptoms

Symptoms of blepharitis include itching, burning, red-rimmed eyes; swelling of the lids; loss of eyelashes; and irritation of the underside of the lid, as if dirt or sand were underneath. The eyes may tear and be sensitive to light. In ulcerous blepharitis, the tough, dry crusts that form leave a bleeding surface when re-

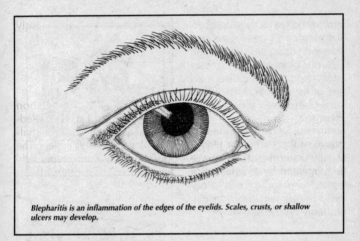

Blepharitis is an inflammation of the edges of the eyelids. Scales, crusts, or shallow ulcers may develop.

moved. In nonulcerous blepharitis, greasy, easily removed scales appear on the edges of the lids.

Treatment

Blepharitis caused by a bacterial infection can be treated with an antibiotic ointment, such as erythromycin or bacitracin, that is specially formulated for use around the eyes. The medication is usually applied three times a day to the eyelash margins. Before applying the medication, scrub the lids gently with a cotton-tipped swab that's been dampened with water. Crusts should be gently removed. Medicated eyedrops may also be used to treat blepharitis.

If an allergy to a cosmetic is the cause, use of the product should be discontinued. If there is scaling on the eyebrows and scalp from seborrheic dermatitis, your doctor is likely to recommend a special sulfur or tar shampoo to control dandruff and a cortisone lotion or cream to be rubbed into hairy areas. Careful attention to cleanliness of hair, scalp, eyebrows, and eyelid margins is necessary during treatment.

If the blepharitis is caused by lice, the nits (lice eggs) should be carefully removed with tweezers, and steps should be taken to keep the patient free of lice.

Both the ulcerous and nonulcerous varieties are difficult to

189

cure and often recur. Nonulcerous blepharitis causes no permanent damage. However, ulcerous blepharitis, if it recurs often enough, can cause scarring of the eyelids, loss of eyelashes, and even ulcers of the cornea.

Prevention

Meticulous cleanliness may help prevent the disease. If it is treated promptly when it occurs, permanent damage can probably be prevented.

Cataract

A cataract is a clouding of the lens of the eye that results in obscured vision. People with this defect see their environment as if they were looking through a waterfall.

Normally, the lens is clear. Its function is to focus light onto the light-sensitive cells lining the back of the eye, so that objects at various distances can be seen clearly. If the lens becomes hazy, however, incoming light is scattered and vision blurs.

Causes

The exact cause of cataracts is unknown. Aging may play a role, but the condition also occurs in some newborns whose

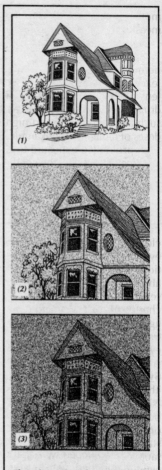

The main symptom of cataract is painless blurring of vision. Vision with early cataract may be close to normal (1). As cataract progresses, vision gradually blurs (2) and eventually may become extremely blurred (3).

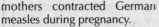

mothers contracted German measles during pregnancy.

Diabetes, glaucoma, and detachment of the retina (the innermost layer of the eye) may lead to cataracts. Injury to the lens, prolonged use of certain drugs (including steroidal drugs such as prednisone), and high doses of radiation (for example, from prolonged exposure to X rays) may also trigger the condition.

Although the condition is usually curable, cataracts can cause blindness. In addition, the shadowy lens prohibits a clear view of the interior of the eye. Because of this obstruction, a physician may not be able to detect other potentially serious eye disorders, such as changes in the retina and damage to the optic nerve (which transmits information from the eye to the brain).

Symptoms

The main symptom of cataracts is painless blurring of vision, occurring most often in only one eye. During the initial stages of development, cataracts can cause the person to experience glare in bright light, since the clouded lens scatters, rather than focuses, incoming light. As the condition progresses, the lens becomes milky white, and vision continues to worsen.

Treatment

Successful treatment begins with surgical removal of the affected lens. With the aid of a microscope, the surgeon opens an area in the front of the eye and removes the lens. The use of local anesthetic eyedrops makes this usually out-patient procedure relatively painless.

After the patient has recuperated for a few weeks, special cataract eyeglasses or a contact lens can be prescribed to help correct the vision. These aids are by no means perfect and require an adjustment period. Another option, one that most doctors now recommend, is the implantation of an intraocular lens in the eye after cataract surgery. The lightweight plastic lens is relatively free of distortion. It affords vision that is closer to normal than cataract eyeglasses or contact lenses can provide, because it occupies the exact position of the natural lens. (Eyeglasses may still be necessary, however.)

In the vast majority of cases, surgery for cataracts is without complications. Restoration or substantial improvement of vision usually results after surgery. If vision remains unimproved, a disorder that was not detected due to the presence of the cataract may be the cause.

Color blindness

Color blindness is an inability to distinguish certain colors. By far the most common type is inherited red–green color blindness, which affects 8 percent of men and boys but only 0.5 percent of women and girls. Total color blindness, which is very rare, and pastel-shade color blindness are believed to be inherited. Other types, including blue–yellow color blindness and red–green color blindness, can be either inherited or acquired. Disease or injury affecting the retina may also be the cause of color blindness.

Description
Color blindness results from a defect within the cone-shaped light-sensitive cells of the fovea (the tiny, yellowish pit in the retina, which is the center for perceiving color). The 7 million cone cells differ from the 130 million rod-shaped cells in the rest of the retina. While the rod cells register only black and white, the cone cells contain pigments for red, green, and blue—the colors that can combine to produce all the colors of the spectrum. The pigments become more vivid or fade in response to colors that the eye sees. The changes in pigmentation produce tiny flashes of electricity, which are carried by means of the optic nerve to the visual center of the brain. There, the electrical signals are combined into a full-color picture. In the color-blind person, the cones are missing or defective. No cure is known.

Inheriting red–green color blindness
Why is red–green color blindness inherited by boys more often than by girls? The reason is that the defective gene that directs production of the defective pigment is carried on the same pair of chromosomes that determines the sex of the child. In a female child (who has two X sex chromosomes), a defective gene on one X chromosome is almost always counteracted by a normal gene on the other X chromosome; as a result, the girl is born with normal color vision. In a male child (who has an X and a Y sex chromosome), there is no matching normal gene to block the defect on the only X chromosome the boy has; the boy is, therefore, born color-blind.

Red–green color blindness cannot be passed from a father to his sons, nor will his daughters be color-blind, unless the mother carries the defective gene as well. However, his daughters will all be carriers of the defective gene, and the daughters' sons will have a 50 percent chance of being color-blind.

Conjunctivitis

Conjunctivitis, or pinkeye, is an inflammation of the conjunctiva. The conjunctiva is a delicate membrane that lines the inner surface of the eyelid and covers the exposed surface of the eye.

Causes

Most cases of conjunctivitis result from disease-causing microorganisms such as bacteria and viruses. Allergies, chemicals, dust, smoke, and foreign objects that irritate the conjunctiva may also lead to conjunctivitis. Swimming may be associated with conjunctivitis, because of exposure to chlorine or contaminated water. Occasionally, a sexually transmitted disease can cause pinkeye if the eyes are rubbed after the hands have touched infected genitals.

Children are most often affected by conjunctivitis. Measles, a viral disease, may be accompanied by this eye inflammation. In addition, those people, both children and adults, who have allergies such as hay fever or who work and live in areas where they are exposed to chemicals or other irritants are more susceptible to noninfectious conjunctivitis.

Symptoms

Conjunctivitis may cause redness, a grating sensation, burning, itching, and light sensitivity. Occasionally, tearing occurs, or a discharge containing pus will be present. Symptoms can last a few days or up to two weeks.

Conjunctivitis usually produces no permanent damage. However, if left untreated, the infection may lead to more serious eye problems. Ulcers (eroded areas) may form on the cornea (the clear "window" in front of the iris and pupil of the eye). If these ulcers persist, they can scar the eye and interfere with vision.

Treatment

Treatment depends on the cause and resulting symptoms of the conjunctivitis. If the inflammation is environmentally caused, simply removing the ir-

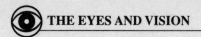

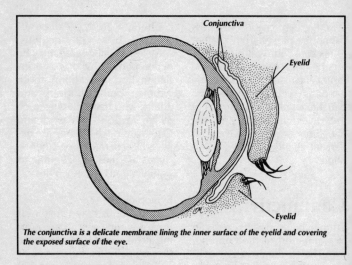

The conjunctiva is a delicate membrane lining the inner surface of the eyelid and covering the exposed surface of the eye.

ritant may be sufficient to eliminate the condition. For more difficult cases, a physician may prescribe antibiotics, steroids, or combination eyedrops. Frequent use of eyedrops is usually necessary because the drops tend to be washed away by the natural cleansing action of the tears.

Sensitive eyes should be shielded from bright lights. If the discharge glues the eyelids closed, bathing them with warm water and wiping with a clean cloth will help loosen them.

Conjunctivitis in its infectious form is highly contagious. Individuals with infectious con-junctivitis should not share handkerchiefs, towels, or wash-cloths and should be careful to avoid touching the unaffected eye after contact with the infected eye.

Detached retina

Normally, the retina is firmly attached to the choroid, an underlying layer of tissue that is rich in blood vessels. If blood or other fluid collects between the retina and the choroid, the retina may become partially or totally detached. Fluid from the vitreous cavity (the fluid-filled space within the eye) may penetrate beneath the retina via a small hole. Fluid leaking out of certain blood vessels in the eye may also penetrate beneath the retina to cause detachment.

Causes
Cataract surgery, severe myopia (nearsightedness), and injury can cause retinal detachment. Although injury can cause this condition, it is more likely to accelerate a detachment that has already begun. Conditions that increase susceptibility to retinal detachment are inflammation or tumors of the eye, high blood pressure, and vitreous hemorrhaging.

Symptoms
Initial symptoms include seeing floating dark spots or streaks of light and experiencing blurring of vision. As the condition progresses, a veil seems to fall over part or all of the field of vision.

Treatment
A detached retina can be treated by using a laser to fuse the retina to the choroid. It can also be treated by diathermy (repair using heat), cryotherapy

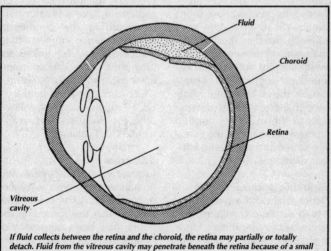

If fluid collects between the retina and the choroid, the retina may partially or totally detach. Fluid from the vitreous cavity may penetrate beneath the retina because of a small hole in the retina.

(repair using extreme cold), or microsurgery (surgery using a microscope). Left untreated, the detachment may increase and lead to the loss of sight.

Glaucoma

Glaucoma is an eye disorder caused by increased pressure within the eyeball, which builds up because fluids are unable to drain normally.

Cause
Although glaucoma is understood to be a problem with the fluid-regulating mechanism of the eye, its precise cause is unknown. In the healthy eye, aqueous fluid in the anterior chamber of the eyeball (between the lens and the cornea) is under a slight degree of pressure. If the delicate fluid balance changes, internal pressure rises in the eye. This buildup produces damage to the sensitive structures and nerve endings within the eye.

Forms of glaucoma
Depending on the type of defect in the fluid-regulating system, one of two primary forms of glaucoma results. Chronic, or open angle, glaucoma develops when pressure increases gradu-

ally, and normal fluid drainage slows but is not obstructed at the drainage angle (the network of tissue between the iris and the cornea, through which fluid can normally pass). Acute, or closed angle, glaucoma occurs when pressure mounts suddenly and forces the iris into contact with the cornea, thereby blocking fluid drainage from the anterior chamber of the eye.

Those at risk
Glaucoma occurs more commonly in adults over 40 years of age. Statistics indicate that people with a family history of glaucoma have a greater risk of acquiring the condition. Some evidence suggests that glaucoma may be linked to long-term use of various medications, especially steroids, which can alter body fluid levels. Glaucoma can also follow other eye disorders, such as infections and cataracts.

Symptoms
Chronic glaucoma begins with no noticeable symptoms. Vision deterioration is so gradual and painless that this form of glaucoma has been termed the "sneak thief of sight." Sometimes, loss of peripheral vision slowly progresses as central vi-

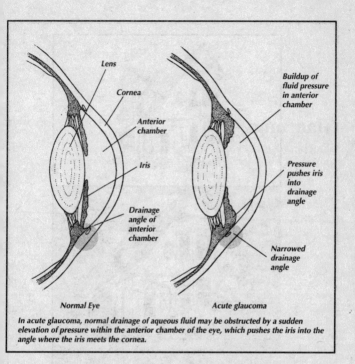

In acute glaucoma, normal drainage of aqueous fluid may be obstructed by a sudden elevation of pressure within the anterior chamber of the eye, which pushes the iris into the angle where the iris meets the cornea.

sion remains normal. As the disorder advances, other symptoms (which can be intermittent or constant) include foggy or blurred vision, difficulty in adjusting to brightness and darkness, and slight pain in or around the eye, usually on one side. The one symptom indicative of chronic glaucoma is the perception of a faint white circle or halo surrounding a light, which is most easily visible when looking at a distant light while in the dark.

Acute glaucoma brings sudden and severe symptoms of extreme eye pain and abrupt vision blurring. Frequently, the pain can be so intense that it causes nausea and vomiting. Fortunately, acute glaucoma is rare, but when it does occur, medical attention is needed immediately to prevent permanent blindness. Usually, however,

197

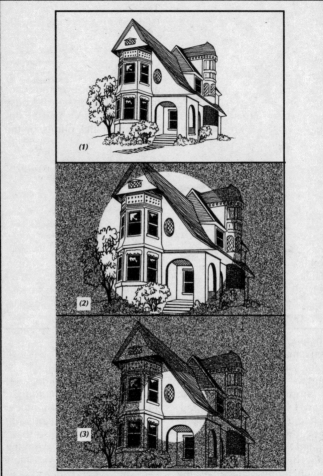

Normal vision (1) will deteriorate gradually if glaucoma is not treated. Loss of peripheral vision may slowly progress as central vision remains normal (2). Untreated glaucoma can lead to partial or complete vision loss (3).

the symptoms are so severe that medical help is sought promptly.

Diagnosis

If left untreated, glaucoma can lead to partial or complete vision loss. However, if diagnosed early, treatment can usually halt the process. Because chronic glaucoma has no warning signs, it is particularly important that people over the age of 40 be tested for glaucoma every two or three years. In addition, physicians recommend that people with a family history of the disease be screened every year beginning even before the age of 40.

Glaucoma testing is a relatively simple office procedure. The doctor uses a special device called a *tonometer* to measure the amount of pressure within the eyeball.

The doctor also inspects the interior of the eye through an instrument that allows a view of the angle where the iris and the cornea meet. This part of the examination shows whether there is blockage in the drainage system or damage to the optic nerve. The doctor also tests peripheral vision by measuring the point at which objects can be seen in the patient's field of vision.

Treatment

Glaucoma treatment is usually effective if started early in the course of the disease. Oral drugs work by decreasing production of eye fluid, while daily applications of eyedrops promote fluid drainage. Because some medications cause constriction of the pupils of the eyes, which can be misconstrued as a symptom of drug overdose, many glaucoma patients carry an identification card that describes their medical history in case of medical emergency.

Beta-blocker eyedrops reduce production of eye fluid without altering the size of the pupil. However, beta-blockers can affect the heart rate and cause narrowing of the breathing passages, which may make these drugs unsuitable for patients with heart or respiratory disease. Other antiglaucoma medications are also available.

Although chronic glaucoma responds to medication, some patients require surgery to open new pathways for fluid drainage. Laser therapy is a relatively new surgical technique under investigation. The laser uses an intense light beam to slightly modify tissues in the region in order to allow better fluid drainage.

Prevention
The best way to prevent serious complications of glaucoma is to undergo periodic screening for early diagnosis.

Keratitis

Keratitis is an inflammation of the cornea (the clear "window" in front of the iris and pupil of the eye), which commonly produces redness, tearing, tenderness, sensitivity to light, and blurred vision.

Interstitial keratitis
Interstitial keratitis is often caused by congenital (present at birth) syphilis in children or by tuberculosis. This type of keratitis produces deep deposits of scar tissue, which cause the cornea to become hazy and give it a ground-glass appearance. There is little that can be done for this condition, although the inflammation and redness usually diminish after a month or two. Vision may or may not be impaired thereafter.

Herpes simplex keratitis
A common type of keratitis is caused by the herpes simplex virus, the same virus that produces cold sores. Herpes simplex keratitis is usually not painful, although at first there is a sensation that foreign matter may be present. If the infection is left untreated, all feeling in the cornea will eventually be lost. Like a cold sore, the infection tends to come and go, but it should be taken care of when the first sign—a whitish lesion on the cornea—appears. Treatment usually consists of applying eyedrops or ointment, but some specialists prefer to scrape the cornea, after which they cover the affected eye temporarily.

Traumatic keratitis
Traumatic keratitis occurs when scar tissue remains after a corneal injury has healed. If a considerable amount of scar tissue covers the pupil, blindness may result. This condition can generally be cured by corrective surgery or corneal transplantation.

Macular degeneration

Macular degeneration is the deterioration of the macula (the yellowish depression in the central part of the retina). The macula is the part of the eye with the greatest density of visual receptor cells. As light enters the eye, the image that is focused on the macula is the one that is most clearly perceived in the brain. The function of the macula is to distinguish fine detail in the central visual field. Consequently, degeneration of the macula leads to blurring of central vision; peripheral vision remains intact.

Causes

The exact cause of macular degeneration is unknown. In many cases, it may be a result of another disorder, atherosclerosis, which causes a narrowing of the blood vessels, including those that supply the macula with blood. In these cases, the macula wastes away. This form is often referred to as the "dry" form. In another less common form of the disease, tiny blood vessels proliferate around the macula and leak blood or fluid, causing blurred or distorted central vision. This is often called the "wet" form of macular degeneration.

Symptoms

Macular degeneration, in its dry form, usually develops slowly and painlessly. Therefore, the blurring of central vision is gradual. In the wet form of macular degeneration, the blurring and loss of central vision may occur much more rapidly.

If both eyes are affected—as is almost always the case—activities requiring sharp vision, such as reading and driving, usually have to be curtailed. Eventually, all central vision disappears, although peripheral vision is unaffected.

Treatment

There was no treatment for macular degeneration until recently. It has now been found that some individuals who have the wet form of macular degeneration may be helped with laser beams if the treatment is initiated early in the disease process, before significant damage has occurred. There is no treatment for the dry form of macular degeneration, although early in the course of the condition, vision may be improved by special powerful eyeglasses.

Myopia

Myopia, or nearsightedness, is a common optical defect in which close objects can be seen clearly but faraway objects look blurred. About one in every five persons is myopic. The condition tends to be

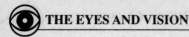

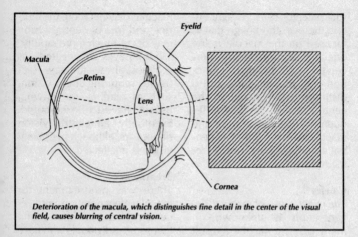

Deterioration of the macula, which distinguishes fine detail in the center of the visual field, causes blurring of central vision.

hereditary, developing in childhood around age 12 and progressing until the late teen years or early adulthood.

Cause
The defect occurs if the eyeball is too long from front to back. Normally, the cornea and the lens (the disk-shaped structure just behind the front of the eye) refract (bend) light coming from a viewed distant object so that the image is focused on the retina (the layer of specialized, light-sensitive cells that line the back of the eyeball). In myopia, the focused image falls short of the retina because of the greater length of the eyeball, resulting in a fuzzy image.

Types
There are several kinds of myopia. *Curvature myopia* occurs when there is an excessive curve of the refractive surfaces of the eye, which causes light to enter the eye in an abnormal path. The curvature is in the front surface of either the cornea or the lens. In *index myopia,* there is an increase in the light-refracting properties of the lens. It is sometimes associated with future development of cataracts or iritis (inflammation of the iris). *Progressive myopia* is an uncommon form in which the eyeball continues to elongate throughout a person's life, eventually leading to degeneration or detachment of the retina.

Diagnosis

Blurred or fuzzy vision should be evaluated by an ophthalmologist, who will look inside the eyes with a special instrument called an *ophthalmoscope,* diagnose any disorders, and test the acuity (sharpness) of vision.

Treatment

Nearsightedness is easily corrected with a concave lens that pushes the images back toward the retina and focuses them clearly.

A surgical procedure known as *radial keratotomy* also has been used to correct myopia. It involves cutting numerous "spokes" into the corneal surface, coming out from the center; the cornea flattens as it heals, which counteracts the problem. This procedure, however, is considered controversial by many ophthalmologists.

Myopia rarely progresses after age 30. In fact, the onset of middle age sometimes lessens the severity of the condition.

Night blindness

Night blindness, or nyctalopia, is a condition in which a person

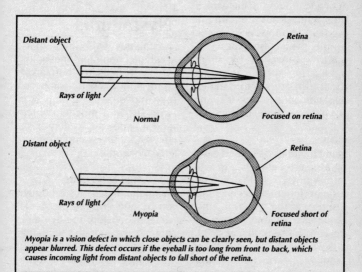

Myopia is a vision defect in which close objects can be clearly seen, but distant objects appear blurred. This defect occurs if the eyeball is too long from front to back, which causes incoming light from distant objects to fall short of the retina.

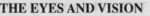

can see well in good light but not in dim or fading light.

The retina contains a layer of photoreceptors (specialized, light-sensitive cells) that lines the interior of the eyeball. These photoreceptors make the adjustments that are responsible for adaptation to varying degrees of light. There are two types of photoreceptors—cones and rods. Cones, concentrated in the center of the retina (the region called the *macula*), distinguish fine detail and color, while rods, which predominate around the edges of the retina, are sensitive to the intensity of light and do most of the work in dim light. Rods contain the pigment rhodopsin, or visual purple, which becomes temporarily bleached by bright light. The speed at which rhodopsin adjusts to darkness depends on a sufficient supply of vitamin A in the body.

Causes
Night blindness is caused either by a severe deficiency of vitamin A or by retinitis pigmentosa, an inherited degenerative disorder of the retina. In cases of extreme vitamin A shortage, the cornea may soften or start to dissolve (a condition called *keratomalacia*), or the eyes may become excessively dry.

Treatment
A vitamin A deficiency can be treated with doses of the vitamin. However, consuming large doses of vitamin A without a doctor's recommendation and without documentation of a deficiency can be extremely dangerous.

Prevention
The only preventive measure for nyctalopia is to obtain enough vitamin A in your diet (for example, from liver, egg yolks, and yellow and dark-green vegetables).

Nystagmus

Nystagmus is the involuntary, rhythmic, and rapid movement of the eyeballs in a horizontal, vertical, or rotary direction. The eye movements of a person who sits in a moving vehicle and watches the scenery flashing by are an example of normal nystagmus.

Abnormal nystagmus
Abnormal nystagmus is brought on by one of three problems: defective vision (the eye does not receive enough stimulation to concentrate on one object); disturbances in the elaborate mechanisms responsible for

balance in the inner ear; and diseases relating to the nervous system, especially those affecting the parts of the brain responsible for eye movement and coordination. Generally, the only symptoms of abnormal nystagmus are double vision, vertigo, and dizziness. Treatments will vary, depending on the underlying cause.

Retinitis

Retinitis is an inflammation of the retina, the light-sensitive innermost lining of the eye.

Types and causes

There are several types of retinitis. Toxoplasmic retinitis, which can be either acquired or congenital (present at birth), is caused by a microorganism. If the condition is congenital, the microorganism was passed to the fetus in the uterus through the placenta. A similar type of retinitis is caused by a blood-borne infection that settles in the eye. Exudative retinitis stems from unknown causes but can result in detachment of the retina from the internal surface of the eyeball. Retinitis pigmentosa is an inherited disorder in which excessive amounts of a substance called *phytanic acid*

accumulate and cause extensive damage to the retina. This form of retinitis also usually accompanies the rare inherited disorder of fat metabolism called *Refsum syndrome*.

Symptoms

The symptoms of retinitis pigmentosa are night blindness, inflammation of the retina, marked limitation of the field of vision (tunnel vision), loss of kinesthetic sense (sense of body movement), shrinkage of the retina, clumping of retinal pigment, and dislodging of the blood vessels of the retina. Many of the same symptoms are found in the other forms of retinitis. They are sometimes accompanied by cloudiness of the vitreous humor (liquid filling the eyeball). This can be detected by a special instrument called an *ophthalmoscope*.

Treatment

In the case of retinitis pigmentosa, there is little that can be done. If the retina is detached (a condition often caused when a hole in the retina allows fluid to seep into the eye and create a pocket), surgery is usually the treatment. The pocket is eliminated either by freezing or by heat, sometimes with a laser. If retinitis is the result of blood-borne infection, that condition must be treated first.

Prevention
Other than genetic counseling for persons with a family history of retinitis pigmentosa, there are no preventive measures.

Retinopathy

Retinopathy is a condition in which deterioration of the retina is caused by damage to or overproduction of the blood vessels in the retina.

Causes
The vast majority of cases of retinopathy are due to diabetes.

Although fewer than 5 percent of all people with diabetes completely lose their sight because of retinopathy, diabetes is one of the leading causes of irreversible blindness today. Other conditions that increase susceptibility to retinopathy include high blood pressure; hemorrhaging due to sudden vessel blockage by a blood clot, fat globule, or cholesterol plaque; and chronic kidney failure.

If a sudden hemorrhage is triggered, total blindness in the eye can strike swiftly; immediate medical attention is necessary. In cases of retinopathy due to high blood pressure or diabetes, vision usually worsens over time.

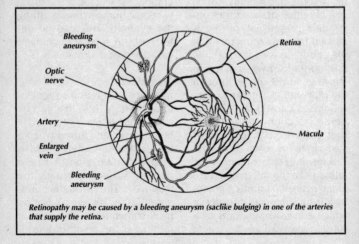

Retinopathy may be caused by a bleeding aneurysm (saclike bulging) in one of the arteries that supply the retina.

Treatment

Hypertensive retinopathy is primarily treated by strict control of the blood pressure through diet and, in many cases, medication. Diabetic retinopathy is also treated through diet and medication; if people with diabetes continually allow their glucose levels to exceed normal bounds, retinal damage can be extensive and may require laser treatments to seal off leaking blood vessels.

Sty

A sty is an inflamed or infected swelling of the sebaceous (oil-producing) glands in the eyelid.

Causes

The infection is commonly caused by *Staphylococcus* bacteria. An external sty appears on the surface of the skin at the edge of the eyelid. An internal sty is on the inner surface of the eyelid. This type of sty appears as a protrusion or lump on the eyelid without visible pus or redness.

Symptoms

Initially, a sty feels like a foreign object in the eye. Tearing, redness, swelling, and tenderness in or around a particular area of the eye soon follow. In addition, pustules (small, yellow bumps filled with pus) may develop. These pustules often burst, release the pus, and begin to heal. Once the pressure has been released, the pain usually subsides.

Treatment

Treatment for a sty often involves antibiotic eyedrops or ointments. Applying warm, moist compresses to the eye for about ten minutes three or four times a day may encourage the sty to burst. In some cases, surgical opening may be needed to cure the condition. One should never attempt to open or squeeze a sty on his or her own, as the risks of spreading and worsening the infection are quite high.

EARS, NOSE, AND THROAT

The ear, nose, and throat are interconnected. Because they are joined, infection in one structure often spreads into one of the others.

Ear
The ear consists of three parts: the outer ear, the middle ear, and the inner ear.

The outer ear consists of both the pinna, or external ear, which captures sound waves and directs them inward, and the ear canal, which leads to the eardrum. In the middle ear, sound waves vibrate through three tiny bones commonly called the hammer (malleus), the anvil (incus), and the stirrup

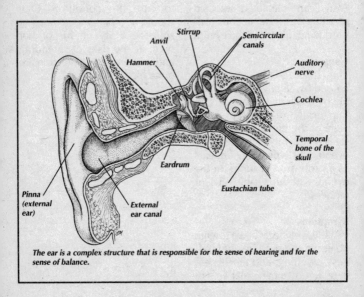

The ear is a complex structure that is responsible for the sense of hearing and for the sense of balance.

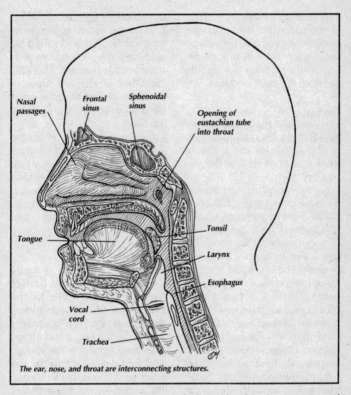

Nasal passages

Frontal sinus

Sphenoidal sinus

Opening of eustachian tube into throat

Tongue

Tonsil

Larynx

Esophagus

Vocal cord

Trachea

The ear, nose, and throat are interconnecting structures.

(stapes). The vibrations continue into the inner ear, where a spiral structure called the cochlea transforms them into nerve impulses. These impulses are conveyed to the brain via the auditory nerve.

The semicircular canals (also called the *labyrinth*) within the inner ear serve as the organ of balance by detecting motion of the head and conveying this information to the brain.

The eustachian tube in the middle ear connects the ear with the nasopharynx (the upper part of the throat). This tube allows the air pressure in the middle ear to equalize with the pressure outside the body,

209

thus helping to prevent rupture of the eardrum. However, the eustachian tube also provides a passageway for infecting microorganisms to enter the middle ear from the nose or throat.

Nose

The nose is a specialized structure that serves dual functions as the organ for the sense of smell and as an entry to the respiratory tract.

Nerve receptor cells within the nose detect odors that enter via the nostrils and transmit signals to the brain through the olfactory nerve. The sense of smell also enhances the sense of taste. The ability to smell is more refined than the ability to taste; therefore, when a cold blocks nasal passages, food may seem bland and tasteless.

As part of the respiratory tract, the nose moisturizes and warms incoming air and filters out foreign materials. Small glands within the lining of the nose secrete mucus, a sticky substance that lubricates the walls of the nose and throat. Mucus humidifies the incoming air and traps bacteria, dust, and other particles entering the nose. Many bacteria are either dissolved by chemical elements in the mucus or transported to the entrance of the throat by tiny, hairlike structures called *cilia*. In the throat, bacteria are then swallowed and killed by acids and other chemicals produced in the stomach. This efficient line of defense protects the body against the billions of bacteria that continually enter the nose.

Connected to the nose are the sinuses—air-filled cavities lined with mucus-secreting glands that are located within certain facial bones. There are four groups of sinuses—frontal, sphenoidal, ethmoidal, and maxillary.

Throat

The throat, or pharynx, is a passageway connecting the back of the mouth and nose to the esophagus (the tube between the mouth and the stomach) and to the trachea, or windpipe (the tube between the mouth and the lungs). Because air and food pass through the throat, the throat is considered part of both the respiratory and the digestive systems.

Three sections make up the five-inch throat tube. The nasopharynx is the upper part of the throat, which opens into the nose. The oropharynx is the middle portion, which opens into the mouth. The lower section of the throat, or laryngopharynx, connects the other sections with the larynx, or voice box.

Within the throat are two small, almond-shaped masses of lymphoid tissue called *tonsils*. Tonsils help fight disease by destroying bacteria that enter the throat.

Adenoids

Adenoids are masses of protective lymphoid tissue located in the lining of the nasopharynx. Like the tonsils located below them, the adenoids (technically known as the *nasopharyngeal tonsils*) are lymph nodes containing the specialized white blood cells that help localize and destroy harmful bacteria and viruses. The adenoids provide an important defense against diseases of the respiratory system.

Enlarged adenoids
It is normal for adenoids to become enlarged during throat infections, just as the tonsils do, and then to diminish in size after the infection has passed. Sometimes, however, as a result of continuing infection or allergies, the adenoids remain enlarged. The resulting obstruction of the nasal passage may cause

mouth breathing, the characteristic "nasal" voice, and continuing drainage of pus-filled mucus down the throat. It may also cause a blockage of the eustachian tubes, which connect the throat to the ears, resulting in retention of fluid in the middle ear, impaired hearing, earache, and recurring ear infections.

Treatment
Antibiotics are used to treat infection of the adenoids. Surgery may be recommended when the infected or enlarged adenoids themselves are the source of the disease (usually the tonsils beneath are infected as well and are removed in the same operation). This would be the case if recurrent or continuing infection of the adenoids could not be eliminated with antibiotics, if the adenoids caused repeated ear infections, or if cancer or an abscess (a mass of pus in a cavity) was present.

Surgical removal of the adenoids may also be recommended if chronically infected adenoids increase susceptibility to a serious condition, such as rheumatic fever or nephritis (a kidney disease). Surgery is generally not performed during an acute attack of tonsillitis, however, because it actually may

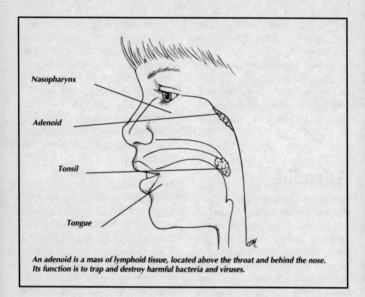

Nasopharynx

Adenoid

Tonsil

Tongue

An adenoid is a mass of lymphoid tissue, located above the throat and behind the nose. Its function is to trap and destroy harmful bacteria and viruses.

worsen the infection. Surgery is also not recommended to prevent snoring, mouth breathing, or the nasal voice caused by enlarged adenoids because the enlargement usually diminishes after childhood.

Prevention

Adenoid infection and enlargement cannot always be prevented. In fact, enlarging in order to trap and fight infectious organisms is a normal function of the adenoids. Good general health measures can help, however, as can the use of antibi-

otics prescribed by a physician when the adenoids become infected and enlarged.

Common cold

A simple common cold is a collection of familiar symptoms signaling an infection of the upper respiratory tract, which includes the nose, throat, and sinuses.

Colds are self-limiting diseases, meaning that their symptoms last a certain length of time (or "run their course") and then disappear without leaving lasting ill effects. A cold is a mild but commonplace disease, contracted by adults about two to four times a year and by children about six to eight times a year. Adults with children at home are more likely to catch colds than are those who do not have children. Children are especially susceptible to colds because they have not yet developed immunity or resistance to the many viruses that can cause colds. Small children gradually build up immunity to the viruses in their homes, but when they go to school and have close contact with many other children, they are exposed to new viruses. Similarly, adults who travel frequently or have a high number of close contacts outside their community are more likely to contract colds or encounter new cold viruses.

Complications

A cold can be a minor irritation, but it can increase susceptibility to more serious conditions, especially in the very young, the very old, and the very weak. Pneumonia, an inflammation of the lungs, is probably the most serious condition. Ear infections, sinus infections, and bronchitis are other possible complications. A few days after a cold, children sometimes develop croup, which is recognized by a harsh, barking cough that signals swelling of the airways to the lungs.

Causes

At least five major categories of viruses cause colds. One of these groups, the rhinoviruses, includes a minimum of 100 different types of viruses. Various combinations of symptoms and possible complications can develop from each of these viruses. It is not known exactly how viruses spread, but it seems to be a combination of physical contact and the presence of both virus particles and moisture in the air. A virus can be spread by hand-to-hand contact, for example, or by the passage of droplets from an infected person's nasal passages and throat into the air. Colds have an incubation period of 48 to 72 hours, meaning that it takes that long after the virus enters the body for early symptoms to appear.

Symptoms

Early symptoms of the common cold include a stuffy or runny nose, sneezing, a sore or scratchy throat, a cough, and occasionally a mild fever. Usually, as the cold progresses, other symptoms—burning or watery eyes, loss of the senses of taste or smell, pressure in the ears or sinuses, nasal voice, and tenderness around the nose—may also appear.

Symptoms vary in type and severity from one viral infection to another, so a cold can begin with any symptom or combination of symptoms. Most colds last about a week, but about 25 percent of all colds last two weeks. Smokers and those with chronic respiratory diseases tend to have more severe symptoms and longer-lasting colds. They also experience complications more readily than do those who do not fall into these categories.

Diagnosis
Since common colds are mild diseases, the physician, in diagnosing a cold, will actually be looking for symptoms indicating a condition more serious than a common cold. Material from the patient's throat or nasal passages may be tested for bacterial infections. A blood test may be recommended to check for mononucleosis, a disease characterized by a long-lasting sore throat and swollen lymph nodes. An X-ray examination of the sinuses may be necessary if sinusitis (an infection of the sinuses) is suspected.

Treatment
Getting plenty of rest, drinking lots of fluids to prevent dehydration, and using a humidifier or vaporizer can help relieve the irritating symptoms of a cold. Nevertheless, the common cold cannot be cured, and no known treatment will actually hasten recovery. Many over-the-counter (nonprescription) medicines and preparations are available that will at least ease the discomfort of a cold. However, it is best to take specific medications only for the symptoms actually present and to follow directions on the medication package carefully. Overuse of an otherwise effective remedy can backfire and actually make the symptoms worse, and treating symptoms that are not there can complicate matters. For example, the use of a nasal decongestant for more than three days can actually increase congestion, because the blood vessels tire and relax, causing rebound congestion. Anyone who is pregnant or has a chronic disease should check with a doctor before using cold preparations, even seemingly harmless over-the-counter drugs.

Prevention

There is no known preventive for the common cold. Vitamin C has been said to help prevent colds, but many studies have shown that it has no measurable effect in this regard. Avoiding exposure to viruses, when possible, may be the only means of avoiding the common cold.

Deafness

Deafness is a term used to describe complete or partial loss or absence of the ability to hear.

Types

There are three major types of deafness:

Conductive deafness is caused by a defect in the outer or middle ear, which prevents normal transmission of sound. It may be present at birth as the result of an inherited defect, an abnormality in development, or an infection of the fetus in the womb. It may also be produced by an injury that perforates the eardrum or that breaks up the linkage of the three tiny bones—the hammer, the anvil, and the stirrup—that normally transmit sound from the eardrum through the middle ear to the inner ear. Inflammation of the middle ear, a condition known as *otitis media,* is another important cause of conductive deafness. Infection from an upper respiratory tract ailment, such as strep throat or the flu, can produce a buildup of pus in the middle ear so great that it ruptures the eardrum. Also, a plugged eustachian tube (the tube leading from the back of the throat to the ear) may trap fluid in the middle ear, creating temporary deafness. Conductive deafness in the middle and later years is most often caused by otosclerosis. In this inherited condition, new spongy bone grows over the stirrup bone, preventing it from vibrating when sound travels to it through the hammer and anvil bones.

Sensorineural deafness is a type of hearing loss that occurs because of damage to the structures of the inner ear, to the auditory nerve carrying sound messages to the brain, or to the hearing center of the brain itself. It can be caused by a head injury during birth, the effects of a rubella infection on the developing fetus, a skull fracture affecting the inner ear or the auditory nerve, fever, bacterial or viral infections (such as mumps or meningitis), syphilis, Ménière disease, tumors, multi-

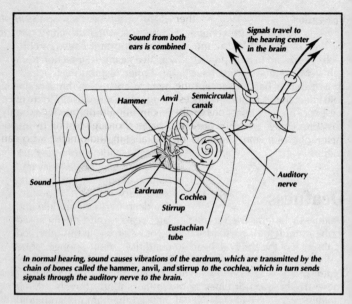

Sound from both ears is combined

Signals travel to the hearing center in the brain

Hammer   Anvil   Semicircular canals

Sound

Eardrum   Cochlea

Stirrup

Auditory nerve

Eustachian tube

In normal hearing, sound causes vibrations of the eardrum, which are transmitted by the chain of bones called the hammer, anvil, and stirrup to the cochlea, which in turn sends signals through the auditory nerve to the brain.

ple sclerosis, a hemorrhage or blood clot in the inner ear, drug side effects, normal aging, prolonged or repeated exposure to intense noise, or edema (fluid buildup) caused by a thyroid deficiency. Most sensorineural deafness is not nerve deafness. It is usually sensory deafness, caused by defects in the structure of the inner ear, especially in the fluid-filled cochlea. The cochlea contains sensory cells that convert sound waves into electrical impulses, which can then be transmitted via the auditory nerve to the brain.

Mixed deafness is a relatively common form of deafness. It is a combination of conductive and sensorineural deafness.

People with pure conductive deafness simply need louder volume to hear all sounds. Those with defects in the inner ear usually can hear low-pitched sounds more easily than high-pitched sounds, and some sounds may be distorted. When there is damage to the hearing center in the brain, the person may be able to hear sounds but has trouble recognizing them and understanding words. (This can also occur with the other types of deafness.)

Diagnosis

When hearing loss is suspected, a complete examination of the ears, nose, and throat is necessary to identify infections or abnormalities that may be present. Infections of the adenoids or tonsils, as well as sinus or nasal infections, may be linked to ear infections.

Testing of hearing is important for all ages, but especially for infants. Many times, partial deafness in a baby is not discovered until the child fails to learn to talk, a direct result of the hearing loss. Babies who were born prematurely or ill or whose mothers had certain viral infections, such as rubella, during pregnancy are in special need of testing.

Treatment

Although inborn hearing defects usually cannot be corrected, deaf children can be helped to deal with their handicap. Starting very early, they can be fitted with hearing aids and can be instructed in lipreading, speaking, and sign language.

Surgery to correct conductive hearing loss includes operations to replace the stirrup bone or all three tiny bones with tissue or synthetic material, to repair a punctured eardrum, and to clean a chronically infected middle ear.

A hearing aid can often help to restore hearing. However, one should be purchased only after thorough testing by a specialist in audiometry, who can suggest the most appropriate type. Classes in lipreading can also be helpful.

Prevention

It is far easier to prevent deafness than to cure it. Antibiotics have made it possible to eradicate most of the middle ear infections that have been the major source of conductive hearing loss in children. Middle ear problems are sometimes eliminated by treating allergies that cause the eustachian tubes to close up or by removing infected adenoids. Nerve deafness caused by continued exposure to intense industrial noise, gunshots, rock music, or aircraft engines can be avoided by wearing earplugs or other ear protectors. (Some lost hearing returns after several months of relief from intense sound.) Drugs that can cause hearing loss, including some antibiotics and certain diuretics (drugs that stimulate production of urine),

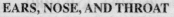

need to be used with care, and signs of hearing loss should be brought to a doctor's attention.

Glossitis

Glossitis is an acute (short-term) or chronic (long-term) inflammation of the tongue. The condition may exist either as a primary disease or as a symptom of another disorder.

Causes
The causes of glossitis can be either local or systemic (affecting the entire body). Local causes include immediate irritants, such as jagged or broken teeth, badly fitting dentures, poor oral hygiene habits, biting of the tongue (such as during convulsions), and external irritants, such as alcohol, tobacco, hot or spicy foods, and even mouthwashes, toothpastes, and breath fresheners. Local infections, burns, and injuries may also produce symptoms of glossitis. Systemic causes may include certain vitamin deficiencies, anemia, syphilis, and generalized skin diseases.

Symptoms
Symptoms vary widely, ranging from simple redness of the tip and edges of the tongue (if the cause is pellagra, anemia, or irritation from smoking or a tooth with a rough surface) to painful ulcers and whitish patches. In the later stages of pellagra, the entire tongue may be fiery red, swollen, and ulcerated. In iron-deficiency and pernicious anemia, the tongue is pale and smooth. Painful ulcers on the tongue may indicate a number of diseases, including herpes, tuberculosis, and streptococcal infection. White patches suggest candidiasis (a type of yeast infection), syphilis, or mouth breathing (which dries out the mucous membrane of the tongue). Very smooth and painless areas may be what is called *geographic tongue,* or benign (harmless) glossitis. Hairy tongue often follows antibiotic therapy, a high fever, excessive use of certain mouthwashes, or a simple reduction in saliva secretion.

Severe acute glossitis, which can result from local infection, burns, and injury, can cause tenderness, pain, and swelling sufficient to make the tongue protrude from the mouth into the back of the throat—creating the danger of airway obstruction and even suffocation. In severe cases, the patient may not be able to chew, swallow, or speak. Steroid drug treatment usually reduces the swelling and helps relieve symptoms.

Patients may also complain of a painful burning tongue without other symptoms of inflammation. This complaint is common among postmenopausal women. Diabetes, anemia, nutritional deficiencies, and malignant conditions should all be considered as possible primary causes.

Treatment

The patient should be reassured that redness and most lesions of the tongue are usually harmless and respond well to treatment. Ulcers and hairy tongue often recur periodically; however, if an ulcer does not respond to treatment after several weeks, a biopsy (removal of a tissue sample for examination under a microscope) may be performed.

In treating glossitis, specific causes, such as jagged teeth and ill-fitting dentures, should be corrected. Irritants, including hot or spicy foods, tobacco, alcohol, mouthwashes, and toothpastes, should be avoided if they have been identified as the source of glossitis. A bland or liquid diet, preferably cool or cold, will often have a soothing effect.

Tiny brown growths on the tongue are usually caused by contact with tobacco or certain bacteria; the treatment is to stop smoking or otherwise correct the underlying cause and also to brush the tongue with a toothbrush.

Symptomatic relief for large lesions includes rinsing the mouth with a medicated mouthwash before meals. Application of topical anesthetics, such as lidocaine and benzocaine, can also bring relief. Patients should be tested to rule out vitamin B_{12} deficiency, diabetes, and anemia.

Prevention

Prevention of glossitis involves avoiding irritants, correcting nutritional and vitamin deficiencies, treating primary infections that produce glossitis, and practicing good oral hygiene.

Laryngitis

Laryngitis is an inflammation of the mucous membrane lining the larynx (voice box), which is located in the upper part of the respiratory tract. It causes hoarseness and possibly a temporary loss of speech.

Causes

Laryngitis may result from a bacterial or viral infection, such as a cold or the flu; from an irritation of the mucous membrane of the larynx, such as that caused by smoking; or from overuse of the voice.

Chronic or persistent laryngitis is most often caused by smoking, air pollution, or dust. It may also stem from tonsillitis, tuberculosis, the early stages of some forms of cancer, or paralysis of the vocal cords. Because laryngitis may be a symptom of a more serious condition, persons who consistently suffer from it should consult their physician.

Symptoms
Hoarseness, loss of the voice, dryness and scratchiness of the throat, coughing, and pain on speaking are common symptoms for laryngitis.

Treatment
Laryngitis is best treated by completely resting the vocal cords. The pain of laryngitis may be eased with throat sprays, steam inhalations, and mild pain relievers, such as aspirin and acetaminophen.

Mastoiditis

Mastoiditis is a bacterial infection of the mastoid air cells (small, air-filled cavities located in the mastoid process, which is the bulge in the skull behind

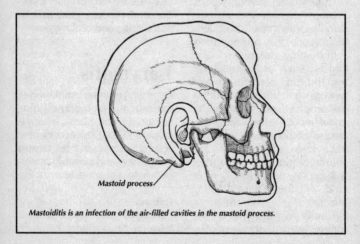

Mastoid process

Mastoiditis is an infection of the air-filled cavities in the mastoid process.

the ear). Mastoiditis is most often a complication of a middle ear infection.

Symptoms

Mastoiditis is characterized by ringing in the ear, a discharge of pus from the ear canal, and fever. Other indications of mastoiditis include swelling and tenderness over the mastoid process.

Complications

In severe cases, an abscess may develop in the mastoid process. This is a serious complication, because it carries the risk that infection will spread to the interior of the skull and cause meningitis.

Treatment

Because antibiotics are so effective against ear infections and mastoid infections, mastoiditis is now a rare condition. Sometimes, however, surgery is required to remove the infected cells if antibiotic treatment is started too late or if the treatment is not effective.

Ménière disease

Ménière disease is a disease of the inner ear that affects balance and equilibrium.

Causes

The cause of Ménière disease is unknown, although it is thought that pressure changes in the ear may be brought on by an infection, a small hemorrhage in the ear, or an allergic response. Ménière disease occurs most commonly in men and women aged 40 to 60.

Symptoms

The symptoms of Ménière disease include recurring and violent attacks of vertigo or dizziness, ringing in the ears, muffling or distortion of noises, and nausea that is sometimes accompanied by vomiting. Deafness in one or both ears may eventually develop.

Mild attacks of Ménière disease can last from a half hour to several days before fading away naturally. They may recur regularly at intervals of weeks, months, or years.

Severe attacks of Ménière disease may last for several weeks, requiring the person to be confined to bed. In such cases, almost any movement of the head will result in bizarre and disturbing sensations that the floor and the furniture in the room are spinning around. Severe cases may also be accompanied by anxiety attacks and migraine headaches.

Treatment

The use of certain drugs, such as diuretics and antihistamines, may help to relieve severe and recurrent attacks. In severe cases, surgery may be necessary to treat the condition.

Middle ear infections

The ear can become infected in any one of its three parts—the inner ear, the middle ear, or the outer ear. However, ear infections most commonly settle in the middle ear. The medical term for middle ear infection is otitis media.

Ear infections are much more likely to affect children than adults; children are most susceptible between the ages of six months and six years. Children who contract ear infections in their first year are more likely to have chronic (long-term) ear infections later in life. By the age of eight, almost every child has had at least one ear infection.

Causes

Middle ear infections develop when viruses or bacteria in the nose or throat travel to the ear through the eustachian tube, which connects the middle ear to the nose and throat. The middle ear also can become infected when infection spreads from a severe outer ear infection or injury.

Symptoms

Middle ear infections can be recognized by severe throbbing pain in the ear, fever as high as 105°F (102°F in adults), hearing loss, and dizziness, nausea, vomiting, or sore throat. The eardrum may bulge out or may even burst, oozing blood and pus into the outer ear. Symptoms may worsen over a period of hours or days. A child too young to talk may seem ill or feverish or may pull on an ear as an indication of discomfort.

Diagnosis

Ear infections are diagnosed by an inspection of the eardrum. If it is red and swollen or bulging, middle ear infection can usually be confirmed.

Treatment

Middle ear infections are usually quickly eliminated by treatment with an antibiotic, often a form of penicillin. Decongestants may also be used. If a viral infection is present, however, antibiotics are not used, because viruses do not respond to antibiotics. If the eardrum is

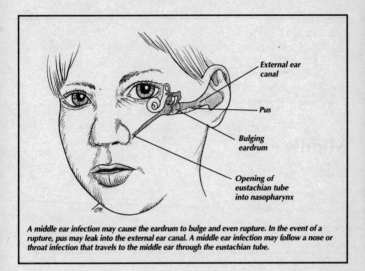

A middle ear infection may cause the eardrum to bulge and even rupture. In the event of a rupture, pus may leak into the external ear canal. A middle ear infection may follow a nose or throat infection that travels to the middle ear through the eustachian tube.

bulging and the pain is severe, the doctor may make a small cut in the eardrum (called a *myringotomy*) to relieve the pressure. If the eardrum bursts, the outer ear must be kept clean to prevent infection from spreading.

The development of more effective antibiotics has lessened the need for surgery. In rare cases, however, the infected tissue may have to be surgically removed.

Middle ear infections usually clear up quickly, but the more severe or persistent infections can lead to a variety of serious complications, including temporary or permanent hearing loss, infection of the semicircular canals in the inner ear, facial paralysis, brain abscess, meningitis (inflammation of the membranes covering the brain and spinal cord), and infection of the mastoid process (the bulge in the skull behind the ear).

Nosebleeds

A nosebleed occurs when there is a break in the blood vessels in the inner lining of the nose. Nosebleeds seldom require medical attention, but it is possible, although relatively rare,

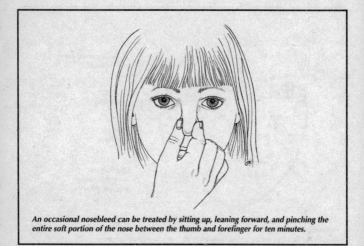

An occasional nosebleed can be treated by sitting up, leaning forward, and pinching the entire soft portion of the nose between the thumb and forefinger for ten minutes.

for nosebleeds to be a symptom of serious illness.

Causes

Nosebleeds can be caused by an injury to the nose, breathing dry air for prolonged periods, repeated blowing or picking of the nose, tumors in the nose, high blood pressure, and certain blood diseases.

Treatment

Very persistent or frequently recurring nosebleeds will require the attention of a doctor, who may cauterize (use heat or the chemical silver nitrate to seal off) the blood vessels in the back of the nose.

However, occasional nosebleeds can be treated simply by sitting up and leaning forward, so as not to swallow the blood, and pinching the entire soft portion of the nose between the thumb and forefinger for ten minutes. If the bleeding does not stop, cold packs can be applied to the bridge of the nose for 15 to 20 minutes. If bleeding still persists, a doctor should be notified.

Frequent nosebleeds from breathing dry air may be relieved by the use of a humidifier. Also, those who have frequent nosebleeds should not blow the nose too harshly nor blow through only one nostril.

When nosebleeds occur along with colds or other respiratory infections, a nasal decongestant may help to temporarily shrink the blood vessels in the nose. However, these decongestants should not be used by anyone with high blood pressure, heart disease, diabetes, or thyroid disorders, because decongestants also shrink blood vessels in parts of the body other than the nose, which can lead to complications for these patients.

Otosclerosis

Otosclerosis is a condition in which an abnormal spongy overgrowth of bone in the middle ear leads to totally or partially muffled hearing or deafness. The excess bone grows at the entrance to the middle ear, where it immobilizes the base of the stirrup, or stapes (one of the three tiny, interconnected bones that transmit sound waves to the inner ear). As a result, sound-conducting vibrations are diminished, and hearing is impaired. In most cases, both ears are eventually affected by otosclerosis. The cause of otosclerosis is unknown, but the condition tends to be hereditary.

Symptoms

Hearing loss generally begins in the late teens or early 20s; the rate of deafness may accelerate and stabilize several times, but ordinarily the loss is complete within 10 to 15 years of onset— sooner if the disease begins in childhood. In some cases, the hearing loss stops just short of deafness, and the affected person can still hear loud sounds. Otosclerosis usually affects one ear before the other and is preceded by tinnitus (ringing in the ear).

Treatment

The only way to halt or reverse otosclerosis is surgery, which is successful about 70 percent of the time. (Although a hearing aid can help, most doctors prefer to operate.) In a procedure called a *stapedectomy,* a surgeon folds back the eardrum, removes the affected stirrup, and replaces it with a synthetic or wire substitute that restores the conductive vibrations of the middle ear. Because the bones involved are the tiniest in the body, the surgery is very delicate and entails a risk of failure. In most cases, the operation is done on only one ear at a time.

After surgery, the hearing of most patients is greatly improved within two to three weeks. In some cases, a residual blood clot at the site of the surgery temporarily blocks hearing until it dissolves. Patients with advanced otosclerosis in both ears are usually advised to undergo stapedectomy as soon as possible.

Sinusitis

Sinusitis is an infection (usually bacterial) of one or more of the sinuses. In general, it occurs more commonly in adults than in children.

The sinuses are air-filled cavities located within the facial bone structure and connected to the nose. There are four major groups of sinuses: frontal, ethmoidal, sphenoidal, and maxillary.

The sinuses are lined with a mucous membrane and are normally kept clear when mucus drains through them into the nasal passages. If they are obstructed, normal drainage cannot occur, and infection can result.

Complications
It is rare but possible for long-lasting sinusitis to lead to more serious disorders. A persistent infection can travel to the brain, causing meningitis (inflammation of the membranes covering the brain and spinal cord), or to the bone, resulting in osteomyelitis (inflammation of a bone).

Causes
A sinus infection may be triggered by anything that prevents the mucus in the sinuses from draining properly into the nasal passages. Possible causes include swimming and diving, injuries, abnormal structure of the facial bones, allergies, or an abscess (inflamed pocket of pus) in a tooth, which may penetrate the sinuses and allow bacteria to enter them. Many different types of bacteria can also cause sinusitis, including some of the same strains that lead to pneumonia, laryngitis, and middle ear infections.

Symptoms
Sinusitis is characterized by pain and tenderness above the infected sinus, which is felt in the face and forehead, behind the eyes, in the eyes, near the upper part of the nose, and even in the upper teeth. This facial pain may be accompanied by headache, slight fever, chills, sore throat, and a discharge of pus from the nose.

Sinusitis usually lasts about two weeks, with the pain often

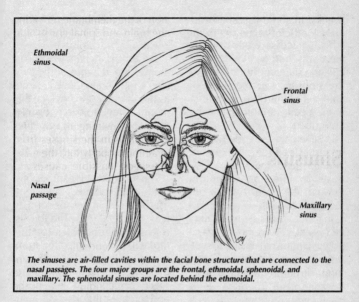

Ethmoidal sinus

Frontal sinus

Nasal passage

Maxillary sinus

The sinuses are air-filled cavities within the facial bone structure that are connected to the nasal passages. The four major groups are the frontal, ethmoidal, sphenoidal, and maxillary. The sphenoidal sinuses are located behind the ethmoidal.

subsiding in the morning and worsening as the day goes on. The pain tends to fluctuate as the patient moves about and changes positions, especially when bending forward from the waist.

Diagnosis

The sinuses cannot be seen directly by a doctor, so diagnostic evaluation may include an X-ray examination to check for the presence of fluid or abnormalities in the sinuses and to determine which of the sinuses are infected. Computed tomography is an excellent tool for evaluating serious sinus problems.

Treatment

Sinusitis is treated by encouraging drainage of the sinuses. Nasal decongestants and moist heat work to aid sinus drainage. The doctor will usually prescribe an antibiotic that will kill the bacteria that most commonly trigger sinusitis.

If these treatments bring no relief, the doctor may perform a sinus puncture to determine exactly which bacteria are present. In this procedure, a needle

227

is inserted into the sinus, and a sample of the fluid is removed. (This is necessary because the nasal discharge may contain bacteria different from those in the sinuses.) On the basis of analysis of the fluid sample, a more specific antibiotic may be prescribed.

In severe cases, codeine may be prescribed to dull the pain, and the doctor may clear the sinuses by injecting a solution through the nose to flush out the sinus cavities.

In some cases, surgery may be necessary to remove a nasal polyp (a mass of swollen tissue), repair abnormal bone structures, or remove infected sinus tissue.

Prevention
There is some evidence that smokers are more likely to suffer from sinusitis than are nonsmokers. Those who frequently have colds are also more susceptible to sinusitis. Avoiding smoking and exposure to persons with colds may help to prevent sinusitis.

Tonsillitis

Tonsillitis is an inflammation or infection of the tonsils. It occurs most commonly in children from 5 to 15 years old and only rarely in those under the age of 2 years.

The tonsils are two small, almond-shaped lumps of specialized lymph node tissue located in the throat at the back of the mouth. They are barely visible in infants, increase in size during the preschool and early school years, and shrink by adulthood.

The function of the tonsils has not been pinpointed, but scientists believe that they perform at least two vital jobs. The tonsils release antibodies into the throat to prevent infection from spreading into the lungs (a useful service to children, who are highly susceptible to ear, nose, and throat infections).

The tonsils also attract bacterial infection, thereby stimulating the production of antibodies, which accumulate in the body and are then available to prevent future, and potentially much more serious, infections. (Antibodies normally do not develop unless infection is present.) If the tonsils do indeed perform these two functions, then each attack of tonsillitis may help immunize a child against disease; once resistance has been developed, the function of the tonsils is complete.

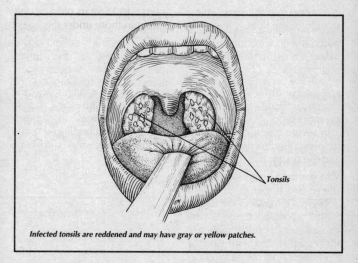

Infected tonsils are reddened and may have gray or yellow patches.

There are two types of tonsillitis: acute tonsillitis, in which the infection flares up and then disappears in a short time; and chronic tonsillitis, in which the tonsils seem to be permanently inflamed and have abscesses (pus-filled cavities) on them.

Causes

Tonsillitis is caused by many different infectious agents, both viral and bacterial. *Streptococcus* bacteria are the most common bacterial cause; acute tonsillitis is usually a "strep" infection. Chronic tonsillitis, however, is more of a mystery; it is not yet known why chronic tonsillitis occurs.

Symptoms

The symptoms of acute tonsillitis are a sore throat, fever (up to about 101°F), chills, headache, and muscle aches. These symptoms worsen for one to three days and then subside. Nausea, vomiting, stomachache, and swelling of lymph nodes in the neck may also occur.

The symptoms of chronic tonsillitis include a persistent or recurrent sore throat, difficulty in swallowing or breathing, and foul breath.

Diagnosis

Tonsillitis is diagnosed by examination of the tonsils for redness, swelling, and the pres-

229

ence of infectious material. The doctor will take a sample of this material with a cotton swab in order to identify the infectious organism.

Treatment

Bed rest or reduced activity and the use of antibiotics, often penicillin, are recommended to treat tonsillitis if the inflammation is due to bacteria. Gargling with warm salt water can help relieve sore throat.

Surgical removal of the tonsils (called a *tonsillectomy*) is performed only if the tonsils are abscessed (filled with pus) or so enlarged that they are blocking the air passages. Tonsillectomies were commonplace at one time but are seldom performed today because research has found that even when tonsils are enlarged, they almost always shrink over time. Furthermore, removing the tonsils does not necessarily prevent recurrent sore throats and colds, as was once believed.

Complications

Complications resulting from tonsillitis seldom occur today because of effective, fast-acting antibiotics. Complications such as rheumatic fever and infections of the sinuses, ears, and kidneys are rare.

Prevention

Since it is not yet known why some people suffer from chronic tonsillitis, preventive measures have not been established. Because episodes of acute tonsillitis may be useful in developing the body's immunities, prevention of tonsillitis may not be appropriate.

THE LUNGS AND RESPIRATORY SYSTEM

The respiratory system includes the nose, throat, larynx, trachea, bronchi, and lungs. The function of the respiratory system is to supply the blood with necessary oxygen and to relieve it of the waste product carbon dioxide. This exchange of oxygen and carbon dioxide occurs in the lungs. Air from the outside enters through the nose, where it is warmed, moistened, and filtered before it passes through the throat and past the larynx (voice box) into the trachea (windpipe). The trachea divides into two main bronchi (the airways connecting the windpipe and the lungs). Within each lung, the bronchi divide and subdivide, forming progressively smaller passageways called bronchioles. The smallest bronchioles end in small, cup-shaped sacs called alveoli. It is in the alveoli that the exchange of gas takes place. Each alveolus is served by numerous tiny blood vessels called capillaries. Oxygen in the alveolus crosses the thin alveolar and capillary walls to enter the blood, while carbon dioxide passes from the blood through the capillary walls into the alveolus. The oxygen is then carried by the blood to cells throughout the body, and the carbon dioxide is exhaled.

During inhalation and exhalation, the lungs are expanded and contracted by movements of the rib cage and the diaphragm (the large muscle separating the chest and abdominal cavities). During inhalation, the diaphragm contracts. This causes the diaphragm to descend and the chest cavity to expand. At this point, the air pressure inside the chest cavity is less than that of the air outside the body; consequently, air from the outside rushes into the lungs. During exhalation, the diaphragm relaxes and moves upward, reducing the chest capacity and pushing air out of the lungs. The friction caused by expansion and contraction of the lungs is eased by the pleurae (thin, moist membranes that cover the lungs and line

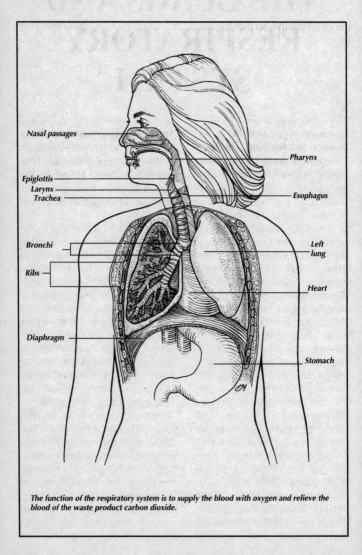

Nasal passages

Epiglottis
Larynx
Trachea

Bronchi

Ribs

Diaphragm

Pharynx

Esophagus

Left
lung

Heart

Stomach

The function of the respiratory system is to supply the blood with oxygen and relieve the blood of the waste product carbon dioxide.

the chest cavity), so that the surfaces of the lungs and chest cavity can move past each other smoothly.

Apnea

Apnea is strictly defined as the absence of breathing. The term is also used to refer to an interruption in breathing that occurs in some infants and during the sleep of some children and adults.

Apnea in infants

The usual cause of apnea in infants is immaturity of the brain centers that regulate breathing. From time to time, the infant suddenly stops breathing completely and turns blue. If the baby is stimulated in some way (for example, by a flick of the finger on the bottom of the foot), he or she will usually start breathing normally at once. Seldom is it necessary to use first-aid measures or a mechanical respirator to restart breathing. However, because a history of apnea is one of the factors that may be associated with sudden infant death syndrome (SIDS), physicians sometimes recommend monitoring high-risk infants with equipment that sounds an alarm if any stoppage of breathing is detected (for more on SIDS, see page 548). In some cases, the tendency toward apnea disappears a few weeks after birth, when the breathing control centers have matured.

Apnea in children and adults

Apnea in children and adults is generally less immediately life-threatening than apnea in infants, but it can be physically exhausting and, in a severe form, can cause cardiovascular and respiratory problems. In some patients, episodes of sleep apnea can cause the concentration of carbon dioxide in the blood to build up to a dangerously high level.

Recognition of the problem generally cannot be made by the patient. A spouse or parent may be the first to notice an abnormal sleep pattern—for example, loud snoring, followed by silence (when the breathing stops), and then a loud choke or gasp as the sleeper partially awakens, clears the air passage, and resumes breathing. Such a pattern may be repeated many times during the night. As a result, people with sleep apnea are likely to be drowsy during the day and irritable due to lack of sleep, with decreased memory and attention span. A definitive diagnosis can be made after observation in a hospital sleep laboratory.

In children and adults, apnea may occur because of a disorder in the breathing control centers in the brain, or it may be a result of physical abnormalities of the chest, neck, and back due to obesity, the presence of a disease, or an inborn structural defect. The most common treatment for adult sleep apnea is a device called continuous positive airway pressure (CPAP). With CPAP, a mask is worn over the nose and mouth; air is forced through the mask to keep the airways open while the individual is sleeping. If apnea is due to an abnormality of the breathing control centers, drugs may be prescribed or stimulation of the diaphragm (the large muscle separating the chest and abdominal cavities, which is instrumental in breathing) with an electronic pacemaker may be tried. Obesity is a common cause of sleep apnea in adults, because the presence of excess tissue can block the airway in certain sleeping positions; the disorder may disappear after weight loss. If a physical abnormality due to disease or a structural defect is the cause, surgical treatment may be necessary; for example,

enlarged tonsils and adenoids that are partially obstructing the upper airway may be removed. In extreme cases, the only solution may be tracheostomy (surgical creation of a hole in the trachea and neck, through which the patient can breathe).

Asthma

Asthma is a respiratory disorder marked by unpredictable periods of acute breathlessness and wheezing. Asthma attacks can last from less than an hour to a week or more and can strike frequently or only every few years. Attacks can occur at any time, even during sleep.

The difficult breathing occurs when the small respiratory tubes called *bronchioles* constrict or become clogged with mucus or when the membranes lining the bronchioles become swollen. When this happens, stale air cannot be fully exhaled but stays trapped in the lungs, so that less fresh air can be inhaled.

Causes
Asthma attacks can result from oversensitivity of the bronchial system to a variety of outside substances or conditions. About half of all attacks are triggered

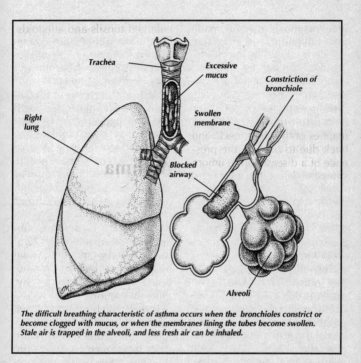

Trachea

Excessive mucus

Constriction of bronchiole

Swollen membrane

Right lung

Blocked airway

Alveoli

The difficult breathing characteristic of asthma occurs when the bronchioles constrict or become clogged with mucus, or when the membranes lining the tubes become swollen. Stale air is trapped in the alveoli, and less fresh air can be inhaled.

by allergies to such substances as dust, smoke, pollen, feathers, pet hair or dander, insects, mold spores, and a variety of foods and drugs. Attacks not related to allergies can be set off by strenuous exercise, breathing cold air, emotional stress, and infections of the respiratory tract. Heredity may play a part in the tendency to develop asthma; if one or both of a child's parents have asthma, the child has up to a 50 percent chance of developing the condition.

Asthma is rarely fatal, but it can be a very serious condition, especially in young children. Attacks often become less frequent and less severe as a child grows older.

Symptoms

Common symptoms of an asthma attack include tightness

in the chest, difficulty in breathing, coughing, and wheezing, which is caused by the effort to push air through the narrowed bronchioles. As the attack progresses, muscles surrounding the bronchioles constrict further, breathing becomes even more difficult, and mucus collects in the airways.

Diagnosis
Diagnostic procedures may include a complete physical examination and medical history, chest X ray, and allergy testing.

Treatment
Asthma, for the most part, cannot be cured, but it can be controlled with a variety of drugs. Corticosteroids can control asthma very effectively, but patients can experience such undesirable side effects as weight gain, ulcers, and high blood pressure. Stunting of growth has been reported in children. Consequently, corticosteroids such as prednisone are usually used in large doses in an acute attack and then are tapered as rapidly as possible. Some individuals, however, need relatively low doses chronically. Frequently, aerosol forms of corticosteroids are used to keep the asthmatic as attack-free as possible. Since there is less absorption of corti-

sone into the body with these forms, the likelihood of side effects is lessened.

Epinephrine or isoproterenol may be given by injection or inhaled as an aerosol during an acute attack in order to enlarge the bronchioles; however, these drugs may overstimulate the heart and so cannot be used for long periods or by many people with heart conditions. Similar drugs, such as metaproterenol, albuterol, and terbutaline, exert much less of a stimulating effect on the heart. These drugs can be taken in an oral tablet form but are more commonly used in their aerosol form, which delivers the greatest effect in the bronchial system itself. They act by dilating or relieving the spasm of the bronchial tubes.

For long-term therapy, the drug theophylline can be used to help keep the bronchioles open. Its dosage, however, must be closely supervised because its rate of absorption into the body varies widely among patients; some people eliminate the drug so quickly that it is almost ineffective, whereas in others, the drug accumulates in the body, at times to toxic levels. Nausea, vomiting, and agitation are common side effects.

Cromolyn, a drug that actually prevents attacks, acts to inhibit the release of histamines (the substances produced by the body during an allergic reaction). Cromolyn, however, cannot relieve an attack already in progress.

If an allergy is causing the attacks, the troublesome substance must be removed from the patient's environment. If the substance cannot be removed or if there are multiple allergies, injections of minute amounts of the allergen may help the body build tolerance to the substance.

Prevention

Although there is no way to prevent asthma, several precautions can be taken to reduce the possibility that asthma attacks will occur. Allergy testing to determine sensitivity to common environmental agents such as dust, mold, pet hair, and pollen can be done by a physician. Once the allergy is determined, desensitization injections can be tried. Rapid treatment of upper respiratory tract infections can help prevent severe attacks. Chronic preventative medication can lessen the frequency and severity of attacks. With proper medical therapy and supervision, most people with asthma can lead normal lives.

Bronchiectasis

Bronchiectasis is a lung condition in which some of the bronchi and bronchioles have lost their elasticity and have expanded and filled with fluid.

Causes

Most often, bronchiectasis follows pneumonia, whooping cough, tuberculosis, or another lung disease. (Fortunately, the use of antibiotics has reduced the number of cases due to lung infection.) Other causes include obstruction; clogging of the airways by the thick, mucous secretions of cystic fibrosis; and Kartagener syndrome, a condition in which the cilia (hairlike projections that line the bronchial walls and wave mucus, pus, and dirt upward) do not work properly.

Symptoms

Bronchiectasis is a chronic condition that persists for life. The individual almost always has some symptoms, which will worsen if an acute infection occurs. The most typical symptom is a chronic cough that produces thick, white or green sputum (discharge). The sputum may be foul-smelling and abundant and may also contain blood. The individual generally

237

coughs up large amounts of sputum after changing position (for example, after rising from bed).

Diagnosis

The doctor, listening to the chest with a stethoscope, can hear abnormal sounds inside the lungs as the patient breathes. Chest X rays or a computed tomography (CT) scan can be used to confirm the diagnosis. Chronic bronchitis must be ruled out as a cause, along with tuberculosis, certain fungal infections, a tumor, and the presence of an inhaled object that is lodged in a bronchi.

Treatment

Treatment of an active case of bronchiectasis includes fighting the infection with an antibiotic, such as penicillin or tetracycline, and eliminating the fluid with postural drainage. In the latter procedure, the patient lies face down in bed, with pillows elevating the hips, and a therapist strikes the back with cupped hands to loosen mucus. The treatment, which can be taught to a family member, requires two to four ten-minute sessions a day. Inhaling warm mists may also help to moisten the thick mucus clogging the airways, so that it can be more easily expelled. The patient

should avoid anything that can irritate the lungs, such as tobacco smoke, fumes, and dust.

In the relatively few cases in which the infection is confined to a small part of the lung and is progressing despite antibiotics and other forms of therapy, it may be best to surgically remove the affected portion of the lung.

Prevention

Progression of the disease can be prevented by being immunized against flu and pneumonia, avoiding contact with anyone with a cold or cough, and stopping smoking. Prompt treatment with antibiotics can help to control new infections.

Bronchitis

Bronchitis is a respiratory illness characterized by inflammation and swelling of the bronchi (the main airways connecting the windpipe and the lungs). When the mucous membranes lining these tubes become inflamed, the mucous glands in the membranes expand and release more mucus. The bronchi, already narrowed by the swelling, become further clogged by the excess mucus. This mucus must then be coughed up to keep the breathing tubes free for normal airflow into the lungs. This illness is characterized by frequent coughing, production of sputum, and shortness of breath.

When the condition is of short duration, it is called *acute bronchitis* and is often accompanied by fever and production of thick, foul-smelling sputum. This condition is difficult to distinguish from pneumonia, and chest X rays are usually needed to establish a diagnosis.

When the symptoms linger for months or years, it is called *chronic bronchitis*. In either case, the coughing stops only when the source of inflammation has been removed or overcome and the inner linings of the bronchi have returned to normal.

Complications

Bronchitis alone is rarely fatal, but it can lead to another condition that proves fatal. For example, the functioning of lungs that have been severely damaged by chronic bronchitis may be so limited that the heart is deprived of adequate oxygen, ultimately resulting in death. Also, bronchitis can be very serious when combined with other respiratory diseases. Such is the case for people who suffer from a category of respiratory conditions called *chronic obstructive pulmonary disease* (*COPD*). Bronchitis, emphysema, and several other diseases are included in this category. Patients may suffer from two or three of the COPD conditions, or one may lead to another.

Causes

Bronchitis occurs when the bronchial tubes are infected or irritated. A cold or the flu may lead to acute or, less often, chronic bronchitis. Chronic bronchitis is more commonly triggered by the constant irritation of environmental substances such as cigarette smoke and occupational dusts.

Cigarette smoking is the predominant cause of chronic bronchitis. Seventy-five percent of all those who suffer from bronchitis are cigarette smokers. When tobacco smoke reaches the bronchial linings, it stops the action of the cilia (the hairlike projections that line the bronchial walls and wave mucus, pus, and dirt upward). When the cilia are stilled by smoke, particles remain trapped in the stagnant mucus, irritating the delicate bronchial tubes and eventually creating a breeding ground for infection.

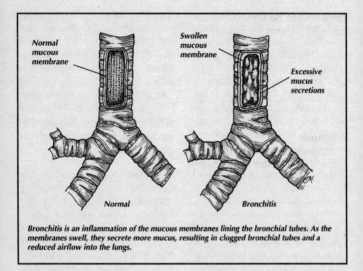

Normal mucous membrane

Swollen mucous membrane

Excessive mucus secretions

Normal

Bronchitis

Bronchitis is an inflammation of the mucous membranes lining the bronchial tubes. As the membranes swell, they secrete more mucus, resulting in clogged bronchial tubes and a reduced airflow into the lungs.

Bronchitis occurs in about 90 percent of all smokers who live in polluted environments or who are exposed to occupational dusts. Babies and young children with chronic bronchitis usually overcome the condition.

Symptoms

Bronchitis can be recognized by its major symptom, the persistent cough in an effort to bring up the excess mucus. Acute bronchitis may be accompanied by hoarseness, chest discomfort, slight fever, wheezing, and shortness of breath. In children, chronic bronchitis may establish itself after several short-term infections. In adults, the beginning of chronic bronchitis is signaled by regular coughing and clearing of the throat the first thing each morning; the coughing will become more persistent and the mucus more plentiful as the disease progresses, and these symptoms may be accompanied by wheezing, shortness of breath, chest infections, and heavy panting after exercise.

As the years pass, chronic bronchitis may cause the bronchial tubes to become severely obstructed and the breathing to be irreversibly impaired. The heart sometimes becomes enlarged because it must pump harder than normal to deliver needed oxygen to the rest of the body. The nails, lips, and skin may develop a blue tinge due to lack of oxygen.

Diagnosis

To diagnose bronchitis, the doctor will obtain the individual's medical history, do a physical examination of the chest with a stethoscope, and perhaps order a chest X ray. Special machines can measure the amount of air flowing in and out of the lungs and can measure how well oxygen is being transported from the lungs to the bloodstream.

Treatment

Bronchitis is treated by removing the irritants from the patient's surroundings, clearing the lungs of mucus, and trying to prevent infections. A patient with chronic bronchitis will need to quit smoking and to avoid exposure to pollutants or hazardous dusts. Humidity plays a large part in treating bronchitis; patients should drink plenty of liquids, and breathe warmed, humidified air from a vaporizer or humidifier. Humidity acts to moisten mucus trapped in the airways,

allowing it to be brought up from the lungs and thereby promoting what is known as a *productive cough*. A bronchodilator drug, which relaxes the walls of the air passages, also may be prescribed. The use of antibiotics to treat bronchitis is somewhat controversial but appears to be helpful, particularly in acute cases.

Prevention

Bronchitis can best be prevented by avoiding the irritants that cause the illness, namely cigarette smoke, air pollutants, and dusts. Patients with chronic bronchitis can prevent further irritation by maintaining good health habits to avoid infections. Other lung disorders may precipitate the condition; therefore, antibiotics may be prescribed to treat bacterial infections, and vaccinations against influenza and pneumonia are strongly recommended in those with chronic bronchitis.

Dyspnea

Dyspnea is a sensation of "air hunger." It is usually accompanied by difficult, labored breathing and discomfort. Dyspnea is a symptom that occurs in a variety of diseases and conditions, ranging from congestive heart failure to emotional upset.

Causes

Dyspnea may be caused by inadequate delivery of oxygen to the tissues, as in severe anemia; by failure of the heart to keep up with the needs of the body, as in congestive heart failure; by overexertion; by obstruction of the airways; by narrowing of air passages, such as occurs in asthma; or by restriction of lung capacity which may be caused by a chest deformity. Emphysema is commonly associated with dyspnea. Dyspnea can also occur if there is fluid in the lungs, as in pneumonia or congestive heart failure, because the entry of oxygen into the alveoli (the tiny air sacs in the lungs, where gas exchange takes place) is blocked by the fluid, thereby preventing oxygenation of the blood.

In a nighttime form of dyspnea called *paroxysmal nocturnal dyspnea,* the patient awakens gasping for breath and can breathe only by sitting up or standing. Usually this type of dyspnea is caused by congestive heart failure.

Another type of dyspnea, called *psychogenic* or *hysterical hyperventilation,* is a physical response to stress, anxiety, or emotional upset. In this condition, excessive breathing results in exhalation of too much carbon dioxide, which causes light-headedness, numbness and tingling of the hands and toes, and fainting.

Symptoms

Signs of dyspnea include noisy breathing; an anxious, distressed expression; dilated nostrils; gasping; a protruding abdomen; an expanded chest; and blue lips and fingertips.

Treatment

Treatment involves controlling whatever condition is causing the dyspnea.

Emphysema

Emphysema is a chronic, progressive lung disease that develops when the small air passages leading to the alveoli (the tiny air sacs in the lungs, where gas exchange takes place) become distended and the walls dividing the alveoli are injured or destroyed. Spaces form where alveoli had been, and lung tissue becomes nonfunctional and stiff rather than elastic. Emphysema is commonly associated with chronic bronchitis, in which the airways

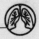
become inflamed, causing specialized cells within them to secrete abnormally large amounts of mucus. The inflammation, swelling, and excessive mucus production result in obstruction of airflow and entrapment of air within the lungs.

Effect on the body

As the disease progresses, many complex changes take place, ultimately leading to diminishment of the amount of oxygen in the blood, frequently associated with an increased amount of carbon dioxide. As the lung tissue deteriorates and loses its elasticity, changes also occur in the blood vessels carrying deoxygenated blood to the lungs for a fresh supply of oxygen. The net effect is that the right side of the heart, which is responsible for collecting deoxygenated blood from the veins of the body and pumping it through the lungs, must work much harder. As the process continues, the muscle of the right side of the heart is weakened by this extra work and becomes less able to pump blood into the lungs. The blood "backs up," causing increased pressure in the veins. This, in turn, causes fluid to recede into the tissues, resulting in severe swelling of the feet, ankles, and legs. If this right-sided heart failure (also known as *cor pulmonale*) is very severe, the abdomen will become distended with fluid.

Causes

External factors that irritate the lungs, such as tobacco smoke and air pollutants, are commonly linked to emphysema. Unlike many respiratory diseases, emphysema is not caused by a viral or bacterial infection. However, it is often aggravated by a case of bronchitis or another lung infection.

In a minority of cases, emphysema is a result of a genetic deficiency or an inherited lack of a specific blood protein, which leads to loss of elasticity in the alveoli.

Those afflicted with emphysema are most likely to be white men over the age of 50, although the number of women who are susceptible has risen dramatically because of an increase in smoking among women during recent years. The overwhelming majority of emphysema cases have been directly linked to cigarette smoking.

Symptoms

Emphysema is characterized by one major symptom—shortness

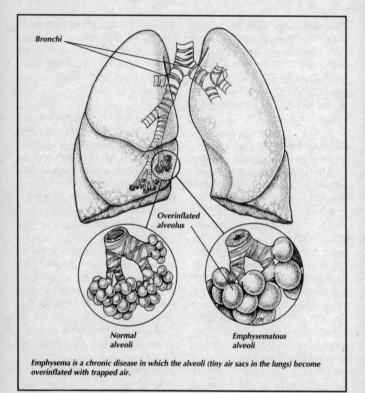

Bronchi

Overinflated
alveolus

Normal
alveoli

Emphysematous
alveoli

Emphysema is a chronic disease in which the alveoli (tiny air sacs in the lungs) become overinflated with trapped air.

of breath. Patients may also have a persistent, racking cough, which either brings up mucus or is overly dry. Patients experience difficulty in breathing, often taking twice as many breaths as others to get enough oxygen. It has been found that advanced emphysema sufferers exert tremendous amounts of energy just to breathe. They also tire quite easily and require more calories to maintain their weight than healthy individuals do. An enlarged, rounded "barrel" chest often develops due to overinflation of the lungs and excessive growth of the chest muscles due to the increased stress placed upon them to inflate stiff lungs. Lips, ear lobes, skin, and fingernails may be tinged blue from lack of oxygen in the blood.

Diagnosis

With the exception of cases caused by genetic disorder, there is no single test that can pinpoint the condition. Breathing tests to measure the amount of air being inhaled and exhaled can reveal the disease in its early stages. A blood test may be performed to determine the red blood cell count (when emphysema causes diminished oxygenation of the blood, more red blood cells are produced in an effort to increase oxygen transport). A chest X ray may be taken to search for specific changes in the lungs that may point to advanced stages of the disease; however, a chest X ray is not diagnostic of early emphysema. Thus, emphysema is diagnosed by putting together a collection of findings.

Treatment

There is no known cure for emphysema, nor is it reversible. However, the progress of the disease can be checked by removing irritants, particularly tobacco smoke, from the patient's environment. Patients are encouraged to drink large amounts of fluids to help thin out the mucus that may block the airways. Adequate rest, a balanced diet, and moderate regular exercise are recommended. Vaporizers, humidifiers, and air conditioners help to moisturize and filter the air. A respiratory therapist can teach an emphysema patient how to use his or her chest and abdominal muscles to breathe more efficiently.

Several drugs aid the emphysema patient. They act to loosen mucus or to relax and expand the air passages. Antibiotics are sometimes prescribed if infection exists. Cortisone drugs (corticosteroids) are sometimes prescribed as well. Drugs such as albuterol and terbutaline are also used both in inhalation aerosol and oral forms.

In advanced cases of emphysema, oxygen may have to be administered continuously. However, an emphysema patient must be particularly careful to use only the amount of oxygen prescribed. Too much oxygen may suppress the drive to breathe, thereby causing respiratory failure. In addition, sedatives and sleeping medications should be avoided by patients with severe emphysema, as these can also lead to a dangerous slowing of breathing.

245

Emphysema is a very serious condition. However, with the help of modern treatments, breathing aids, and medications, patients can lead a reasonably comfortable life. It is, however, necessary for these individuals to stop smoking and avoid air pollutants as much as possible.

Legionnaires disease

Legionnaires disease is a severe bacterial infection of the respiratory tract. The first identifiable outbreak occurred in 1976 in Philadelphia. More than 180 people at the state convention of the American Legion became afflicted with the disease, and 29 of them died. Other outbreaks have since occurred in the United States and Europe. Studies have also shown that outbreaks of respiratory diseases later identified as Legionnaires disease occurred as early as 1947.

Cause
Legionnaires disease is caused by the bacteria *Legionella pneumophila,* which was not identified until the 1976 outbreak. The major environmental source of the infection is water from reservoirs and cooling units of air-conditioning systems. Lakes, creeks, and areas of excavation also may harbor the bacteria. Transmission occurs when one breathes in droplets of contaminated water. Person-to-person transmission has not been documented.

Those at risk
Cigarette smokers, the elderly, and people receiving drugs that depress the immune system are more likely to contract Legionnaires disease than are other people. People who have another medical problem—heart trouble, cancer, respiratory illness, or kidney disease—are also believed to be particularly susceptible.

Symptoms
Legionnaires disease has symptoms similar to those of many other respiratory diseases, making it difficult to differentiate and diagnose. Symptoms include dry coughing, high fever, chills, diarrhea, shortness of breath, chest pains, headaches, excessive sweating, nausea, vomiting, and abdominal pain. Occasionally, bloody sputum is produced. Lethargy and confusion may occur in progressive, serious cases.

Although Legionnaires disease is uncommon, it should be considered in the case of anyone (particularly an elderly or chronically ill person) who has a respiratory tract infection that worsens over a period of about four days. The disease can initially be mild and have the same appearance as an episode of the flu. The diagnosis is made from the individual's medical history and physical examination, chest X rays, and special tests of the blood and sputum that determine the presence and changing numbers of antibodies (protective substances that fight off infection).

Treatment

If an antibiotic (usually erythromycin) is given early in the course of the illness, the outlook for recovery is excellent.

Prevention

There is no preventive vaccine against Legionnaires disease. If an outbreak is suspected, public health officials may search for and attempt to eliminate the source of infection.

Pleurisy

Pleurisy, or pleuritis, is an inflammation of the pleurae (thin, moist membranes that cover the lungs and line the chest cavity). The pleurae normally reduce the friction between the chest structures as the lungs expand and contract. Inflammation of the pleurae causes breathing to become painful and less effective, however.

Types and causes

There are two types of pleurisy: "dry pleurisy" and "wet pleurisy." In dry pleurisy, the more common condition, the inflamed pleurae rub directly against each other. In wet pleurisy, or pleurisy with effusion, fluid oozes from the inflamed tissue into the space between the lungs and the chest wall. This fluid compresses the lungs, making breathing difficult.

Both types of pleurisy often occur as complications of respiratory tract infections, such as pneumonia, viral infections, and tuberculosis, and are more likely to develop in people who are highly susceptible to such infections. They can also be caused by a tumor or an injury. Some cases are due to certain gastrointestinal tract diseases, particularly of the liver and pancreas, which can inflame the diaphragm (the large muscle separating the chest and

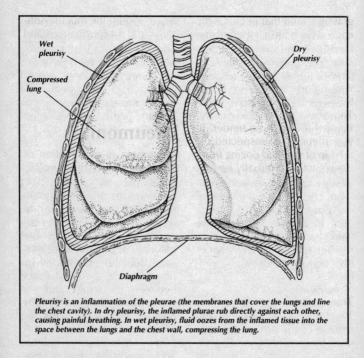

Pleurisy is an inflammation of the pleurae (the membranes that cover the lungs and line the chest cavity). In dry pleurisy, the inflamed plurae rub directly against each other, causing painful breathing. In wet pleurisy, fluid oozes from the inflamed tissue into the space between the lungs and the chest wall, compressing the lung.

abdominal cavities) and the portions of the pleurae that cover it.

Symptoms

The major symptom of dry pleurisy is a sharp, stabbing pain toward the side and lower part of the chest. The pain may also be felt along the shoulders, neck, and abdomen. Any movement involving the chest, such as breathing or coughing, will aggravate the pain, which may be accompanied by shortness of breath, a dry cough, and fever. Wet pleurisy is characterized by similar symptoms, but breathing may also be difficult.

Diagnosis

A diagnosis of pleurisy usually begins with a physical examination, during which the doctor listens to the chest with a stethoscope for the low-pitched grating sound that occurs with each breath in a case of dry pleurisy. If fluid in the lungs is suspected, the physician may percuss, or tap on, the chest wall (usually on the back) to determine the level or amount. The skin near the affected area is often found to be tender. If wet pleurisy is suspected, a sample of the fluid oozing from the pleurae will usually be obtained (by inserting a needle directly into the pleura) and analyzed. A tuberculin skin test may be done to learn whether tuberculosis is a factor. An X-ray study is very helpful in detecting the presence of pleural fluid.

Treatment

To treat pleurisy, the doctor will first need to treat the underlying infection or disease, often with antibiotics. The symptoms of pleurisy can be relieved somewhat by resting. Strapping the chest firmly with a nonadhesive elastic bandage is sometimes recommended; however, it may prevent deep breathing and coughing up of mucus, both of which are necessary to clear the respiratory tract. Painkillers help to relieve chest discomfort at least enough so that the patient will not need to stifle the painful coughing that is neces-

sary to loosen the mucus. Anti-inflammatory medications and even cortisone drugs are very effective in relieving the inflammation and pain, particularly in dry pleurisy.

Pneumonia

Pneumonia is an infection of the lungs in which the alveoli in one or more sections of the lungs become inflamed and filled with fluid and white blood cells, which try to fight off the infection. Pneumonia can be fatal, especially in the very young and the very old.

Types

There are several types of pneumonia, distinguished by the location, causative agent, and extent of infection. Lobar pneumonia is an infection in only one lobe (section) of the lungs. Double pneumonia occurs in all or parts of both lungs. Bronchial pneumonia is an infection in the areas of the lungs near the bronchi (the airways connecting the windpipe and the lungs). Walking pneumonia is an infection that an individual may have for a week or more with no symptoms other than cough. When eventually seen by a physician, the individual is sent for a chest X ray, which shows pneumonia. This type of pneumonia is often caused by the organism *Mycoplasma pneumoniae*. Although often mild, it can be quite serious if left untreated.

Pneumonia most often strikes the individual whose resistance is lowered, frequently by an upper respiratory tract infection or a systemic disease. It is commonly a secondary disease stemming from inadequate defense mechanisms, from a cold or the flu, or from long-term diseases, such as chronic bronchitis, emphysema, asthma, diabetes, cancer, or sickle-cell anemia. In the elderly, pneumonia may be a consequence of being bedridden for long periods of time.

Causes

Viruses, bacteria, fungi, and other microorganisms can cause pneumonia. It may also develop if a person inhales certain chemicals or if food, vomit, or a foreign object passes through the trachea (the windpipe) instead of the esophagus (the passageway from the mouth to the stomach) and settles in a lung (called *aspiration pneumonia*). Smoking, excessive drinking, a prolonged period of being bedridden, anesthesia, and use of sedatives and drugs that suppress the immune system may make an individual more susceptible to pneumonia if he or she is exposed to an infectious organism. Pneumonia is most common during flu and cold epidemics and during the winter months, when people are more likely to be indoors where bacteria and viruses are easily spread.

Symptoms

Pneumonia is generally characterized by four major symptoms: chest pain, a sudden rise in temperature, coughing, and difficulty breathing. Viral pneumonia is signaled by coughing and other cold symptoms and fatigue. Bacterial pneumonia generally comes on suddenly with shaking chills; a rapid, steep rise in temperature; shallow breathing; and a cough that brings up bloody, dark-yellow, or rust-colored sputum. An oxygen shortage that is sometimes a result of fluid and debris blocking small airways in the lungs will be indicated by headache, nausea, vomiting, and bluish discoloration of the lips and fingertips.

Diagnosis

Pneumonia is diagnosed by listening to the chest with a

stethoscope to detect the presence of fluid in the lungs. An analysis of the sputum and an X-ray examination are also done to identify the type and location of the infection.

Treatment
Viral pneumonia is generally treated by bed rest, drinking lots of fluids, maintaining a light diet, and using painkillers to combat discomfort. Hospitalization is not usually necessary. Viral pneumonia, however, can be quite serious and even fatal, particularly in those with underlying diseases affecting the immune system and in premature newborns. Newer antiviral drugs, in both intravenous and aerosol form, have been helpful in select cases.

Bacterial pneumonia is treated with antibiotics, such as penicillin. Patients also need to rest or, in severe cases, to enter the hospital for care, supervision, and intravenous drug therapy. If breathing is difficult, oxygen may be administered.

Prevention
There are vaccines that help prevent some types of pneumonia. Pneumococcal pneumonia caused by certain bacteria may be prevented with a vaccine, which is especially recommended for the elderly or for those with chronic diseases that weaken the respiratory system. Pneumonia caused by one type of influenza virus may also be prevented with a vaccination.

Psittacosis

Psittacosis is a rare form of pneumonia caused by a microorganism *Chlamydia psittaci*, which can be transmitted to humans by certain birds. It is often called *parrot fever,* because it was first found to be transmitted by members of the parrot family, including parakeets and lovebirds. It may also be transmitted by other birds, such as seagulls, pigeons, canaries, and poultry, in which case it is called *ornithosis.*

Causes
Infection usually takes place when a person inhales dust from the feathers or droppings of infected birds. It can also be transmitted directly to a person by a bite from an infected bird. Eating poultry has not been reported as a source of infection.

Symptoms
The incubation period (the time between exposure to the microorganisms and the appear-

251

ance of symptoms), is one to two weeks. The disease usually begins with fever, chills, headache, muscle aches, and loss of appetite. Nausea, vomiting, and enlargement of the spleen may also be present. The patient's temperature continues to rise, and a dry cough develops.

Coughing brings up mucus and pus in the later stages of psittacosis. Chest X rays made during the first week of noticeable symptoms often show inflammation of the lungs. During the second week, the typical symptoms of pneumonia develop. The patient's temperature will remain above normal for at least two weeks and then begin to fall slowly. A steady increase in the pulse and breathing rate may be serious. About 30 percent of untreated cases end in death.

Treatment
The drug most commonly used to treat psittacosis is oral tetracycline, an antibiotic. Complete bed rest is necessary in most cases. Cough preparations with codeine are also advised. In severe cases, tetracycline may be given intravenously.

Prevention
Flocks of infected pigeons or other birds, dust from feathers, birdcage contents, and sick domestic birds or fowl should be avoided. Specially treated feed is often used to prevent the spread of infection among imported birds and among turkeys raised for market.

Pulmonary embolism

Pulmonary embolism is a potentially fatal condition that occurs when an embolus (a clump of matter originating elsewhere in the body and traveling via the blood) blocks a blood vessel in the lungs.

Causes
Emboli (the plural of embolus) may be solid (detached blood clots, clumps of tumor cells, or bits of foreign objects), liquid (globules of fat), or gaseous (air). Pulmonary emboli are venous thrombi (blood clots that form in the veins) that have originated most often in the lower extremities and pelvis, usually as the result of injury, surgery, or blood-vessel diseases. Such thrombi are common in people on prolonged bed rest, particularly after surgery, due to the lack of movement of blood in the legs.

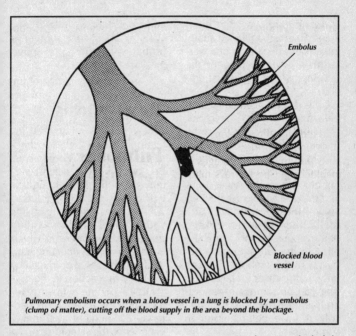

Pulmonary embolism occurs when a blood vessel in a lung is blocked by an embolus (clump of matter), cutting off the blood supply in the area beyond the blockage.

Embolus

Blocked blood vessel

Symptoms
The presence of a pulmonary embolus is indicated by the sudden development of dyspnea (labored or difficult breathing), chest pains, and hemoptysis (spitting up of blood).

Diagnosis
Diagnostic procedures for detection of pulmonary embolism may include an electrocardiogram and analysis of arterial blood obtained from the wrist, arm, or groin. Radioisotope scanning is also very helpful. The definitive diagnostic procedure is pulmonary angiography, which is an X-ray scan of the lungs done after the introduction of a special dye into the pulmonary circulation (via a catheter inserted into the groin and floated up to the right side of the heart).

Treatment
Initial treatment may include administration of oxygen, pain-relievers, and medication to

253

maintain cardiovascular functions. An anticoagulant (usually intravenous heparin or oral warfarin) is given to prevent the development of additional emboli.

If it is determined that the embolism was caused by a venous thrombus, and there is some reason why anticoagulants should not be used, the inferior vena cava (the main vein draining blood from the lower limbs and the pelvis) may be deliberately blocked with an "umbrella filter" or a clip to keep other venous thrombi from traveling to the lungs. Surgical removal of the embolus is done only in rare cases for large clots that can be removed immediately after detection. Clot dissolvers have been helpful in some cases.

Prevention

The best prevention of pulmonary embolism is prevention of venous thrombosis. People predisposed to embolism may be given injections of heparin or low doses of oral warfarin to prevent the formation of thrombi. Recently, "compression boots," soft plastic bags or sacks wrapped around the legs and rapidly inflated and deflated, have been shown to prevent clot formation in postoperative and bedridden individuals. Walking soon after surgery is probably the best preventive measure.

Tuberculosis

Tuberculosis is a bacterial infection caused by *Mycobacterium tuberculosis* organisms. Because the body's defense system has difficulty fighting this type of bacterium, it attempts to wall off invading organisms within small nodules, called *granulomas* or *tubercles,* which contain both the infecting bacteria and the tissue produced by the body in reaction to them.

Of all people who are infected by the tuberculosis bacteria, 80 percent will never experience the symptoms of the disease. Usually, the body is able to surround the offending bacteria with granulomas; the tuberculosis bacteria then lie dormant in the body, and active disease does not develop. However, because the body cannot kill the bacteria, the infection can become active at a later time, often when some other disease has already weakened the body's defenses.

Of the 20 percent of infected people in whom an active case of tuberculosis does develop,

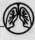

only half will become sick within three months of contracting the infection; the other half will suffer from the disease at some other time in their lives, perhaps years later. Tuberculosis usually affects the lungs, but it can also involve other parts of the body, such as the spine, the kidneys, the digestive tract, and the lining of the heart.

Causes

Tuberculosis is contracted when a person breathes in droplets containing *Mycobacterium tuberculosis* organisms that have been coughed or sneezed into the air by an infected person. Tuberculosis is contagious, especially for people living in crowded conditions. Also highly susceptible to this disease are those who are undernourished, in poor health, or living in poor urban areas, as well as the very young, the very old, and those in the medical professions.

Anyone who has been in close contact with a tuberculosis patient should be tested for the infection.

Symptoms

Early signs include fever, fatigue, loss of appetite, and weight loss. Later signs include coughing up of blood-tinged sputum, chest pain, and shortness of breath.

Diagnosis

The symptoms of tuberculosis are similar to those of many other diseases, and its characteristic symptoms do not appear until the disease is in its advanced stages. For these reasons, coupled with the fact that the incidence of tuberculosis has been declining in recent years in the United States, this disorder often remains untreated or misdiagnosed for some time. Tuberculosis may be accompanied by an infection due to *Streptococcus* bacteria, which often further complicates diagnosis.

Patients can be tested for tuberculosis with a tuberculin skin test. If the bacteria are present, whether active or inactive, the patch of skin that has been treated with dead tuberculosis bacteria will swell. Chest X rays or sputum analysis may also help to identify the site of infection.

Treatment

Tuberculosis is treated with a variety of antibacterial drugs simultaneously. Each type of medication acts individually on a different portion of the tuberculosis bacterium; only in combination do these drugs have the greatest probability of eliminating the infection. The drugs are prescribed for a long period of time, perhaps 6 to 18 months, but usually after two weeks the patient is no longer contagious and can resume normal activities. With this type of treatment, the disease is rarely fatal. (When an infected individual does not complete drug therapy, however, new, drug-resistant strains of tuberculosis may develop.) Severe side effects, such as liver or hearing damage, can result from certain antituberculosis drugs.

Prevention

An active case of tuberculosis can be prevented in some high-risk people by the administration of certain antituberculosis drugs, but these drugs are likely to have undesirable side effects with many who are taking them. (High-risk people include those under the age of 35, especially children, who have been exposed to the disease, as well as those with chronic diseases that have weakened their respiratory systems.) Liver damage that can be caused by these drugs is more likely to occur in those over the age of 35, so people in this age group seldom receive these drugs.

Regardless of age or physical condition, anyone who has been in close contact with a person who has an active case of tuberculosis should be tested for the disease.

THE HEART AND CIRCULATORY SYSTEM

The body's circulatory system, which includes the heart, blood vessels, and blood, brings nutrients and oxygen to every part of the body and carries away waste.

Heart
The heart is a hollow, muscular organ that maintains blood circulation throughout the body. It lies behind the sternum (breastbone), between the lungs. Its

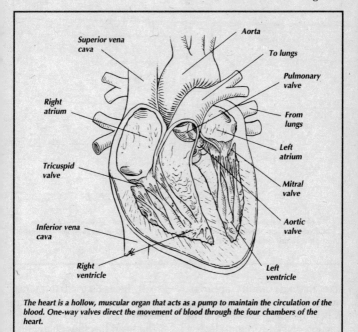

The heart is a hollow, muscular organ that acts as a pump to maintain the circulation of the blood. One-way valves direct the movement of blood through the four chambers of the heart.

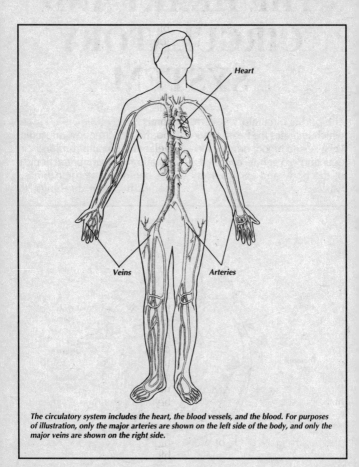

Heart

Veins

Arteries

The circulatory system includes the heart, the blood vessels, and the blood. For purposes of illustration, only the major arteries are shown on the left side of the body, and only the major veins are shown on the right side.

size in most adults approximates that of the clenched fist. A heartbeat is a rhythmic contraction of the heart muscle as it pumps blood. A normal heart usually beats 60 to 90 times per minute when the person is at rest.

The heart has four chambers, through which the blood passes.

Valves control the movement of blood between these compartments. The blood flows from two large veins (the superior vena cava and the inferior vena cava) into the right atrium (upper chamber). The blood continues down to the right ventricle (lower chamber). From this chamber, the blood is pumped to the lungs, where carbon dioxide (a waste product from the cells) is exchanged for oxygen (an element necessary for cell life). The rejuvenated blood then returns to the left atrium. From there, the blood passes to the left ventricle, which forces the blood away from the heart through the aorta (the main artery of the body, which extends through the chest and abdomen) to the other arteries and thereby to all the tissues of the body.

Blood vessels

Blood vessels form the network of passageways that transport blood throughout the body. The blood leaves the heart and passes through arteries of progressively smaller diameter. When the blood reaches the smallest blood vessels, called *capillaries,* the oxygen and nutrients it carries are exchanged for carbon dioxide and other waste products. The "used" blood then continues on its journey back toward the heart through veins of progressively greater diameter.

Blood

Blood is the fluid that courses through the blood vessels of the body. It consists of plasma (a yellowish liquid composed of water, proteins, salts, and other substances) and three formed elements—red blood cells, white blood cells, and platelets—that are visible only under a microscope. These elements are manufactured by the bone marrow (the soft tissue in the center of some bones).

Red blood cells carry oxygen from the lungs to the various body tissues. Oxygen travels attached to hemoglobin, a pigmented substance in red blood cells that contains iron. When the amount of hemoglobin in each red blood cell or the total number of red blood cells falls below a certain level, anemia is said to be present. Normally, there are about 25 billion red blood cells in one teaspoon of blood.

The job of the white blood cells is to protect the body from invasive organisms. Whenever the body becomes wounded or infected, white blood cells attack and kill disease-causing agents in the affected area. In addition, certain white blood cells produce antibodies. These substances counteract harmful agents by destroying or inactivating them. Because the body produces more white blood cells than usual in response to infection, an increase in their number signals disease. From 25 million to 45 million white blood cells are normally present in one teaspoon of blood.

Platelets are small, colorless, irregularly shaped bodies numbering approximately 1.5 billion in a single teaspoon of blood. They work to stop excessive bleeding by forming clots.

Antigens and blood types

An antigen is a substance that can provoke an immune response from the body. An antigen promotes the manufacture of antibodies that will interact only with that antigen. On the surface of all cells are numerous antigens, which cause production of different antibodies. The major blood groups (types A, B, AB, and O) are differentiated on the basis of the presence of two of those surface antigens: Type A blood has antigen A, type B has antigen B, type AB has both antigen A and antigen B, and type O has neither. A person's blood type must be identified before a blood transfusion can be given because his or her blood may reject transfused blood of the wrong type. For example, if a person who has type A blood were to receive a transfusion of type B blood, the body would not recognize the type B antigens and would treat the type B blood as an invader. The recipient would produce anti-B antibodies and destroy all of the blood cells that exhibit type B antibodies.

Anemia

Anemia is a general term referring to a shortage of red blood cells or a reduction in their hemoglobin content. (Hemoglobin is the pigment in the blood that carries oxygen in the red blood cells.) A shortage of red blood cells or hemoglobin indicates that the blood is unable to transport adequate amounts of oxygen to all parts of the body.

Causes

Anemia can be caused by vitamin or mineral deficiencies or the inability to absorb certain vitamins, the destruction of red blood cells, blood loss through bleeding, inherited abnormalities in the blood, or the failure of the bone marrow to manufacture enough red blood cells. Such diverse conditions as bleeding ulcers, drug allergies, cancer, and exposure to radioactivity can also lead to anemia. People with poor diets or histories of alcoholism are likely to suffer from one of the types of anemia caused by vitamin and mineral deficiencies. A tendency toward certain types of anemia (for example, sickle-cell anemia) can also be inherited.

Symptoms

Among the many symptoms of anemia are fatigue, shortness of breath, pounding heartbeat, rapid heart rate, headaches, loss of appetite, dizziness, ringing in the ears, weakness, and faintness. Burning of the tongue or a change in its appearance may also be a clue. Another sign of anemia may be paleness in the creases of the palms, under the fingernails, and in the lining of the eye. Very severe cases may be signaled by swollen ankles; rapid, weak pulse; pale, clammy skin; and a feeling of fullness in the neck or abdomen.

Diagnosis

Diagnosis is based on the findings from a physical examination and tests of the blood (and sometimes the bone marrow) to detect shortages of red blood cells or hemoglobin. A specific diagnosis is necessary because each type of anemia has a different cause and, therefore, needs a different medical treatment.

Iron-deficiency anemia

Iron-deficiency anemia is caused by a shortage of the mineral iron, which is necessary to produce hemoglobin. This shortage can be caused by a variety of conditions, including a drastic blood loss, such as from an accident; chronic blood loss, such as from a bleeding ulcer; hookworm infestation; and a diet lacking in good sources of iron. Women are particularly susceptible to iron deficiency anemia because of the regular loss of blood during menstruation and the depletion of iron by the fetus during pregnancy. This type of anemia can be treated with iron supplements (ferrous sulfate or ferrous gluconate tablets).

Folate-deficiency anemia

Folate-deficiency anemia is caused by either insufficient dietary folate, which is necessary for hemoglobin production, or insufficient absorption of folate from food. This deficiency may be caused or aggravated by malnourishment or alcoholism. Some disorders of the small intestine, such as inflammatory bowel disease, may also cause it. It is treated with folate and sometimes additional supplements.

Pernicious anemia

Pernicious anemia arises if the body is unable to absorb vitamin B_{12}, which is necessary for the production of red blood cells in the bone marrow. *Intrinsic factor,* a substance which helps to absorb vitamin B_{12}, is lacking in the stomach of a person suffering from pernicious anemia. Inability to absorb vitamin B_{12} can also be caused by some parasites, inflammatory bowel disease, and diseases of the small intestine. Pernicious anemia is treated with vitamin B_{12} injections directly into the bloodstream, so that the vitamin is not destroyed by stomach acid.

Aplastic anemia

Aplastic anemia is a serious condition caused by the inability of the bone marrow to produce white and red blood cells and platelets. Bone marrow function can be inhibited by cancer or exposure to radioactivity, hazardous chemicals, or some drugs. This variety

of anemia is treated with blood transfusions and bone marrow transplants.

Hemolytic anemias

Hemolytic anemias are caused by the destruction of red blood cells. These anemias can be either acquired (developed over time) or congenital (present at birth).

Acquired hemolytic anemias can be caused by mismatched blood transfusions, a drug allergy, cancer, or a serious infection. Treatment of the primary condition is necessary to treat the resulting anemia. Blood transfusions can be used to treat the condition temporarily.

Congenital hemolytic anemias are caused by an inherited abnormality in the red blood cells. The most common type is sickle-cell anemia, a disorder that predominantly affects black people. In this form of anemia, the red blood cells, which are sickle shaped instead of disklike, cannot carry enough oxygen. These cells are also very fragile and hemolyze (break down) easily. This disease is characterized by crisis periods of severe joint or abdominal pain and can lead to complications, such as kidney disease, gallstones, and heart failure. Sickle-cell anemia is treated with painkillers, oxygen, and transfusions. Avoiding situations in which oxygen may be scarce, such as high altitudes, is advisable.

Prevention
There are no specific methods to prevent anemias other than selecting a balanced diet to prevent those anemias caused by vitamin and mineral deficiencies. Individuals may also obtain genetic counseling if a hereditary condition appears to be a possibility.

Aneurysm

An aneurysm is a bulge in a blood vessel, usually an artery, due to a weakness in the vessel wall, particularly in the elastic, muscular middle layer of the artery wall. An artery has three layers: the intima, which is the smooth inner layer; the media, or middle layer; and the adventitia, which is the tough outer layer. A true aneurysm involves all three layers, whereas a false aneurysm is a disruption or clot in one or two of the layers, causing a bulge in the vessel. A dissecting aneurysm occurs when blood separates the layers, thereby creating an extra channel, sometimes extending

the full length of the artery, through which blood flow is diverted from the organs or tissues served by the blood vessel. This dangerous condition can develop in a matter of hours or days.

The main danger of most untreated aneurysms is that they may rupture, or dissect, causing death due to loss of blood. Even if death does not occur, the failure of blood to reach vital organs can cause those organs to fail.

Causes
There are various causes of aneurysms. Those occurring in the arteries of the brain are often due to an inherited defect—a weakness or lack of elastic tissue in the media. If an aneurysm in the brain ruptures, a stroke can result. Aneurysms in the small arteries may be caused by infections that weaken the vessel wall. Penetrating wounds can occasionally cause aneurysms.

The sexually transmitted disease syphilis may also cause aneurysms. Syphilis can cause vasculitis (inflammation of the smaller arteries that feed a large one). When this occurs, these small arteries are lost, thereby denying nourishment to parts of the large arterial wall and caus-

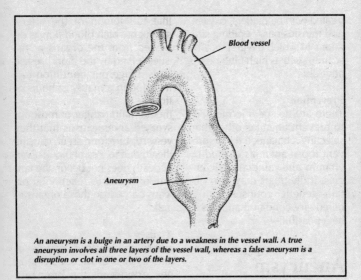

An aneurysm is a bulge in an artery due to a weakness in the vessel wall. A true aneurysm involves all three layers of the vessel wall, whereas a false aneurysm is a disruption or clot in one or two of the layers.

ing scarring and death of tissue. This leads to weakness of the wall and formation of an aneurysm.

Dissecting aneurysms usually occur in the aorta. Atherosclerosis (hardening of the arteries) is the most common cause, especially in the elderly. If a young person is affected, the condition is usually caused by an inherited defect.

Symptoms

Symptoms of dissecting aneurysms of the aorta, if in the chest, include sudden, severe pain in the area of the aneurysm, often resembling a heart attack. There may be pain under the breastbone or in the back of the neck, difficulty in swallowing, shortness of breath, hoarseness, or a heavy cough. An aneurysm in a neck artery may create a pulsating, swishing sound that the patient can detect.

Evidence of an aneurysm can be a tender, pulsating mass in the abdomen or a painful, tender mass at the back of the knee (the latter can lead to blood clots that can travel downward and result in death of tissue in the toes). Symptoms of a dissecting aneurysm in the abdomen can include sudden, severe central or low abdominal pain radiating to the back; a loss of blood flow to the legs; and shock (collapse of circulation, signaled by fainting, pale and clammy skin, and rapid, weak pulse). Death can result quickly.

Diagnosis

Computed tomography and ultrasound studies (see chapter 24) of affected areas are used to locate aneurysms and determine their extent. The most reliable and definitive test is an angiogram (also called an *arteriogram*). In this procedure, a thin catheter is inserted into an artery in the arm or leg and advanced to the site to be studied; a special dye is then injected through the catheter to outline the area so that X rays may be taken.

Treatment

Treatment of most aneurysms, especially dissecting aneurysms, should begin as soon as possible. Patients with dissecting aneurysms belong in an intensive care unit. Drugs are given to lower high blood pressure (which worsens a dissecting aneurysm) and thus reduce the chances of rupture. Occasionally, a dissecting aneurysm heals itself if pressure is lessened. Long-term medication that keeps blood pressure low is standard treatment for those who cannot undergo surgery. Surgery, however, is by far the most satisfactory solution when it is possible. The damaged portion of the blood vessel is removed and replaced with a synthetic vessel or a natural vessel taken from elsewhere in the body. Patients with ruptured aortic aneurysms need emergency surgery, as do most patients with dissecting aneurysms. Rapid replacement of blood is necessary, as is intensive monitoring. Surgery for aneurysm repair is usually long and difficult. However, with newer methods of diagnosis, many more people are being spared the risks of surgery by correction of the aneurysm before it becomes a life-threatening problem.

Angina pectoris

Angina pectoris, or simply angina, is a dull constricting pain usually in the center of the chest that indicates that the heart muscle is not getting enough blood and, as a result, is not getting sufficient oxygen. When, during a period of stress or exertion, the oxygen needs of the heart muscle are greater than the blood supplied from the coronary arteries, angina occurs. Angina, therefore, is a mechanism for warning the body.

An angina attack is not a heart attack and the pain is usually not as severe or as long-lasting. Angina does not destroy heart muscle, as does a heart attack. However, those who suffer from angina are probably more prone to heart attacks than those who do not.

Causes

Angina can be caused by any number of factors that prevent the heart muscle from getting enough blood. By far the most common cause of angina is coronary artery narrowing due to atherosclerosis. The coronary arteries supply the heart muscle with blood. When the body places an increased demand on the heart (by exercise, for example), the heart must work harder to supply blood—and thereby oxygen—to keep the muscles and organs nourished. This increased work effort causes the heart muscle itself to require more blood. When narrowing of a coronary artery is present, the areas of the heart muscle that are supplied by that artery cannot get enough blood to keep up with the body's de-

mand. When this occurs, the muscle reacts by causing the sensation of angina. Exercise, stress, and even cold weather can trigger an angina attack.

The sensation usually occurs during or after physical exertion or emotional stress, lasts only three to five minutes, and is relieved by resting or relaxing. If the pain does not go away within five minutes or if the pain increases, it may not be angina. It may be another disorder unrelated to the heart, or it may be a heart attack.

Overeating and smoking can also trigger and aggravate angina—overeating, by drawing much-needed blood to the full stomach to aid in digestion; smoking, by causing the coronary arteries to constrict, thus reducing their capacity.

Risk factors

Several risk factors are associated with coronary artery disease and angina. A family history of heart disease, diabetes, smoking, high blood cholesterol levels, and high blood pressure are among the best known. There is much controversy in medicine regarding the degree of impact these factors have. It has not yet been clearly established whether alteration of the last three factors

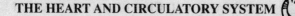

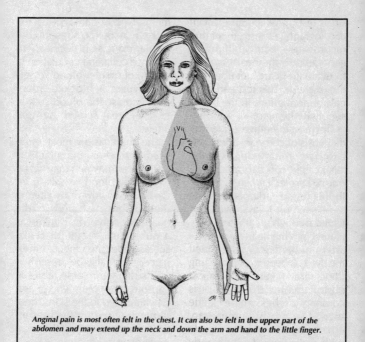

Anginal pain is most often felt in the chest. It can also be felt in the upper part of the abdomen and may extend up the neck and down the arm and hand to the little finger.

will definitely prevent or delay the onset of heart disease. However, there is much evidence favoring their reduction.

Symptoms

The major symptom of angina is the sensation of pressure, squeezing, or burning in the center of the chest behind the breastbone. This pain is often compared to the discomfort felt from indigestion. Angina pain may also be felt along the neck, in the jaw or gums, in the upper part of the abdomen, or extending down the arm (most often the left) and hand to the little finger. The location and severity of the pain vary among angina sufferers, but in a given patient, the same symptoms usually recur with each episode.

Diagnosis

The doctor will take a complete medical history and perform a physical exam and probably a stress test, in which an electrocardiograph (an instrument that records the electrical impulses generated in the heart) is used to evaluate heart function during exercise. This test can indicate abnormalities in the blood supply to the heart.

The most definitive test for the diagnosis of coronary artery disease is coronary angiography (also called *coronary arteriography* or *cardiac catheterization*). In this test, a radiopaque (able to be seen on X rays) dye is injected through a catheter (tube) placed into the heart through an artery in the leg or arm. Once the dye has been injected, X-ray films are taken, and areas obstructing the dye within the coronary arteries can be clearly seen. During this procedure, other important information, such as the overall condition of the heart muscle and its chambers, can also be obtained.

Treatment

Angina is often treated by recommending changes in the patient's lifestyle to reduce the strain on the heart and by administering medication to modify the relationship of the heart muscle and its blood supply.

A change in lifestyle will be necessary for patients who smoke, overeat, or overexert themselves. Certain types of exercise may be too stressful, but regular exercise is necessary to improve collateral circulation (a system of smaller blood vessels that bypass a blocked artery and increase the blood supply to the area served by that artery).

The medication most often used to treat angina attacks is nitroglycerin, which may act by expanding blood vessels to increase blood flow or by altering the volume of blood in the heart. Nitroglycerin is taken as a sublingual tablet that dissolves under the tongue. Nitroglycerin can also be prescribed as a sustained release tablet or capsule, as an ointment, or as a patch applied to the skin. These forms are used for the prevention of attacks, not for the treatment of an acute episode.

Pain should stop within three or four minutes; if it does not, the pain may not be due to simple angina. The possibility that the pain is originating from some other disorder, such as gallbladder disease, rib injury, muscle spasm, or pleurisy (an inflammation of the membrane surrounding the lungs and lining the chest cavity) must be investigated.

Surgery to bypass the obstructions in the coronary arteries is performed only in specific circumstances. (For more on coronary bypass surgery, see pages 200–201.)

In recent years, the technique of angioplasty has become widely used to treat obstructions that are causing angina pectoris. This procedure consists of inserting a balloon-tipped catheter into an artery and inflating the balloon at the site of narrowing, thereby decreasing the obstruction (the balloon is then deflated and removed). The advantage of this technique is that it saves the patient from having to undergo surgery. Unfortunately, it is not useful in all types of coronary artery disease and can be associated with complications that necessitate emergency surgery. Also, the artery frequently becomes obstructed again, and another angioplasty or surgery must be performed.

Prevention

Incidents of angina can be prevented with several drugs: aspirin; nitrates (such as nitroglycerin); calcium antagonists (such as diltiazem and verapamil), which act by blocking the constricting action of calcium on arterial muscle; and beta-blockers (such as propranolol), which decrease the work of the heart, thereby lessening its oxygen needs.

Atherosclerosis

Atherosclerosis is a slow, progressive disease of the arteries in which fatty deposits partially clog or totally block blood flow. Atherosclerosis occurs when the normally smooth, firm linings of the arteries become roughened, thickened, and clogged by deposits of fat, fibrin (a protein involved in blood clotting), calcium, and cellular debris. The condition develops gradually. Lipids (fats) are necessary as an energy reserve and for the production of certain hormones and tissues. Lipids are constantly present in the bloodstream. When the lipid concentration is greatly increased, however, fatty streaks form along the artery walls. These streaks can cause the development of small nodules of fatty deposits of cholesterol to jut out from the normally smooth linings of the artery walls. Fibrous scar tissue grows under these nodules and attracts calcium deposits. Accumulated calcium develops into a hard, chalky film (called *plaque*) that cannot be removed. This permanent lining

269

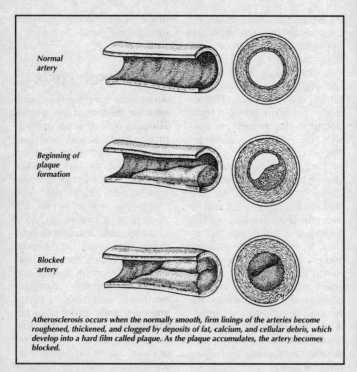

Normal
artery

Beginning of
plaque
formation

Blocked
artery

Atherosclerosis occurs when the normally smooth, firm linings of the arteries become roughened, thickened, and clogged by deposits of fat, calcium, and cellular debris, which develop into a hard film called plaque. As the plaque accumulates, the artery becomes blocked.

inside the arteries hampers their ability to expand and contract properly and slows the blood flow through the narrowed channels. Clots may then form easily, hindering or preventing the blood from traveling through the artery.

Causes

The exact cause of this process has not been pinpointed, but major risk factors have been identified: hyperlipidemia (abnormally elevated concentrations of fats in the blood), hypertension (high blood pressure), a history of smoking, and a family history of atherosclerosis (occurring before the age of 60) or diabetes mellitus. Hyperlipidemia, which promotes the formation of fatty streaks, seems to result from choosing a diet high in saturated fats (fats that are usually solid at room temperature, including all animal fats, such as those found in butter and meats) and cholesterol. Hypertension increases the risk of atherosclerosis because it puts constant strain on the arteries, which speeds up the clogging and hardening process. Smoking narrows the arteries, thus restricting blood flow and setting the stage for atherosclerosis. Diabetes is associated with accelerated atherosclerosis, particularly of small arteries.

Symptoms and complications
Atherosclerosis alone has no visible symptoms. The disease often remains undetected until the arteries leading to a vital organ are blocked. The symptoms that then become apparent are those of the specific condition caused by arterial blockage in that organ. For example, if an artery supplying the heart is partially blocked, angina pectoris may be felt; if the artery is totally blocked, heart attack (the death of heart tissue that is supplied by the artery) can result. If atherosclerosis affects an artery in the head, the person may experience dizziness, blurred vision, and faintness or may suffer a

stroke (death of brain tissue supplied by the blocked artery, causing neurologic damage such as paralysis of the limb or limbs controlled by that part of the brain). Kidney failure can develop from obstruction in the arteries leading to the kidneys. Blindness can result from obstruction of vessels leading to the eyes. Diseases of the extremities can result from blockage of their arteries.

Diagnosis
Diagnostic evaluation begins with a medical history, physical examination, and analysis of the blood. An exercise tolerance test, or stress test, using an electrocardiograph (an instrument that records the electrical impulses generated in the heart) can indicate whether areas of the heart muscle are damaged or have inadequate blood supply. Nuclear medicine studies and angiography can pinpoint obstructions in blood vessels or areas of the body that are insufficiently supplied with blood. Nuclear medicine studies use the injection of radioisotopes into the bloodstream. Angiography is a procedure in which a thin catheter is inserted into an artery in the arm or leg and advanced to the site to be studied; a special dye is then injected

through the catheter to outline the area so that X rays can be taken.

Treatment

Treatment of atherosclerosis is aimed at reducing the strain on the heart and increasing blood flow. Medications, changes in lifestyle and eating habits, and surgery can each be helpful in treating the disorder.

Anticoagulants may be prescribed to prevent clotting of the blood. If atherosclerosis has led to angina, nitrates (such as nitroglycerin) and calcium antagonists (such as diltiazem, nifedipine, and verapamil) may provide relief by expanding the arteries and increasing blood flow. If high blood pressure contributes to the problem, antihypertensive medication is prescribed. There are not yet any medications that will actually dissolve deposits that are clogging arteries.

Lifestyle changes include quitting smoking, reducing saturated fat and cholesterol intake, losing weight (obesity puts a strain on the heart), and maintaining a moderate (but not strenuous) exercise program (exercise helps develop the collateral circulation, a system of smaller blood vessels that bypass a blocked artery and increase the blood supply to the area served by that artery).

Delicate surgical procedures, called *endarterectomies,* may be performed to remove deposits that are blocking arteries to vital organs. These procedures can be performed on relatively large vessels entering the brain, heart, kidneys, and legs but cannot remove deposits in small blood vessels. If the patient suffers from severe and recurrent chest pain that is not relieved by medication, surgery may be performed to bypass major obstructions in arteries.

Recently, angioplasty (the opening of a vessel via inflation of a tiny balloon at the end of a catheter) has been successful in opening arteries to the kidney and legs. Prior to angioplasty, an angiogram must be performed to determine if the individual is a good candidate for the procedure.

Congestive heart failure

Congestive heart failure (also called *left ventricular failure* or simply *heart failure*) is a condition in which the heart weakens and fails to keep the blood moving adequately. As a result, the supply of blood to the body's tissues decreases, lowering efficiency and endurance. With poor circulation, the kidneys fail to remove enough water, salt, and wastes from the blood. In addition, the kidneys, because of the decreased blood flow presented to them, retain even more salt and water in an effort to increase blood volume. The increased blood volume makes more work for the already overworked heart, which may enlarge and beat faster in an attempt to satisfy the body's hunger for oxygen-rich blood. The veins distend with fluid, and the balance of pressures between fluids inside and outside the veins shifts, which causes fluid that normally stays in the bloodstream to leak into surrounding tissue. This fluid leakage, the reduction of forward blood flow, and the backflow of blood are primary factors responsible for the pulmonary edema (accumulation of fluid in the lungs) and the swelling of the abdomen and legs that often accompany this condition.

Causes

The usual cause of congestive heart failure is a diseased heart that cannot pump enough blood. The most common reason is severe coronary artery disease, which decreases blood flow to the heart muscle. If the person has suffered a heart attack, the resultant nonworking scar tissue further reduces the efficiency of the heart as a pump. Leaky or narrowed heart valves, due to a birth defect or rheumatic fever, can also cause heart failure. A large cardiac aneurysm (a bulge caused by the thinning of the wall of the left ventricle of the heart) may also decrease the pumping ability of the heart.

Less frequently, the root of the problem is one of several heart muscle diseases; some are caused by poisons like excessive alcohol, some by a viral infection, and others by the deposition in the heart tissue of iron or a protein called *amyloid*. Cardiac arrhythmias (disturbances of the normal rhythm of the heart) can also lead to heart failure.

Symptoms

Early signs of congestive heart failure include unexplained rapid heartbeat, unusual fatigue during exertion, shortness of breath during stair climbing or other mild exercise, and inability to withstand cold. Attacks of shortness of breath and coughing when lying in bed that are relieved by sleeping with pillows under the back to tilt the chest are also early symptoms. Sometimes, a person is actually awakened by a sensation of "air hunger" and must sit or stand to breathe more easily. These symptoms are caused by increased fluid pressure in the lung circulation. The relief obtained by assuming a more erect position is due to a shift of blood volume to the lower half of the body, easing the burden of the heart. In advanced congestive heart failure, shortness of breath and a severe cough with reddish-brown or brownish sputum are common. There may also be swelling of the legs and ankles and a feeling of fullness in the neck or the abdomen.

Diagnosis

Usually, congestive heart failure can be diagnosed by a physician on the basis of symptoms. However, a chest X ray is commonly taken to determine how much the heart has become enlarged by its overload and to see if fluid has accumulated within the lungs. An electrocardiogram (a recording of the electrical impulses generated in the heart) can reveal damage from a previous heart attack as well as irregularities in the heart rhythm.

Treatment

Treatment for congestive heart failure includes rest, oxygen, medication (such as digitalis) to strengthen the pumping ability of the heart, and medication to prevent irregular heart rhythms. Diuretic medications are given to help the kidneys remove more salt and water from the blood and thus decrease the volume of blood the heart must pump. A low-salt diet is prescribed to prevent water buildup in the blood and tissues (salt tends to cause fluid to accumulate in the body). In more severe or chronic cases, a drug may be given to expand the blood vessels and thus make it easier for the heart to pump blood through them. Newer drugs known as *angiotensin-converting enzyme (ACE) inhibitors* have been very effective in treating congestive heart failure.

In some cases, the original cause of the congestive heart failure can be corrected. For example, bypass surgery may be performed on the coronary arteries to improve blood supply to the heart muscle. Surgery may also replace or correct a faulty heart valve or repair an aneurysm. Contributing factors to be controlled or eliminated include high blood pressure, anemia, excess salt or alcohol intake, fever, an overactive thyroid gland, and stress due to overexertion.

Prevention
The prevention of congestive heart failure rests on good health habits that help prevent heart disease in general: choosing a well-balanced diet with moderate or low intake of fats; maintaining appropriate body weight; getting plenty of exercise, rest, and sleep; avoiding tobacco and excess alcohol intake; and having periodic medical checkups to detect conditions, such as high blood pressure, that might eventually overload or injure the heart. Salt restriction in those suffering from mild congestive heart failure is also very important.

Coronary bypass surgery

Coronary bypass surgery is performed on one or more of the coronary arteries, which lie on the outer surface of the heart and supply the heart muscle with the oxygen and nutrients it needs. In coronary artery disease, a section or sections of the arteries gradually become obstructed by a buildup of cholesterol, calcium, and scar tissue. The purpose of the operation is to bypass the obstructed area to permit free blood flow. Without the procedure, heart muscle beyond the obstruction is starved for blood and oxygen, especially during exercise. This condition causes the chest pains known as *angina pectoris*. If one or more of the coronary arteries become completely obstructed, the result may be a heart attack, in which a portion of heart muscle becomes so starved for blood that it dies.

Indications and alternatives
Bypass surgery is usually considered when a person suffers frequent, severe chest pains from angina. However, not all persons with angina need bypass surgery. Advances are being made in using medication to control angina. Furthermore, some angina is caused by spasms (sudden, violent contractions) of the coronary arteries, which bypass surgery may not prevent or ease. Obstructions in the coronary arteries can now sometimes be eliminated by methods that do not require cutting open the chest,

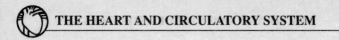

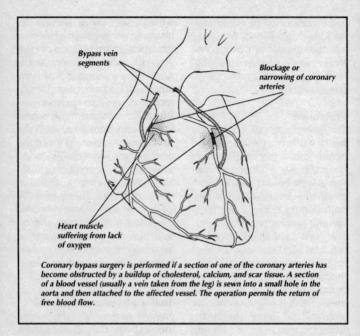

Bypass vein segments

Blockage or narrowing of coronary arteries

Heart muscle suffering from lack of oxygen

Coronary bypass surgery is performed if a section of one of the coronary arteries has become obstructed by a buildup of cholesterol, calcium, and scar tissue. A section of a blood vessel (usually a vein taken from the leg) is sewn into a small hole in the aorta and then attached to the affected vessel. The operation permits the return of free blood flow.

such as percutaneous transluminal coronary angioplasty (also called *balloon angioplasty*), which consists of threading a long, balloon-tipped catheter through the arteries to the site of obstruction and inflating the balloon to open a clogged vessel. Even without outside help, the heart may create its own partial bypass via collateral circulation (a system of smaller blood vessels that bypass a blocked artery and increase the blood supply to the area served by that artery).

If a patient has severe chest pains that cannot be controlled by medication, the doctor could order coronary angiography (also called *coronary arteriography* or *cardiac catheterization*). Through a thin, woven plastic catheter inserted into an artery in the arm or leg and passed through large blood vessels to the heart, X-ray contrast medium is injected so that it flows into the coronary arteries, outlining them on an X-ray screen. The pictures show exactly where and to what extent the blood vessels are narrowed or blocked. Thus, the doctor can determine whether bypasses are needed and, if so, where. The most urgent reason to operate is significant obstruction of the left main coronary artery, which supplies blood to 40 percent or more of the left ventricle.

Procedure

First, the surgeon makes one or more incisions in one leg to obtain a long section of a large vein for use as bypass tubing. Next, the surgeon makes an incision down the middle of the chest, divides the breastbone with an electric saw, and separates the two sides of the rib cage enough to expose the beating heart. The heartbeat is then stopped using electric shock, ice water, or certain drugs. A heart-lung machine is connected to the large vessels that carry blood to and from the heart and takes over the job of adding oxygen, removing carbon dioxide, and pumping the blood through the body.

The surgeon then cuts through the pericardial sac (a thin bag of tissue that surrounds the heart) to expose the coronary arteries, which lie on the surface of the heart. A small hole is made in the aorta, and one end of the vein segment to be used as bypass tubing is sewn to it. The other end is attached to the affected vessel beyond the obstruction. Thereafter, blood will flow freely around the obstructed portion of the artery to nourish the heart muscle, which should decrease the patient's chest pains and risk of heart attack.

The bypass surgery operation takes about three to five hours, depending on the number of bypasses. A double bypass operation is one in which portions of two vessels are bypassed, a triple bypass means that portions of three vessels are bypassed, and so forth. Usually the patient can walk about three or four days after the operation and return home in little more than a week.

Results

Considering that the procedure is such a major operation, the death rate is very low—less than 1 percent in most hospitals in which it is performed. In 80 percent of cases, angina pains are eliminated, and the patient can return to a normal life. Life expectancy may improve, but it cannot be guaranteed in all cases. There has been much controversy surrounding coronary bypass surgery, mainly centering on the question of whether this procedure can increase life expectancy for those with coronary artery disease and angina. At present, there is no question that the surgery relieves pain and allows for greater exercise tolerance in the majority of patients who undergo it for severe angina. In certain patterns of disease, such as obstruction of the left main coronary artery, the operation definitely prolongs life expectancy. In other patterns, such as triple vessel disease, in which branches of the coronary arteries (except for the left main coronary artery) are involved, the procedure most likely allows a longer life. In still other patterns, the question remains unsettled. Whether the surgery will prevent a heart attack has also not been determined.

Cyanosis

Cyanosis is a bluish discoloration of the skin and mucous membranes due to inadequate oxygenation of the blood. The abnormal coloration shows up in these areas because of their rich blood supply and their relative transparency.

Blood rich in oxygen from the lungs is bright red. This is because of the red, iron-containing pigment hemoglobin, which is found in red blood cells. When blood passes through the blood vessels of the lungs, oxygen from the air in the lungs combines with the hemoglobin, causing the blood to turn a very bright red. After the blood releases its oxygen to the cells of the body and picks up carbon dioxide and other waste products, the hemoglobin fades and the blood turns dark. However, if the lungs are not working well or if for some other reason the red blood cells are not being oxygenated, the blood appears bluish.

Cyanosis can be due to asthma, choking, pneumonia, or lung collapse. It can also be a sign of certain inborn heart defects, of severe cor pulmonale (right heart failure), or of abnormally excessive production of red blood cells. It is seen most frequently in cold weather when lips, toes, and fingers turn blue from extreme cold, the result of sluggish surface circulation of the blood (in this case, it can be a normal phenomenon and may not indicate disease).

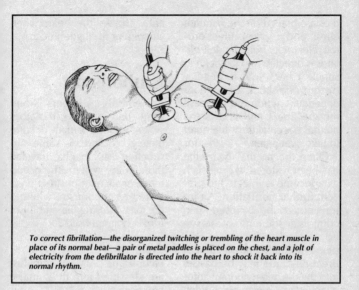

To correct fibrillation—the disorganized twitching or trembling of the heart muscle in place of its normal beat—a pair of metal paddles is placed on the chest, and a jolt of electricity from the defibrillator is directed into the heart to shock it back into its normal rhythm.

Defibrillation

Defibrillation is a technique to correct ventricular fibrillation, a condition marked by very rapid, disorganized twitching or trembling of the heart muscle in place of the normal rhythmic beat. Ventricular fibrillation produces a condition called *cardiac arrest,* in which no heartbeat, pulse, or blood pressure can be detected. Death or permanent brain damage follows within a few minutes unless this condition is corrected or unless first-aid measures maintain blood circulation and breathing until emergency medical treatment is available.

Causes of fibrillation

The most common cause of fibrillation is a heart attack. When this happens, certain parts of the heart will start contracting independently of the normal heartbeat. Other causes of fibrillation are severe electrical shock and prolonged exposure to cold temperatures.

Defibrillation treatment

An electrical device called a *defibrillator* is used to correct fibrillation. A pair of metal pad-

279

dles are placed on the patient's chest, and a jolt of direct-current electricity from the defibrillator is directed into the heart to shock it back into its regular rhythm. The shock stops the independent action of individual muscle fibers and allows the natural pacemaker of the heart to take over again.

Once the normal heartbeat has been restored, a drug such as lidocaine is injected to prevent further fibrillation. An intravenous tube is inserted to administer sodium bicarbonate (to neutralize acids in the blood) and other medication. A breathing tube may be passed into the trachea (windpipe); it is attached to a mechanical pump that forces air in and out of the lungs. Then the patient is taken to a hospital cardiac intensive care unit, where monitoring devices constantly keep track of the patient's condition and sound an alarm if any sign of danger threatens.

Electrical defibrillation is also used to restart a heart that has been stopped for purposes of heart surgery.

In patients with severe heart disease and recurrent episodes of ventricular fibrillation, a defibrillator can be implanted under the skin and attached to the heart. The defibrillator internally shocks the heart when ventricular fibrillation occurs.

Embolism

An embolism occurs when some part of the circulatory system is either partially or completely blocked by some obstructing mass that has traveled through the system. The occurrence of such an obstruction is called an *embolism,* whereas the mass causing the embolism is called an *embolus.*

Types

Emboli (the plural of embolus) are classified into three major groups:
- Solid emboli, which are made up of various substances, such as clumps of tissue, tumor cells, or pieces of blood clots
- Liquid emboli, which are made up of globules of fat or amniotic fluid (fluid that surrounds the fetus in the uterus)
- Gaseous emboli, which are made up of the various constituents of air

Emboli may be further categorized according to their origin and the location of the blockage that they cause:
- Arterial emboli, which originate either from the heart or the artery itself, travel down-

stream and become lodged in a smaller blood vessel, preventing the flow of fresh blood to whatever area or organ is normally supplied

• Paradoxical emboli, which originate in the venous system, pass into the arterial system (usually through a defect in the walls separating the chambers of the heart), and block an artery anywhere in the body

• Pulmonary emboli, which block vessels in the lungs (for more on pulmonary embolism, see pages 252–254)

• Coronary artery emboli, which block the coronary arteries of the heart

• Cerebral emboli, which block vessels in the brain. Cerebral emboli usually originate in the heart or the carotid arteries in the neck

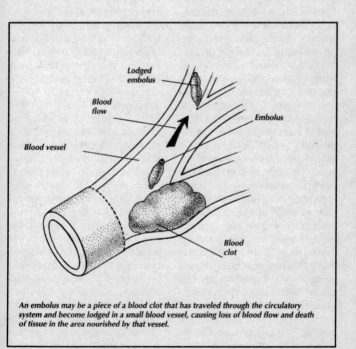

An embolus may be a piece of a blood clot that has traveled through the circulatory system and become lodged in a small blood vessel, causing loss of blood flow and death of tissue in the area nourished by that vessel.

Causes

The most common cause of embolism is blood clots from within the heart or blood vessels. Arterial emboli also commonly originate from plaques or other accumulations on the valves of the heart, from aneurysms, and from plaques or clots within arteries. Fat emboli can result from injury to the bones (particularly the long bones of the legs) or from damage to cells in fat tissue. Air emboli can develop if a very large amount of air is admitted during an intravenous infusion or during surgery, especially in operations on the neck or chest (in the latter cases, air enters vessels that are open because of the surgery). However, the oxygen in air is not the only gas involved in gaseous emboli. When divers ascend from high-pressure levels in deep water to normal-pressure levels too quickly, or when pilots in planes without cabin pressurization climb from normal-pressure levels to low-pressure levels, there is always the possibility that nitrogen bubbles will arise in the bloodstream because of too rapid decompression. If any of these gaseous emboli find their way into the central nervous system, the results can be catastrophic.

Symptoms

The symptoms produced by an embolism vary according to the site at which the embolism occurs. An embolism deprives the affected area of its blood supply, which can cause damage or death of tissue in the area. An embolism in a brain artery may produce the symptoms of a stroke, such as unsteadiness, slurring of speech, and numbness or weakness in the face, arm, or leg on one side. If an embolism occurs in the leg, the area beyond the blockage may become white and painful. Pain may be the first symptom of embolism in other areas.

Treatment

Emboli resulting from blood clots are often treated with a variety of anticoagulants (agents that inhibit normal clotting mechanisms in the blood). Common anticoagulants, such as heparin and warfarin, do not dissolve clots but instead prevent additional clots from forming. There are newer drugs that do dissolve clots but their use is restricted to special situations. If an embolism is in an accessible location, such as an artery in a limb, and tissue is threatened, surgery to remove the clot is the preferred method of treatment to save the limb. In cases of

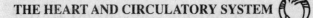
massive embolism in the lung in which life is threatened, surgery can also be attempted. If an individual has clots in the deep venous system of the lower half of the body and anticoagulants cannot be prescribed (for example, because of a recent hemorrhage in the brain or other vital organ), blocking devices, such as clips, can be placed on or in the inferior vena cava (the main vein receiving blood from the lower part of the body) to prevent emboli from reaching the lungs.

Endocarditis

The heart is made up of three cellular layers: the epicardium (outermost layer), the myocardium (middle, muscular layer), and the endocardium (innermost layer). The endocardium lines all of the chambers and valves of the heart, and its cells are continuous with those of blood vessels leaving the heart. Endocarditis is an inflammation of the endocardial layer of the heart.

Causes

The most common form of endocarditis, infectious endocarditis, is caused by microorganisms. *Staphylococcus* and *Streptococcus* bacteria are most often the infectious agents, but viruses, fungi, and other bacteria may also be responsible.

Infectious endocarditis usually occurs in persons with congenital (inborn) or acquired defects in the walls or valves of the heart. An example of a congenital defect would be a hole in the wall between two chambers of the heart. An example of an acquired defect would be damage of the heart valves caused by rheumatic fever or calcium deposition. Such abnormalities make the heart more susceptible to infection.

Bacteria probably circulate through the bloodstream of all people at some time or another. However, certain procedures, such as dental work and surgery, may lead to bacteremia (the presence of large numbers of bacteria in the bloodstream). The bacteria accumulate on these abnormal areas in the heart and cause inflammation or infection that serves as a foundation for the collection of platelets, strands of fibrin (clotting material), and other debris of the circulatory system.

Symptoms

Infectious endocarditis is a serious systemic disease with a wide spectrum of symptoms

283

and signs. Patients may complain of fevers, weakness, and weight loss. Anemia (deficiency of red blood cells) may also be present. Pieces of vegetation may break off and travel through the bloodstream to other areas of the body, causing symptoms of obstruction (for example, a stroke if the brain is affected).

Diagnosis

The diagnosis is made on the basis of the patient's medical history, the physical examination, and the results of laboratory studies, such as blood cultures, to identify the microorganisms present.

Treatment

Once the infectious agent has been isolated, appropriate antibiotics can be administered. Antibiotic administration is by the intravenous route, at least at first, and usually continues for long periods (up to eight weeks). If infection of a heart valve is particularly severe or if a prosthetic (artificial) valve is involved, it may have to be replaced.

Prevention

Persons with abnormal heart valves, prosthetic valves, and other structural abnormalities must be given antibiotics before and after any procedure likely to disperse bacteria (for example, dental work, surgery of the urogenital tract or large intestine, or opening of an abscess). The antibiotics serve either to prevent the passage of microorganisms through the bloodstream or to lessen their number, thereby decreasing the chance that endocarditis will develop.

Extrasystole

An extrasystole is a contraction of the heart caused by a stimulus or impulse somewhere in the heart other than in the sinoatrial node, the natural pacemaker of the heart. In some ways, the condition is like static in an electrical circuit.

While physicians have for years debated the importance of extrasystoles, recent thought on the subject has led to a reassessment of the seriousness of the phenomenon. In many cases of sudden death attributed to severe cardiac arrhythmia (a disturbance of the normal rhythm of the heartbeat) in patients with severe underlying heart disease, the arrhythmia may have actually been triggered by extrasystoles.

Causes

While the immediate cause of an extrasystole is an accidental signal telling the heart muscle to contract, the real causes lie elsewhere. For example, strenuous activity, especially if there are existing heart problems, can trigger extrasystoles, which, in turn, may trigger an episode of heart arrhythmia that leads to more serious complications. Coffee, nicotine, and certain drugs, as well as anxiety and sudden shocks or frights, are thought to play a role in extrasystoles. It is important to note, however, that extrasystoles also occur in healthy hearts and, in these cases, are quite harmless and do not necessarily indicate underlying heart disease.

Symptoms

The symptoms of extrasystoles are familiar to anyone who has ever been startled and felt his or her heart had "skipped a beat." The extrasystole sometimes presents itself as one or two extra heartbeats. On other occasions, there will be a beat followed by a long silence, then a couple of quick beats. Some people experience a feeling of giddiness, shortness of breath, and weakness, with momentary feelings of blacking out. These symptoms, if prolonged (particularly if associated with loss of consciousness), usually indicate that a sustained arrhythmia is occurring, which should be reported to a doctor.

Diagnosis

The primary diagnostic tool is the electrocardiograph (an instrument that records the electrical impulses generated in the heart). One method of documenting the occurrence and nature of extrasystoles is continuous ambulatory electrocardiographic monitoring with a device called a *Holter monitor*. The monitor, which is like a combination tape recorder-electrocardiograph, is worn by the patient for as long as 24 hours. A diary is furnished so that the patient can record his or her activities and symptoms. The patient goes about his or her routine during the test. After the monitor is taken off, the tape is translated into a continuous electrocardiographic record. Comparison of this record with the diary allows a diagnosis to be made as to the presence and type of arrhythmia.

Treatment

Any treatment program must be based on the underlying cause

of the extrasystoles, as revealed by electrocardiographic studies. Treatment may involve medications to regulate the heartbeat, lifestyle changes (such as restriction of tobacco use and caffeine intake), or implantation of an artificial cardiac pacemaker. If the electrocardiographic studies indicate that the extrasystoles do not reflect any disease process, no medical treatment is necessary.

Gangrene

Gangrene is the death of body tissue due to diminishment or loss of blood supply, leading to nutrient and oxygen deprivation. There are three major types of gangrene: moist, dry, and gas gangrene. Although gangrene usually affects the extremities of the body, it can sometimes affect the internal organs.

Causes

Moist gangrene is generally caused by a sudden stoppage of blood flow to a body site, usually resulting from burning by heat or by acid, from severe freezing, from a physical accident that destroys the tissues, from keeping a tourniquet in place too long, or from a blood clot or other blockage. The tissue death that results from loss of blood supply is accompanied by decomposition due to bacterial action. The gangrenous infection is likely to spread rapidly as toxins (poisons) are formed in the affected tissues and absorbed.

Dry gangrene usually occurs gradually and results from a slow, progressive reduction of blood flow in the arteries. There is generally no bacterial decomposition; the tissues simply become dry and shriveled. This type of gangrene occurs only in the extremities. It may occur as a secondary effect of arteriosclerosis in the elderly, of advanced stages of diabetes, or of Buerger disease (an inflammatory condition that affects the blood vessels of the limbs, primarily the legs).

Gas gangrene is often caused by infection of a wound by anaerobic (able to live without air) bacteria, which are found in soil. It can follow rapidly after contamination of deep wounds. The bacteria break down tissues, giving off gas and toxic by-products.

Gangrene in an internal organ can be caused by any condition that cuts off blood supply to an area. For example, if a loop of intestine is caught in

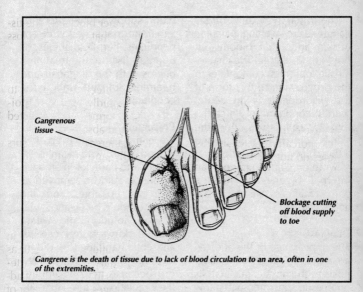

Gangrenous tissue

Blockage cutting off blood supply to toe

Gangrene is the death of tissue due to lack of blood circulation to an area, often in one of the extremities.

an opening in the abdominal wall, the blood supply to that part of the intestine may be cut off (causing what is called a *strangulated hernia*), and gangrene can then occur in that section of the tissue. In acute appendicitis, areas of gangrene can occur in the walls of the appendix, with rupture of the appendix through the gangrenous area. In severe cholecystitis (inflammation of the gallbladder, usually associated with gallstones), gangrene can develop in areas where the stones compress the mucous membrane, cutting off the blood supply.

Symptoms

Moist gangrene is characterized by a purplish-red, bruised appearance; by swelling; and, often, by blisters.

Dry gangrene is marked by gradual shrinking of the tissues, which first grow cold and lack a pulse, then turn brown, then black. Usually there is a sharp line of demarcation where the gangrene stops because the unaffected tissue nearby is continuing to receive blood. This type of gangrene is sometimes called *mummification of tissue* because of the dry, shriveled, and dark appearance.

The initial symptoms of gas gangrene are swelling, paleness of skin, and a thin, bloody (but not foul) discharge. The characteristic foul smell comes later in the progression of this form of the disorder. It is an acute, painful condition in which the muscles and tissues under the skin become filled with gas and a thin, brownish-black fluid.

Symptoms of gangrene in an internal organ may include pain, tenderness over the organ, and fever.

Diagnosis
The appearance of the affected area usually suggests the diagnosis to the physician. Analysis of a tissue specimen will allow the identification of the infective microorganism, which is necessary for selection of an appropriate antibiotic. Areas of gas gangrene may be seen on X-ray studies.

Treatment
Treatment of gangrene generally involves cleaning of the area and administration of antibiotics. The effectiveness of antibiotic therapy seems to depend on the time elapsed between injury or infection and the beginning of treatment.

In the case of gangrene caused by deterioration in the blood supply of the elderly or gangrene associated with appendicitis, hernia, diabetes, or Buerger disease, the treatment begins with the diagnosis and treatment of the underlying condition.

Prevention
Preventing gangrene in an open wound begins with cleanliness. All dirt and particles in an open wound should be removed as soon as possible, and the wound should be cleaned with a soap solution and water. Burned skin requires careful, antiseptic handling to avoid infection. Frostbite is also dangerous because freezing impairs the circulation of the skin, making it tender and easily damaged. Frostbitten skin, especially on the fingers, toes, and earlobes, must be handled with great care to avoid gangrenous infections.

Heart attack

A heart attack, or myocardial infarction, occurs when an area of the heart muscle is damaged or dies because a coronary artery (an artery that delivers blood to the heart muscle itself) has been blocked and the oxygen-rich blood supply to that

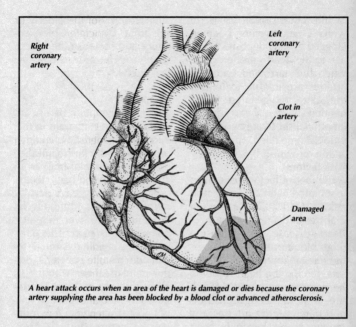

A heart attack occurs when an area of the heart is damaged or dies because the coronary artery supplying the area has been blocked by a blood clot or advanced atherosclerosis.

area of the heart has been drastically reduced. The damaged muscle tissue of the heart is replaced with scar tissue, which does not function as muscle, but rather as a kind of patch. If the area of damage is large enough, the ability of the heart to pump blood is seriously diminished.

Although the chances of surviving a heart attack are now better than ever and complete recovery is common, heart attack is still the number one cause of death in the United States. Heart attacks that do not result in death may lead to serious complications, including shock, cardiac arrhythmia (irregularity of the heartbeat), and congestive heart failure, in which the heart is not able to pump enough blood to meet the needs of the body.

Causes

Heart attack is caused by the blockage of a coronary artery by a thrombus (blood clot) or

289

by atherosclerosis, a disease in which the arteries become clogged by fatty deposits. Damage to the heart muscle occurs when the narrowed coronary arteries are unable to deliver the extra oxygenated blood needed by the heart during emotional stress or physical exertion.

Risk factors

A number of factors have been associated with an increased risk of heart attack, including diabetes and a family history of heart disease. Hypertension (high blood pressure) increases the resistance in the blood vessels, forcing the heart to pump harder to push blood through the body. Smoking constricts and damages the arteries and reduces blood flow to the heart muscle. Stress increases the oxygen requirement of the heart muscle. A diet high in saturated fats (fats that are usually solid at room temperature, including those animal fats found in butter and meats) has been found to increase the serum cholesterol level in the blood and thus the chances of developing atherosclerosis. The lack of moderate, regular exercise results in poor tone of the heart muscle and may also prevent the development of collateral circulation (a system of smaller blood vessels that bypass a blocked artery and increase the blood supply to the area served by that artery).

Symptoms

The major symptom of a heart attack is a crushing pain in the middle of the chest, behind the breastbone; the pain can also extend down one or both arms and into the neck, back, teeth, or jaws. Fatigue, heavy perspiration, dizziness, difficulty in breathing, and fever may accompany this pain. The pain may be somewhat similar to that due to angina pectoris, but the pain of a heart attack is more intense, will not be relieved by nitroglycerin, and will not go away within a few minutes, as angina pain will. Also, a heart attack can take place during sleep, which is uncommon for angina pain.

Heart attacks may be very mild, signaled only by slight discomfort, faintness, and nausea. In very serious cases, a heart attack may be accompanied by cardiac arrest (cessation of the heartbeat) or ventricular fibrillation (degeneration of the normal, steady heartbeat to a useless quivering that prevents blood from being pumped through the body).

Diagnosis

Heart attack is diagnosed on the basis of the individual's medical history, the physical examination, and test results. The electrocardiograph (an instrument that records the electrical impulses generated in the heart) will show disturbed patterns of heart activity, because the impulses must travel around the damaged area. The white blood cell count may also be elevated because the body's immune system increases the number of white blood cells to remove damaged tissue from the heart. Measurements of certain enzymes in the blood may signal that heart muscle has been damaged, although these tests may not confirm that a heart attack has taken place until 24 to 72 hours after the event.

Treatment

There is no home treatment for a heart attack other than emergency first-aid resuscitative measures—cardiopulmonary resuscitation (CPR). If the patient loses consciousness and pulse or respiration are absent, CPR should be initiated immediately and continued until the individual begins to breathe independently.

Many deaths could be prevented if heart attack victims or their families, acting on their behalf, did not delay seeking medical attention. Studies have shown that, on the average, heart attack victims wait three hours before seeing a doctor.

In almost every case, hospitalization will be necessary following a heart attack. Treatment in the hospital will probably begin in the cardiac care unit, with limited physical activity at first and a gradual return to normal activities.

A variety of medications are used to treat heart attack patients: antiarrhythmics, which inhibit irregularities in the heartbeat; diuretics, which reduce strain on the heart by removing excess water from the blood; antianginals, which diminish chest pain; sedatives, which relax the body; and beta-blockers, which ease the strain on the heart by decreasing its work. Another category of drugs, calcium-channel blockers, also appears to be effective in reducing injury to the heart muscle.

Interventional therapy during the first few hours after a heart attack has become common. Usually, an angiogram (also called an *arteriogram* or *cardiac catheterization*) is performed first. In this procedure, a thin catheter is inserted into an artery in the arm or leg and advanced through the large blood vessels to the heart; a special dye is then injected through the catheter into the coronary arteries, outlining them on an X-ray screen.

Once the area of obstruction has been located, it may be possible to inject drugs to dissolve an obstruction. In other cases, percutaneous transluminal coronary angioplasty (also called *balloon angioplasty*) may be performed. In this procedure, a long tube with a balloon tip is threaded through the arteries to the site of the obstruction, and the balloon is inflated to open a clogged vessel (the balloon is then deflated and removed).

Prevention

Prevention of heart attack begins with sensible health and dietary habits. Those who do not smoke and do not overeat or overindulge in saturated fats, but who exercise regularly and eliminate as much stress as possible from their lives, are much less likely to become heart-attack victims. Those who have already suffered one or more heart attacks may be able to prevent further attacks by changing their living habits along these lines.

Heartbeat irregularities

Heartbeat irregularities (also called *cardiac arrhythmias*) are deviations from the normal, steady beating of the heart.

Minor irregularities in the heartbeat are common, but more serious arrhythmias can lead to fainting, angina pectoris, or heart attack. The most devastating heartbeat irregularity is called *ventricular fibrillation*, which occurs when the normally steady pumping action of the heart is reduced to a useless quivering.

Causes

Serious arrhythmias are usually caused by damage to the heart muscle or to specialized heart tissue called the *conduction system*. The first part of the conduction system, called the *sinus node*, serves as the natural pacemaker of the heart; it is responsible for establishing and maintaining a healthy, steady heartbeat.

Heartbeat irregularities can also be caused by improper use of certain drugs (among them, drugs prescribed for arrhythmia, which can actually cause arrhythmia if the dosage is too high), excessive smoking, or

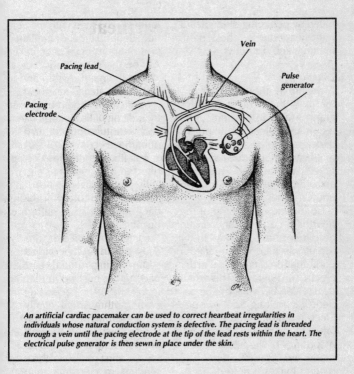

An artificial cardiac pacemaker can be used to correct heartbeat irregularities in individuals whose natural conduction system is defective. The pacing lead is threaded through a vein until the pacing electrode at the tip of the lead rests within the heart. The electrical pulse generator is then sewn in place under the skin.

consumption of large quantities of caffeine (the amounts found in coffee, tea, chocolate, cola, and some cold medicines can overstimulate the heart).

Heartbeat irregularities may also develop as a result of congenital (present at birth) abnormalities, a poorly functioning left ventricle, high blood pressure, or a previous heart attack (because the resulting scar tissue may interfere with transmission of the nerve impulses governing the heartbeat).

Ventricular fibrillation often occurs after a heart attack or some other serious injury, such as a severe electrical shock.

Symptoms

Some heartbeat irregularities have no noticeable symptoms. Other irregularities will be sig-

293

naled by pounding of the heart, light-headedness, chest pain, fainting, and dizziness.

Diagnosis

Arrhythmias are diagnosed primarily with the electrocardiograph (an instrument that records the electrical impulses generated in the heart). A normal heart will produce a record of regular peaks and valleys; an arrhythmic heart will show an uneven pattern.

Continuous recording of the heartbeat can be done on an outpatient basis with a Holter monitor, which is similar to a combination tape recorder electrocardiograph. This small device can be worn by the patient for as long as 24 hours. Electrocardiographic wires are taped to the patient's chest, and recordings of the heartbeat are made on magnetic tape. The patient makes a note of his or her activities and of any symptoms he or she experiences during the testing period, and these reports are later correlated with the recorded heartbeat rhythm.

Treatment

Occasionally, cardiac arrhythmias are so mild that no particular treatment is required. However, more serious irregu-larities are treated with medication, defibrillation, or implantation of an artificial pacemaker. All of these methods act to steady the heart rhythm and to maintain a steady heartbeat.

Medications commonly used include digitalis, beta-blockers, and antiarrhythmics, such as quinidine.

A defibrillator is a device applied to the chest that electrically jolts a quivering heart in a state of ventricular fibrillation back into a normal pattern of beating.

For those whose arrhythmia is caused by a faulty conduction system, an artificial cardiac pacemaker may be implanted in the chest. The pacemaker incorporates a small electrical generator, which causes the heart to beat when its own conduction system fails and steadies an abnormal heartbeat by sending out electrical impulses similar to those emitted by the heart.

Lifestyle changes will probably be recommended to patients suffering from heartbeat irregularities; they may need to quit smoking, lose weight, exercise more regularly, and reduce their caffeine intake. These precautions may also be taken in an effort to prevent arrhythmias.

Heart murmurs

Heart murmurs are extra whishing sounds—in addition to the regular "lub-dub" sounds of the heartbeat—that are made as blood flows through the chambers and valves of the heart. In most cases, heart murmurs are quite harmless and represent no cause for concern. In other cases, however, heart murmurs can be a symptom that first alerts a doctor to the presence of heart disease or a structural abnormality in the heart.

Causes

Heart murmurs can be heard in many healthy persons, especially children, teenagers, and pregnant women. These murmurs are normal sounds caused by the blood rushing through the heart and do not indicate a heart condition. They are called *innocent, functional,* or *insignificant heart murmurs.*

In contrast, organic, or structural, heart murmurs are caused by narrowing or obstruction of the heart valves or by incomplete closure of the valves, which allows blood to seep back into the upper or lower heart chambers. Such heart murmurs can be congenital (existing at birth) or acquired, on account of damage to the heart valves caused by rheumatic fever, atherosclerosis, syphilis, or other ailments. Heart murmurs also occur when there are holes in the walls separating the chambers of the heart.

Symptoms

Heart murmurs can be detected only by physical examination. By listening to the heart through a stethoscope, a doctor can usually distinguish any extra sounds and judge whether they signify a serious problem, such as heart disease.

Diagnosis

If the heart murmur is organic, the doctor will order special studies—for example, chest X ray, electrocardiography, and angiography—to evaluate the cause and extent of the condition.

Treatment

An innocent heart murmur does not require any medical treatment or special care, and a person with such a murmur can live a completely normal life. In fact, it is very important that a child with an innocent murmur be treated as the normal, healthy child that he or she is. Parents are sometimes frightened by the idea of a heart murmur and overprotect a child unnecessarily, which is not good for the child's emotional well-being. Most innocent murmurs detected in children disappear or become undetectable by adolescence; only 15 to 20 percent of such murmurs continue into adulthood.

If a murmur is organic, the underlying condition can usually be corrected through surgery. In cases of heart murmur due to actually diseased valves, taking antibiotics before surgery or dental work may prevent bacterial endocarditis (for more on endocarditis, see pages 283–284).

Hemoglobin

The role of the red blood cells is to carry oxygen through the body. The red blood cells can perform this task because of the presence of hemoglobin, the pigment that is formed when the red blood cells develop in the bone marrow.

Each hemoglobin molecule is made up of a protein molecule called *globin* and four pigmented molecules of a compound called *heme*. Each heme molecule has one atom of iron, and there are four heme molecules in a single molecule of hemoglobin; hence, a single molecule of hemoglobin has four atoms of iron. This structure makes it possible for one hemoglobin molecule to join with four oxygen molecules to form a substance called *oxyhemoglobin*. This reaction is reversible, enabling hemoglobin to pick up oxygen when the blood is in the lungs and to release oxygen in the cells when the blood is pumped to the tissues.

In general, the blood of men usually has a greater concentration of hemoglobin than that of women. Men have about 14 to 16 grams of hemoglobin per 100 milliliters of blood, whereas women have only about 12 to 14 grams per 100 milliliters of blood. (One hundred milliliters is approximately equal to $3\frac{1}{2}$ ounces.)

A number of blood disorders have to do with hemoglobin abnormalities. In many forms of anemia, there is not enough hemoglobin in the red blood cells (for more on anemia, see pages 260–263). In polycythemia, there is too much hemoglobin in the blood (see pages 305–306). In other conditions, such as thalassemia, the abnormal chemical composition or production of hemoglobin molecules reduces both the oxygen-carrying and oxygen-releasing

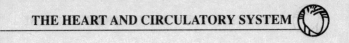
capability of the red blood cells.

Hemorrhage

Hemorrhage is the technical term for bleeding, often referring to substantial blood loss or uncontrollable bleeding, either externally or internally. The effects of hemorrhage depend on the part of the body that is bleeding and the total amount of blood that is lost. Hemorrhage can be a symptom of a number of serious, sometimes fatal, disorders.

Causes
Hemorrhage occurs when blood vessels are torn or broken. Normally, blood will clot within seconds or minutes, stopping the blood flow. However, when serious injuries or other disorders (such as hemophilia, peptic ulcer, or cancer) are involved, the body's normal blood-clotting mechanism may be inadequate or may malfunction. If blood loss is not quickly stopped, death may result.

Symptoms
Severe external hemorrhage is associated with the following symptoms: rapid pulse; dizziness or faintness; collapse; a drop in blood pressure; a rise in pulse rate; and pale, cold, clammy, or sweaty skin.

Internal hemorrhage may also show symptoms, even if the bleeding is slight. Black, tarry stools may signal bleeding in the intestinal tract from a peptic ulcer; blood in the vomitus indicates bleeding in the stomach; and blood in the urine means that bleeding is occurring in the kidneys or urinary tract.

Blood in the stool, urine, or vomitus should always be reported to a doctor at once, as should external bleeding that occurs frequently or that cannot be stopped within minutes.

Treatment
Treatment for internal hemorrhage involves correcting the cause of the bleeding, possibly with surgery. External hemorrhage is treated by applying pressure to the wound with a sterile bandage (or, in an emergency, just pressing it with the fingers) until the bleeding stops. If bleeding cannot be stopped, the patient will almost certainly have to be hospitalized, so that lost blood can be replaced with transfusions of blood products and, in some cases, so that damaged blood vessels can be surgically tied off and sealed.

Hypertension

Hypertension, or high blood pressure, refers to persistently elevated pressure of blood within the arteries, which carry blood from the heart through the body. The exertion of excessive force on the artery walls may cause damage to the arteries themselves and thereby to the heart, kidneys, and brain, leading to heart attack, kidney failure, and stroke.

Causes

Although many people believe that hypertension is caused by extreme activity or tension, this theory has not been proved.

When no underlying cause of hypertension is discovered, the disease is called primary, or essential, hypertension. If another disease, such as kidney or endocrine disease, causes the elevated blood pressure, the condition is called secondary hypertension.

Risk factors

Contrary to popular belief, there is no typical hypertensive person. However, some people are more susceptible to developing high blood pressure than others. Heredity appears to play a role; persons whose parents have hypertension are at greater risk of having it themselves. In the past, hypertension was attributed to aging, but current evidence indicates that age is not a primary factor. The incidence of hypertension in black people, both children and adults, is about twice that in white people.

Overweight, prolonged stress, smoking, drinking, and excessive sodium in the diet (which causes fluid retention) may increase blood pressure, especially in persons prone to hypertension. There are also indications that use of oral contraceptives may contribute to increased blood pressure; however, this is more likely to occur in women who are overweight, who have other hypertensive risk factors (such as smoking), or whose parents have hypertension.

Symptoms

Hypertension has been called the "silent disease" because it often has no obvious symptoms. A person can have high blood pressure for years without noticing any symptoms. Symptoms include headache, fatigue, dizziness, flushing of the face, ringing in the ears, and frequent nosebleeds. However, these symptoms may also result from other conditions.

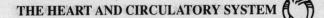

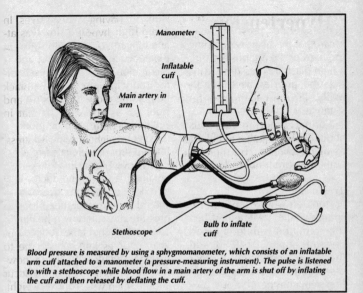

Blood pressure is measured by using a sphygmomanometer, which consists of an inflatable arm cuff attached to a manometer (a pressure-measuring instrument). The pulse is listened to with a stethoscope while blood flow in a main artery of the arm is shut off by inflating the cuff and then released by deflating the cuff.

Diagnosis

To diagnose hypertension, a simple, risk-free, painless test using a stethoscope and a sphygmomanometer is used. Blood pressure is measured in a main artery of the arm by first shutting off and then releasing the flow of blood in the artery with the inflatable cuff of the sphygmomanometer while listening to the arterial pulse with the stethoscope.

The blood pressure measurements are given as the systolic pressure (the pressure at which the first beat of the pulse can be heard as gradual deflation of the cuff begins) over the diastolic pressure (the pressure at which steady flow through the artery can be heard as the cuff is deflated)—for example, 150/95. The systolic pressure essentially measures the pressure of the heart during a contraction. The diastolic pressure is that which exists when the heart is filling between beats. Although diastolic pressure is considerably lower than systolic, there is still pressure in the body when the heart is filling. Both values have diagnos-

299

tic importance. An unusually high systolic pressure may mean that the heart is pumping too hard or the arteries are stiff; a high diastolic pressure means that the arteries have abnormally high muscular tone or resistance.

Normal blood pressure is about 80/46 at birth and climbs as age increases. The normal adult pressure is about 120/80.

Treatment

Fortunately, hypertension responds well to treatment. When the condition is mild (a blood pressure of about 140/90) and there is no indication of other disease, a doctor may suggest lifestyle changes before prescribing medication. These changes may include weight loss, a regular exercise program, and strict limitation of sodium intake, which affects fluid balance and volume and therefore blood pressure. Controlling sodium in the diet requires restriction of table salt as well as careful scrutiny of all food and drug labels. If medication is indicated, a physician may prescribe one or several drugs.

While tension and stress do not directly cause hypertension, these factors do affect the condition. Persons with hyperten-

sion, therefore, are urged to avoid high-pressure situations and to learn to deal with stress. Biofeedback, self-hypnosis, and meditation have proved useful for reducing stress and may help someone with hypertension.

Blood pressure can be monitored at home with a special kit. If three separate elevated readings (above 140/90 in adults) are obtained, a trip to the doctor is in order. Furthermore, everyone should have his or her blood pressure measured by a healthcare professional at least once a year. Persons with a history of hypertension or with any of the risk factors for hypertension should carefully follow their physician's recommendations for periodic blood pressure checks. It is also recommended that children of parents with hypertension begin to receive regular blood pressure measurements early in life.

Hypotension

Hypotension is low blood pressure. Unlike chronic high blood pressure, which can be a serious health problem, low blood pressure usually need not be a cause for concern or even treatment.

Blood pressures vary, depending on such factors as age, race, sex, and environment. On rare occasions, individuals may have medical problems that cause low blood pressure. Among such conditions are some types of heart disease, hormonal deficiencies, and malnutrition. In these cases, the hypotension will usually be corrected by the treatment of the medical problem.

Postural hypotension

Postural hypotension, or orthostatic hypotension, is a form of low blood pressure in which dizziness or faintness occurs when a person stands up abruptly from a sitting or reclining position.

Normally, when an individual stands up, the blood vessels contract to maintain normal blood pressure in the new position. However, in persons with postural hypotension, this mechanism probably does not work properly, and on standing, a temporary reduction in the blood flow to the brain leads to feeling faint. Rising slowly from a sitting or reclining position will usually prevent the symptoms in this situation.

Sometimes postural hypotension results from taking a medication for high blood pressure; in these cases, the physician can reduce the dosage or change the medication.

Fluids, including blood, lost from the body may also cause postural hypotension, as may many diseases. Consequently, although postural hypotension is a benign condition in most individuals, it should be reported to a physician.

Ischemia

Ischemia is a deficiency of blood in a specific part of the body caused by an obstruction of the blood vessels supplying that area. The obstruction may be due to narrowing, compression, or destruction of arteries caused by such conditions as blood clots and atherosclerosis (clogging of the arteries). The resultant oxygen deprivation, if prolonged, leads to tissue death in the affected area.

Ischemia in the brain

An ischemic attack in the brain occurs when the supply of blood to the brain is temporarily reduced. This type of attack resembles a stroke. If the brain is deprived of blood for more than several minutes, the result is irreversible brain damage and often death.

Ischemia in the heart

When the blood supply to the heart is reduced, angina pectoris results. When the blood supply to a region of the heart is cut off, a heart attack occurs. The lower the blood supply that gets through to the heart, the greater the severity of the attack. If a weakened heart is unable to pump an adequate supply of blood to the rest of the body, the other organs will also work at less than capacity.

Treatment

Transient ischemic attacks of the brain are often treated with aspirin or anticoagulant drugs. Angina pectoris is often treated with vasodilator medications, which temporarily widen, or dilate, the blood vessels. In many cases, surgery to remove or to bypass the obstruction is recommended.

Lymphocytes

Lymphocytes are a type of white blood cell. They are produced in the bone marrow and lymph nodes and stored in the thymus gland, spleen, and lymph nodes.

Lymphocytes play an important role in the body's immune system. Lymphocytes make their way through the lymph channels into the bloodstream, where they identify and "memorize" the characteristics of foreign elements called *antigens*. There are two types of lymphocytes—B cells and T cells. B cells manufacture antibodies (highly specialized proteins that destroy the antigens by combining with them). T cells, which make up 70 percent of the lymphocyte total, regulate antibody production and oversee immune responses.

Lymphocytes are the second most numerous type of white blood cell, normally constituting between 22 and 28 percent of the white blood cells in an adult's circulation. In cases of infection, especially those caused by viruses, the percentage of lymphocytes in the blood may increase to above 50 percent.

Pericarditis

Pericarditis is an inflammation of the pericardium (the membranous sac surrounding the heart). The inflammation is often accompanied by development of an effusion (a collection of fluid) between the membrane and the heart, which may lead to serious complications.

Causes

The inflammation commonly stems from an infection, such as bacterial pneumonia, tuberculosis, or a viral infection. Pericarditis can also occur in noninfectious diseases, such as connective tissue disorders and chronic kidney failure. Pericarditis sometimes follows a heart attack or chest injury.

Occasionally, long-term pericarditis arises from a chronic condition, most notably tuberculosis. The chronic inflammation causes thickening and contraction of the pericardium to the point that it restricts the heartbeat. Called *constrictive pericarditis,* this condition is no longer common because of the decrease in the incidence of tuberculosis. When constrictive pericarditis does occur, the condition is severe and calls for immediate attention.

Symptoms

Pain in the center of the chest (and possibly the shoulders, neck, and upper arms) that worsens with coughing, lying flat, or breathing and is relieved by leaning forward may signify pericarditis. Since this type of pain is a symptom of a number of serious illnesses, a doctor should be consulted about any severe chest pain.

Constrictive pericarditis is signaled by difficulty in breathing, swelling of the veins in the neck, and edema (fluid retention) in the legs and abdomen.

Diagnosis

A chest X ray, electrocardiogram, and blood tests, along with the person's medical history and a physical examination, are used to diagnose pericarditis. If an effusion is present, a sample of the fluid may be obtained to identify any infectious agent.

Treatment

When a large effusion exists, the motion of the heart may be restricted, thereby preventing it from filling and pumping effectively. This life-threatening condition must be corrected as soon as possible. The fluid may be drained by inserting a needle through the chest into the pericardial sac.

Once the underlying cause of pericarditis has been identified, the doctor can treat it (for example, by using dialysis in kidney failure or antibiotics for bacterial infection).

Constrictive pericarditis cannot be corrected without a surgical procedure, called *pericardiectomy,* to remove scarred tissue.

Platelets

Platelets (also called *thrombocytes*) are tiny, disk-shaped structures that play a critical role in the process of blood coagulation (clotting). They are manufactured in the bone marrow (soft tissue in the center of some bones) and usually survive for about ten days.

Role in coagulation

Blood coagulation is a complex process requiring the presence of many substances in the blood besides platelets. However, without platelets, coagulation would be impossible. Platelets initiate the coagulation process by aggregating (clumping together). The usual amount of time for adequate coagulation is five minutes or less.

The number of platelets per unit volume of blood plays an important role in proper platelet function. The normal number ranges between 200,000 and 500,000 platelets per cubic milliliter of blood.

Low platelet count

A low platelet count may be seen with many different diseases, including certain liver diseases, uncommon forms of anemia caused by vitamin deficiencies, and certain cancers (such as leukemia) of the blood-forming organs. Use of certain drugs also may cause a low platelet count.

A common cause of a low platelet count is destruction of platelets by the body's immune system. For some unknown reason, the immune system mistakenly identifies the platelets as foreign and forms antibodies to destroy them.

When a lack of platelets causes an increased tendency for bleeding, several types of treatment may be attempted, depending on the cause of the low platelet count. The usual method of immediately increasing the number of platelets in the blood is by transfusion (this procedure is generally reserved for patients with severe platelet deficiencies). Care must be taken to avoid increasing the platelet count too much, however, because emboli (clots that obstruct blood vessels) can develop.

Care should be taken by any patient whose platelet count is low, since bleeding will be prolonged and coagulation will not occur within normal time limits. For this reason, many physicians recommend that until normal platelet counts are attained, patients should not take aspirin and should avoid doing

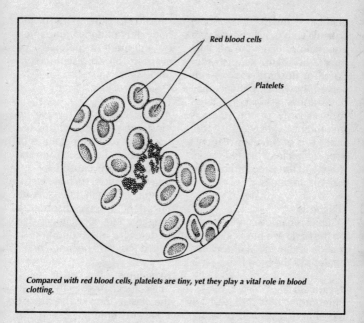

Compared with red blood cells, platelets are tiny, yet they play a vital role in blood clotting.

anything that may cause bleeding, such as vigorous toothbrushing, eating abrasive foods, and having enemas. They should also avoid contact sports and use caution regarding personal injury.

Polycythemia vera

Polycythemia vera is a relatively rare chronic disorder characterized by an increase in red blood cell mass and in the concentration of hemoglobin (the substance in red blood cells that carries oxygen).

Cause
The immediate cause of polycythemia is excessive production of red blood cells by the bone marrow, but the underlying cause remains unknown.

Symptoms
The initial symptoms include fatigue, difficulty in concentration, headache, drowsiness, for-

305

getfulness, and dizziness. Some patients with polycythemia vera complain of itching, especially after a hot bath. Reddish skin color, or flushing, may be observed; however, patients may have normal skin color, with redness only of the mucous membranes, especially the inner lids of the eyes. Patients may complain of blurred vision, ringing in the ears, and circulatory disturbances.

Diagnosis
Diagnosis can usually be made on the basis of a physical examination and medical history and analysis of the blood.

Treatment
Phlebotomy (withdrawal of blood from a vein) to offset the overproduction of red blood cells is probably the safest treatment because it does not interfere with the functioning of the bone marrow. Other treatments, such as drug therapy and radiation, are used when phlebotomy alone fails.

Raynaud disease

Raynaud disease involves spasms of the arterioles (small artery branches), especially in the fingers and hands and occa-

sionally in other parts of the body. It is often accompanied by intermittent paleness or cyanosis (bluish discoloration) of the skin.

Causes
Attacks of Raynaud disease are most often precipitated by exposure to cold temperatures or by emotional stress. When the symptoms are caused by another condition, such as scleroderma (a connective tissue disorder), a nerve disorder, a drug reaction, or pulmonary hypertension, the condition is called *Raynaud phenomenon*.

Symptoms
The color changes in the skin in the classic form of the disease come in three stages—pallor (extreme paleness), cyanosis, and then extreme redness, called *reactive hyperemia*. Sometimes the color changes may go through only two stages, cyanosis and then redness. Normal color and sensation are restored when the hands are warmed. Color changes in the hands do not affect the joints and seldom affect the thumb. Pain is usually not present, but numbness, tingling, and burning are common complaints. Ulcers (open sores) may appear on the tips of the fingers.

A wide range of other symptoms may be associated with Raynaud phenomenon, depending on the underlying disease process.

Treatment

Mild cases of Raynaud disease can be relieved substantially by protecting the body and extremities from exposure to cold. This is extremely important because prolonged spasm of the small arteries leads to severe tissue injury. Mild sedatives, taken orally, can sometimes be of help. The patient is strongly advised to stop smoking, since nicotine acts as a constrictor of blood vessels. Drugs known as *calcium-channel blockers,* such as nifedipine, verapamil, and diltiazem, are of great benefit in relieving symptoms but do not cure the condition.

A more extreme measure, which is not often used, is regional sympathectomy (an interruption of certain portions of the nerve pathways). This operation is reserved for patients with progressive disability; while it abolishes the symptoms, the relief may last only for a year or two. Results of the surgical procedure are usually better in patients with Raynaud disease than in those with Raynaud phenomenon.

Therapy for Raynaud phenomenon depends chiefly on correctly diagnosing and then treating the underlying disorder.

Restless legs syndrome

Restless legs syndrome is a feeling of uneasiness, shakiness, twitching, and restlessness that affects the legs after a patient has gone to bed for the night. Insomnia is almost always a result of the syndrome.

Causes

The precise cause of the syndrome is not known, although some authorities consider it to be brought about, or intensified, by poor blood circulation; others say that it can be brought about by intense physical activity just before bedtime. Restless leg syndrome has also been associated with iron and folate deficiencies, renal failure, and diabetes. The syndrome occurs in up to 25 percent of pregnant women.

Symptoms

The patient often has difficulty falling asleep in the evening because of an uncomfortable feeling or a jerking sensation within the legs, usually located in the thighs and calves. The discomfort is often relieved by moving about, but as a result, normal sleep is largely prevented. Consequently, the person may be excessively tired the next day.

Diagnosis

The diagnosis can generally be made on the basis of the patient's medical history and report of symptoms. The physician will perform a physical examination to rule out more serious disorders.

Treatment

Since the syndrome has been connected with circulatory disorders, drugs that increase the circulation to the lower extremities may prove helpful. A mild sedative at bedtime may also be useful.

Rheumatic fever

Rheumatic fever is the result of a bacterial disease characterized by inflammation, swelling, and soreness of the joints—especially the ankles, knees, and wrists—and inflammation of the heart. Occurring most commonly in children and adolescents, it is a serious illness that can result in permanent dam-

age to the heart. The attacks of fever can recur over a period of years and last from a few weeks to several months.

Cause

The disease is considered to be a complication of a streptococcal infection, such as strep throat; however, not all species of *Streptococcus* bacteria cause rheumatic fever. In some cases, the earlier infection may have been so minor that it cannot be recalled. Some researchers believe that rheumatic fever is an autoimmune disorder, in which the immune system forms antibodies to attack the body's own healthy tissues, such as those of the joints and the heart. The disease is more prevalent in some families than in others, but whether this indicates a hereditary factor or is due simply to sharing the same environment and living habits is not clear. Because only 1 percent of all cases of streptococcal infection in children and adolescents are followed by rheumatic fever, it is believed that a special susceptibility is involved.

Symptoms

Rheumatic fever should be immediately suspected when a child or teenager develops an unexplained fever with joint inflammation a few weeks after a throat infection or tonsillitis, even if that preceding condition was very mild. The joints then become inflamed one after another. A peculiar skin rash of large, reddened, nonitchy areas with irregular borders develops, lasting a day or two. Nodules may emerge over the elbows, kneecaps, and other bony prominences; they may also form within the heart. Chorea (involuntary movement of the limbs and facial features) may occur if the infection spreads to involve the brain. Fortunately, chorea leaves no lasting brain damage and passes after some time.

Effects on the heart

The acute stage of joint involvement leaves no permanent deformity or crippling, but damage to the heart is permanent when it involves destruction of heart valve tissue. Scar tissue is then eventually formed on the valves, so that they cannot open and close properly. The heart, unable to efficiently carry out its function of pumping blood through the circulatory system, must work harder and thus becomes enlarged. Blood clots may form on its inner lining and may be carried in the blood throughout the body, often lodging in a blood vessel and blocking it.

Diagnosis

Joint inflammation, heart abnormalities, chorea, and the appearance of the rash and the nodules are the most common manifestations of rheumatic fever, but these signs may appear alone or in a number of different combinations. Because no single laboratory finding or symptom is common to all cases of rheumatic fever, the diagnosis is made presumptively on the basis of the total clinical picture.

Treatment

The chief treatment for rheumatic fever is the use of antibiotics for an extended period to eliminate any remaining *Streptococcus* bacteria. Aspirin is commonly used to bring down fever and relieve inflammation and pain. Corticosteroid drugs are sometimes given if there are signs of heart involvement, and sedatives may be prescribed if chorea becomes severe. The long periods of bed rest that were once recommended are now believed to be unnecessary, although bed rest during acute attacks may be prescribed. Seriously damaged heart valves can often be repaired surgically or replaced by artificial valves. Long-term penicillin therapy is given to recovering rheumatic fever patients to prevent recurrent strep infections.

Prevention

The only preventive measure is prompt diagnosis and treatment of all streptococcal infections, especially those involving the throat and ears. Since dental procedures can sometimes be a source of bacterial infection, special precautions (such as the administration of antibiotics) may be taken for persons whose heart valves have been injured.

Rheumatic heart disease

Rheumatic heart disease is a variety of abnormal cardiac conditions, including heart valve scarring and endocarditis (inflammation of the lining of the heart).

Cause

This disease is a potential aftermath of rheumatic fever, once one of the prime killers of children. Rheumatic fever may cause inflammation of the heart valves and scarring of the valve leaflets. This scarring can result in valve leakage, allowing blood to flow backward, or severe narrowing of the valve, restricting blood flow out of the heart.

Symptoms

The most common symptom is a heart murmur, caused by abnormal blood flow across a scarred valve. There may be hemorrhaging (excessive bleeding) and impairment of vision if microscopic blood clots that have formed in the heart block tiny blood vessels in the eye. Kidney function may deteriorate in middle or later life. Muscle shrinkage due to inactivity may be accompanied by lack of muscular and cardiovascular endurance. Irregular pulse, shortness of breath, and fainting spells are also common symptoms.

Treatment

Many people who have suffered rheumatic heart disease have gone on to live extremely active lives, despite heart murmurs, heart enlargement, and damaged valves. Although rheumatic heart disease is a serious matter, regular exercise, a sensible diet, and determination can mean the difference between a sedentary and an active life.

Supervision by a physician is a necessity for anyone who suffers from rheumatic heart disease and wants to embark on a regular exercise program. In some cases, however, it may be impossible for a patient to participate in vigorous physical activity, especially if the heart damage is advanced or severe. For some of these individuals, surgery to implant an artificial valve can offer relief.

People with rheumatic heart disease must consult their physicians about antibiotic treatment before undergoing any dental or surgical procedures.

Rh factor

Rh factor refers to a specific antigen present in the blood. (*Rh* is derived from the name of the rhesus monkey, in which the factor was discovered.) An antigen is a substance that can induce the production of antibodies, which are crucial to the functioning of the body's immune system. Rh-positive blood has the antigen on its red cells; Rh-negative blood does not. An estimated 85 percent of the population has Rh-positive blood; that is to say, they possess Rh antigens.

Dangers of anti-Rh antibodies
Blood normally has no anti-Rh antibodies. Anti-Rh antibodies can develop in Rh-negative blood, however, if Rh-positive blood is introduced into the bloodstream. This can come about in two ways: if a person with Rh-negative blood receives a transfusion of Rh-positive blood or if a woman with Rh-negative blood conceives a child with Rh-positive blood (inherited from the father) and some of the Rh-positive cells from the fetus find their way into the bloodstream of the mother. In either case, the Rh-positive red blood cells will stimulate the mother's body to form anti-Rh antibodies. If this happens, the blood will form clumps, and a potentially lethal situation will develop—the clumps may block blood vessels.

If difficulties do not appear with the formation of these antibodies during the first transfusion or the first pregnancy, they will surely appear if Rh-positive blood is ever again introduced into the person's bloodstream. The antibodies are already present, and the introduction of additional Rh-positive blood will result in a mobilization of existing antibodies and the production of even more. In addition to clumping of blood, other problems will arise. For example, hemolysis (the breakdown of red blood cells and release of their hemoglobin) will make it impossible for those cells to carry oxygen, resulting in anemia.

There are potential dangers to the fetus if the mother's blood contains anti-Rh antibodies. If the fetus has Rh-positive cells, anti-Rh antibodies may pass through the placenta from the mother's bloodstream and cause hemolysis of the fetus's blood cells. Once born, the baby may need to have massive, possibly even total, transfusions of Rh-negative blood to prevent clumping of the red blood cells and hemolytic anemia. This situation is now relatively rare because injections of gamma-globulin are routinely given to an Rh-negative mother after every pregnancy. These injections inhibit the formation of the potentially dangerous antibodies.

Stroke

Stroke is a nervous system disorder of abrupt onset caused by interruption of the blood supply to an area of the brain, resulting in malfunction or loss of function in those parts of the body that the damaged area controls. Generally speaking, each side of the brain controls the motor and sensory functions of the opposite side of the body (for example, damage to cells on the left side of the brain will impair function on the right side of the body). Stroke can have a wide range of consequences, among them temporary or permanent loss of memory and difficulty in speaking, walking, and controlling emotions.

Causes

Stroke can be caused by several conditions. One is called *cerebrovascular embolism*, which occurs when a blood clot formed elsewhere in the body (usually in the heart or in one of the carotid arteries in the neck) lodges itself in an artery in the brain or leading to the brain. Interruption of blood flow also occurs when a clot is formed in the arteries that supply blood to the brain, usually due to atherosclerosis (clogging of the arteries).

Stroke can also be caused by cerebral hemorrhage, in which a diseased artery in the brain bursts, depriving the cells that are normally nourished by that artery and flooding the surrounding tissue with blood. This accumulation of blood forms a clot, which displaces and compresses brain tissue and thus interferes with brain function. This type of stroke often afflicts people who have both hypertension (high blood pressure) and atherosclerosis.

A third condition that can lead to stroke is rupture of an aneurysm (a bulge in an artery because of a defect in its wall), which interrupts blood flow to an area of the brain and floods the area with blood. The formation of aneurysms is sometimes associated with hypertension. Congenital (present at birth) aneurysms are often the cause of cerebral hemorrhage in young people.

Those at risk

People who have both hypertension and atherosclerosis are the most likely to suffer a stroke, since both diseases weaken and damage the arteries. Hypertension probably also encourages hemorrhage. Heredity may play a role in stroke, since the tendencies to develop both hypertension and atherosclerosis appear to be inherited. Black people are more susceptible to stroke, because high blood pressure is about twice as common in the black population as it is in the white population.

Smoking, diabetes, and high blood cholesterol levels may also contribute to stroke. Stroke is more likely to occur if there is a history of mild strokelike episodes called *transient ischemic attacks (TIAs)*, which are like mild strokes that clear up within 24 hours, leaving no residual effects.

Symptoms

A stroke can present itself in many ways, but some of the more common symptoms are sudden weakness or numbness in the face, arm, and leg on one side of the body; loss or slurring of speech or difficulty in understanding others; unexplained unsteadiness; and persistent falling to one side. It is possible for an individual to suffer a mild stroke and experience minor degrees of these symptoms.

Diagnosis

Stroke is diagnosed mostly from one's medical history and a physical examination. Sophisticated X-ray techniques are also employed. For example, angiography will show damage or clots in the arteries in the brain or leading to the brain. In this procedure, a thin catheter (tube) is inserted into an artery in the arm or leg and advanced to the site to be studied; a spe-

313

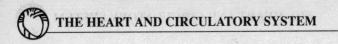

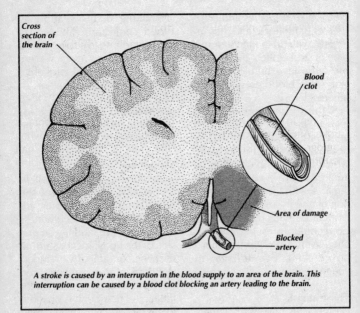

Cross section of the brain

Blood clot

Area of damage

Blocked artery

A stroke is caused by an interruption in the blood supply to an area of the brain. This interruption can be caused by a blood clot blocking an artery leading to the brain.

cial dye is then injected through the catheter to outline the area so that X-ray studies may be taken.

Computed tomography provides cross-sectional images that may indicate whether the stroke was caused by a hemorrhage or by blockage of blood flow. Tumors (abnormal tissue growths), which can cause symptoms identical to those of stroke, are also frequently diagnosed by these means. Magnetic resonance (MR) imaging provides very clear images of

the brain without the use of X rays.

Treatment
Treatment of stroke begins with immediate hospitalization. Blood pressure is normalized, and drug therapy to prevent further damage and to reduce swelling of the brain tissue is often begun. Anticoagulants (drugs that inhibit the clotting of blood) are sometimes administered in the hope of limiting the progress of the stroke or preventing other strokes. After the

acute period, rehabilitation is begun by speech, physical, and occupational therapists.

Prevention

For those who have experienced TIAs or other warning signs of stroke, precautions can be taken to prevent an actual stroke. After a TIA, some form of angiography or MRI is usually performed to locate obstructions or ulcerated areas of the arteries supplying blood to the head. Depending on the results of the angiogram, the general condition of the patient, and many other factors, surgery to "clean out" the arteries or treatment with anticoagulants or other medications may be elected.

Prevention of stroke mainly involves control of high blood pressure and other risk factors, such as smoking and high cholesterol intake.

Thrombocytopenia

Thrombocytopenia is a disorder characterized by a decrease in the number of platelets in the blood. Platelets are tiny components of the blood that act to promote clotting when there is an injury or another problem that requires bleeding to be stopped. Normally, about five to ten times the number of platelets needed for clotting circulate in the bloodstream; this amounts to about 200,000 to 500,000 per cubic milliliter. In general, thrombocytopenia is considered to be present when the platelet count is less than 100,000. Abnormal bleeding commonly does not occur, however, until the count is less than 50,000, and serious or unprovoked bleeding usually does not occur with counts above 20,000.

Causes

There are basically two mechanisms whereby thrombocytopenia occurs: decreased production of platelets and increased destruction of platelets. In the former, the elements in the bone marrow responsible for the production of platelets may malfunction or be severely diminished. Increased destruction of platelets occurs in essential, or idiopathic (of unknown cause), thrombocytopenia. In this disorder, which is most common in children, antibodies are made against the person's own platelets, thereby causing their destruction. Thrombocytopenia can also be due to the use of some medications. Severe, overwhelming infection can also cause increased destruction of platelets. In pregnancy, platelets from the fetus can sometimes enter the circulation of the mother, causing antibody formation and the destruction of fetal platelets, creating abnormal bleeding in the newborn.

Symptoms

An obvious sign of thrombocytopenia is a rash of reddish to reddish-purple spots. These are due to bleeding within and underneath the skin. Abnormal or easily provoked bleeding is the most dangerous symptom of thrombocytopenia. This bleeding may be minor, such as oozing from the gums while simply brushing the teeth or bruising caused by merely leaning on or brushing up against something.

The bleeding of thrombocytopenia can be much more serious, however, as in spontaneous internal bleeding, which, in some cases, may go unrecognized until the individual goes into shock (collapse of the circulatory system).

Diagnosis

Laboratory evaluation of the blood is the basis of a diagnosis of thrombocytopenia. Examination of a sample of bone marrow may also be performed.

Treatment

Treatment depends on the cause. If infection is present, this must be remedied; usually, the platelet count will then return to normal on its own. In essential thrombocytopenia, corticosteroids (cortisone or prednisone) are the initial treatment. In drug-induced thrombocytopenia, the first step is generally to discontinue the drug. This will usually result in improvement; if not, corticosteroids may be helpful. In severe immune thrombocytopenia of the newborn, exchange transfusion (whereby all or most of the blood is exchanged with transfused blood) may be necessary. If the platelet count on any of these conditions is dangerously low (around 20,000), transfusion of platelets may be indicated until the disease process has been controlled.

Prevention

Thrombocytopenia may not be preventable in most cases, but early recognition of symptoms, such as rash and easy bleeding, may lead to prevention of the disorder's serious complications.

Thrombo-phlebitis

Thrombophlebitis is a condition in which a blood clot exists in a vein at the same time that the vein is inflamed. There are many different factors that can lead to the development of such a condition. For example, when a person is immobilized for a long period of time, as is the case in prolonged bed rest or paralysis, blood stagnates in the veins of the legs. Ordinarily, the movement of muscles in the leg aids in returning blood to the heart, but without this help, the blood has a tendency to pool. Stagnation induces the blood to begin clotting as it would in an injury. This clotting, in turn, prevents even more blood from being able to return to the heart. The blood below the clot remains there, and the buildup of pressure causes fluid to be squeezed out of the blood vessels and into the surrounding tissue. These tissues swell with the fluid, and the veins in the area become inflamed and very tender. Partly because of their distance and position relative to the heart muscle, the deep veins of the legs are the vessels most often involved, but thrombophlebitis can also occur in the veins of the pelvis and arms.

Thrombophlebitis itself may not be too serious, but it can lead to other conditions that are life-threatening. If the clot formed in a deep vein of the leg breaks off and travels through the bloodstream, it can cause major complications elsewhere. Because blood returned to the heart is immediately sent to the lungs to pick up oxygen and drop off carbon dioxide, any clot travelling up from a leg vein can become lodged in a small vessel of the lung, causing what is called a *pulmonary embolism*. A pulmonary embolism can lead to chest pain, shortness of breath, coughing up of blood, and even death.

Causes

The development of thrombophlebitis is precipitated by any condition that inhibits the free flow of blood through the veins, such as prolonged bed rest or inactivity, perhaps following illness or surgery; congestive heart failure, which affects the ability of the heart to pump blood throughout the body; and injury or infection that damages a vein. Other factors that may lead to thrombophlebitis are pregnancy, the use of birth control pills by susceptible individuals, occupations that require long periods of standing or sitting, obesity, old age, and chronic infections. Thrombophlebitis may indicate the presence of a blood disorder or a tumor in the pancreas or lung.

Symptoms

Symptoms of deep-vein thrombophlebitis (which often appear only in advanced cases) are swelling, aching, and a feeling of heaviness in the leg or affected area. The skin may appear white and will be painful to the touch. If the veins of the leg are affected, the condition is characterized by increased pain when walking or when the foot is flexed backward or forward.

Diagnosis

Thrombophlebitis of a surface vein (known as *superficial thrombophlebitis*) can be diagnosed by a simple physical examination, which usually reveals a red, warm, tender cord-like vein.

Diagnostic tests for thrombophlebitis include Doppler imaging (a technique used to detect obstructions by changes in the sounds made by flowing blood), nuclear medicine scans, plethysmography (a test to measure the resistance to blood flow in the veins), and venography. Venography involves the injection of a special dye into the veins so that a clot, if present can be seen on an X ray. This is the most sensitive and specific test for thrombophlebitis.

Treatment

Treatment of the superficial form of thrombophlebitis usually begins with bed rest with elevation of the leg. Warm compresses are also helpful, as are anti-inflammatory drugs. Superficial thrombophlebitis rarely, if ever, leads to pulmonary embolism.

Deep-vein thrombophlebitis, because of the potential for pulmonary embolism, is treated much more aggressively. The patient is usually hospitalized and put on bed rest with the leg elevated. Heparin (an anticoagulant that inhibits the normal clotting mechanism of the blood) is given intravenously, usually for about seven days (up to ten days if pulmonary embolism has occurred). The patient is also usually given the oral anticoagulant warfarin for about six weeks (three to six months if pulmonary embolism has occurred). These drugs do not dissolve an existing clot but serve to prevent new clots from

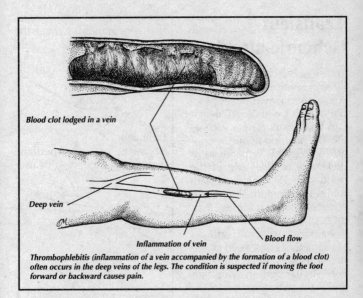

Blood clot lodged in a vein

Deep vein

Inflammation of vein

Blood flow

Thrombophlebitis (inflammation of a vein accompanied by the formation of a blood clot) often occurs in the deep veins of the legs. The condition is suspected if moving the foot forward or backward causes pain.

forming while the old ones are resolving. Newer drugs do dissolve clots but are still used only in special situations.

Prevention

Prevention of thrombophlebitis is a controversial subject. In hospitalized patients who are immobilized for long periods or who are about to undergo major surgery, doing leg exercises, wearing long support stockings or compression boots (soft plastic bags or sacks that are wrapped around the legs and rapidly inflated and deflated), and increasing activity as soon as feasible may be helpful.

Low-dose heparin therapy has also been beneficial in preventing deep-vein thrombophlebitis in certain patients.

For nonhospitalized patients who are susceptible to thrombophlebitis, regularly exercising the legs, elevating the legs when lying down, and wearing support hose may be helpful. In some cases the physician may also prescribe anticoagulant drugs such as heparin or warfarin.

319

Transient ischemic attacks

Transient ischemic attacks (TIAs) are temporary lapses in some aspect of neurologic functioning. This neurologic deficit can take many forms, such as the loss of vision in one eye, inability to speak, or paralysis or weakness of one side of the body. All TIAs have certain things in common: They occur suddenly and last for less than 24 hours.

Transient ischemic attacks are sometimes described as "little strokes." Indeed, they are very similar both in symptoms and in the factors that contribute to their occurrence. Strokes also impair neurologic function, sometimes causing symptoms such as loss of vision and paralysis. And both are caused by a lack of blood supply to part of the brain. However, TIAs, because they are temporary, do not do any discernable lasting damage to brain functioning to the extent that strokes can.

TIAs are usually a major predictor of future strokes. If left untreated, the factors that led to the TIA can lead to a major stroke, resulting in permanent damage to the area of the brain that is affected.

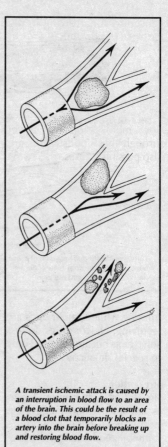

A transient ischemic attack is caused by an interruption in blood flow to an area of the brain. This could be the result of a blood clot that temporarily blocks an artery into the brain before breaking up and restoring blood flow.

Causes

Transient ischemic attacks are probably due to a temporary interruption in blood flow to an area of the brain. They can be caused by a narrowing in the carotid arteries (the arteries in the neck that supply the brain with oxygenated blood). This narrowing is usually due to the presence of atherosclerosis (clogging of the arteries). Blood vessel spasms and showers of tiny emboli (clots that travel through the bloodstream) are also possible causes.

Symptoms

The symptoms of TIAs are both varied and frightening to the victim. They can include weakness on one side of the face, numbness in various parts of the body, blindness in one eye, weakness in the arms or legs on one side, difficulty in speaking and understanding speech, and a prickling ("pins and needles") sensation in parts of the body. Vertigo (a sensation of spinning) combined with any of these or other symptoms can also be due to TIAs, but this is only a rare occurrence. Fainting spells alone and light-headedness are usually not due to TIAs.

Diagnosis

The first step in diagnosis is a complete examination, including a medical history and physical, neurologic, and eye examinations. Bruits (noises caused by narrowing in an artery) may be heard in a carotid artery. Detailed testing, commonly with angiography, is performed to pinpoint the problem. In this procedure, a thin catheter is inserted into an artery in the arm or leg and advanced to the site to be studied; a special dye is then injected through the catheter to outline the area so that X rays may be taken. An ultrasonic examination of the carotid arteries can determine if disease (narrowing) is present.

Treatment

Treatment of TIAs is aimed at preventing more TIAs and stroke. There are two basic methods of treatment: medical, with anticoagulant drugs; and surgical, with the opening and "cleaning out" of the obstructed arteries. Anticoagulation is usually done with aspirin or heparin and warfarin. Whether medication or surgery is more effective in preventing further TIAs or a stroke is dependent on many factors and is a subject of considerable controversy.

Varicose veins

Varicose veins are swollen, stretched veins in the legs, close to the surface of the skin, caused by pooling of blood. Varicose veins alone are not too serious, but they may lead to a more serious condition, such as a skin ulcer, phlebitis (inflammation of a vein), or thrombosis (blood clot formation).

Causes

Blood from the legs must return to the heart uphill, against the force of gravity, so the veins in the legs have one-way valves to prevent blood from flowing back down toward the feet. When pressure on the veins stretches them or when the valves are injured in some way, the valves cannot close properly, and some blood travels back down. This blood accumulates in pools, which stretch the veins even more.

Varicose veins are caused by a number of factors that put excess pressure on the veins in the legs: prolonged standing; prolonged sitting, especially with the legs crossed; lack of exercise; confining clothes; obesity (which puts excess pressure on the legs and contributes to the inability of the muscles to push blood upward); heredity (a tendency toward weak vein walls and valves seems to be inherited); and even height (tall people may be more susceptible

because their blood needs to travel farther in its return trip to the heart).

In general, women are more susceptible to varicose veins than men, largely due to hormonal factors. Pregnancy accentuates this difference because special hormones released at this time tend to relax the walls of the veins. Also, varicose veins often appear during the last few months of pregnancy due to the increased strain from the weight of the growing uterus. The varicose veins may recede, however, after the birth of the baby.

Symptoms

Varicose veins are very noticeable since they form close to the skin. They appear as bulging, bluish, cordlike lines running down the legs. Symptoms that accompany varicose veins are feelings of achiness, heaviness, and fatigue in the legs, especially at the end of the day; itchy, scaly skin covering the affected areas; and, in advanced cases, swollen ankles, pain shooting down the leg, and leg cramps at night.

Diagnosis

Diagnosis can most often be made on the basis of physical examination, because the af-

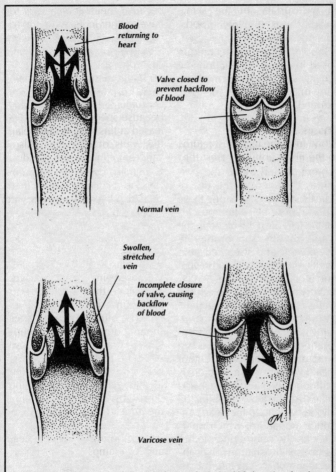

Blood returning to heart

Valve closed to prevent backflow of blood

Normal vein

Swollen, stretched vein

Incomplete closure of valve, causing backflow of blood

Varicose vein

The drawing at the top shows the interior of a normal vein, in which the action of a valve prevents blood returning to the heart from flowing backward. In the drawing of a varicose vein, the valve has been weakened and cannot completely close, causing the blood to accumulate.

fected superficial veins can be readily seen. If involvement of deeper veins is suspected, Doppler imaging (a technique used to detect obstructions by changes in the sounds made by flowing blood) may be performed.

Treatment

Varicose veins can be treated in a number of ways. The most common, and by far the simplest, treatment is the use of elastic stockings. Wearing these special hose helps the muscles of the legs push the blood in the veins up. By supporting the weakened and stretched vein walls, they also help to prevent the blood from pooling.

Very severe cases of varicose veins can be treated by surgery. A procedure called *vein stripping* is very effective. In this operation, the affected veins are tied off and removed. Other, healthy veins whose structure is still sound pick up the slack and take over the job of pushing the blood back up to the heart. Another procedure, which operates on the same principle but is not so invasive, involves injecting a chemical into the affected veins, closing them off and forcing the blood to find other channels back to the heart. The advantage of the lat-

ter treatment is that the varicose veins need not be removed but rather remain in the body without any pooled blood to make them swell.

Those with varicose veins may need to lose weight, exercise regularly, and stretch their legs or put their feet up whenever possible. Exercises to improve circulation in the legs may help relieve pressure.

In many cases, varicose veins tend to recur, particularly if adequate preventive measures are not taken.

THE DIGESTIVE SYSTEM

Digestion is the process by which the body converts food into basic substances that can be either absorbed in the bloodstream as nutrients or passed out of the body as waste. This process of breakdown and assimilation occurs within the digestive tract, a convoluted tube more than 30 feet long that is lined with a mucous membrane. The tract includes several hollow organs—the mouth, esophagus, stomach, small intestine, and large intestine—each of which has a specific function in digestion. The muscles of these organs move the food through the system, while mucus lubricates the tract and prevents irritation. The liver and pancreas are also critical organs in digestion. While not an essential organ, the gallbladder is involved in digestion as well.

Food first enters the digestive tract through the mouth. Movement of the jaws allows the teeth to cut and grind the food into smaller pieces, which are mixed with saliva (a secretion of the glands in the mouth). Saliva moistens food for easier swallowing and contains an enzyme (a special type of protein) that begins the chemical breakdown of starches.

From the mouth, food passes down the throat and into the esophagus, the muscular tube through which the food is conducted to the stomach. The stomach is a large pouch in the abdominal cavity, where food is combined with acid- and enzyme-containing digestive juices secreted by glands located within the stomach walls.

The food becomes semifluid, which allows it to pass easily into the small intestine. The small intestine consists of three portions—the upper section, or *duodenum*; the middle section, or *jejunum*; and the lower section, or the *ileum.*

In the duodenum, digestive juices from the liver and pancreas continue the process of breaking down the food into its constituent nutrients, which can then be absorbed into the

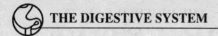

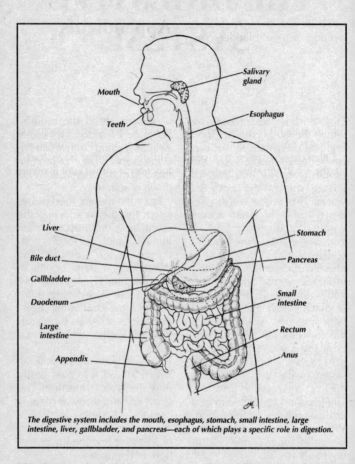

The digestive system includes the mouth, esophagus, stomach, small intestine, large intestine, liver, gallbladder, and pancreas—each of which plays a specific role in digestion.

bloodstream throughout the remainder of the small intestine. The liver aids digestion by producing bile, which is necessary for absorption of fat in the small intestine.

The gallbladder, which can be found on the underside of the liver, is another organ that performs an indirect digestive function. The gallbladder stores the bile that has been manufactured by the liver. As bile is needed, the gallbladder contracts and releases the fluid into the duodenum. If it becomes necessary for the gallbladder to be removed for medical reasons (such as in severe gallbladder disease), however, the liver can compensate for its role, and digestion is not hindered.

Other digestive juices required by the small intestine to digest and absorb food, particularly fats and starches, come from the pancreas, an organ located just behind the stomach. The pancreas also secretes insulin and other hormones into the blood. Insulin is the hormone responsible for aiding absorption and use of glucose.

Whatever substances are not assimilated into the bloodstream through the small intestine move into the large intestine. Within the large intestine, waste material is processed into stool (feces), and water and certain chemicals are absorbed into the bloodstream to preserve the body's fluid balance.

The fecal matter continues to move through the colon to the rectum. Once in the rectum, waste is ready to be passed out of the body through the anus (the opening at the end of the digestive tract), thus completing the process of digestion.

Appendicitis

Appendicitis is an inflammation of the appendix, most frequently caused by some type of hard material getting lodged at its tip.

The appendix is a small pouch located at the juncture of the small and large intestines. Although it may have had a function at some point in evolutionary development, the appendix serves no purpose now.

Causes

Despite its uselessness, the appendix can cause problems when it becomes inflamed. Inflammation occurs when the hollow, tubular structure becomes clogged with masses of waste matter, intestinal worms, or other material that can prevent normal drainage. The blockage provides a fertile environment for bacteria to grow and multiply, causing infection and inflammation.

Symptoms

In the beginning, appendicitis may produce a dull or sharp pain in the navel area of the abdomen. Any movement, such as coughing or sneezing, can intensify the pain. In early stages, patients may also feel nauseated and may be unable to eat.

327

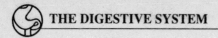

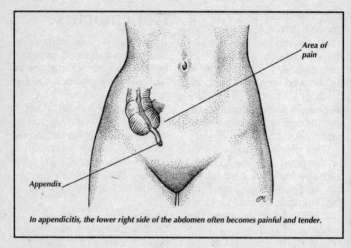

In appendicitis, the lower right side of the abdomen often becomes painful and tender.

Constipation can accompany appendicitis; however, about 10 percent of patients have diarrhea instead. Adults may run a mild fever (up to 101°F), but children generally experience higher fevers. Occasionally, the pulse rate accelerates to about 100 beats per minute.

Within hours, the pain moves to the lower right side of the abdomen over the appendix and becomes continuous. Because the location of the appendix may vary from one individual to another, pain may emanate from the back, side, or pelvis— or even from the opposite side of the abdomen. Soon the entire area around the appendix becomes extremely tender as the abdominal muscles begin to tighten.

As the fever rises and the pain grows more intense, chances of rupture also become greater. Rupture results when the appendix becomes so swollen and filled with pus that it bursts, spreading infection to surrounding organs. One serious complication that may result from rupture is peritonitis (inflammation of the lining of the abdominal cavity).

Any fever with nausea and abdominal pain should be reported to a physician. More severe pain is an immediate medical emergency that must be evaluated and treated to prevent potential complications.

Appendicitis can affect anyone, but the disease is more prevalent among people between 10 and 30 years of age.

Diagnosis

When confirming appendicitis, the doctor checks for tenderness over the appendix. A blood test determines whether there is an elevated white blood cell count (in response to infection, the body produces extra white blood cells to help fight the disease). The doctor may perform additional tests to rule out disorders sometimes mistaken for appendicitis, such as inflammation of the gallbladder, kidney stones, or a kidney infection. In women, a twisted ovarian cyst (the formation on an ovary of a sac filled with fluid or semisolid material) or a ruptured ectopic pregnancy (a pregnancy that develops outside the uterus) may produce symptoms that are similar in appearance to those of appendicitis.

Treatment

Although appendicitis cannot be prevented, prompt diagnosis can lead to effective treatment. Patients who suspect appendicitis should not eat, drink, or take drugs to relieve pain until a doctor has been consulted. Eating or drinking any substance, especially taking a laxative, will stimulate activity in the intestine, which may cause the appendix to rupture.

The most common treatment for acute appendicitis is surgery to remove the inflamed organ. To ensure against further infection, antibiotics may also be prescribed after surgery.

Bile

Bile is a fluid produced by the liver, stored in the gallbladder, and discharged into the small intestine, where it helps in the digestion of food, particularly fats. Bile is made up of water, salts, bile acids, cholesterol, and lecithin (a fatty acid).

Functions

Bile acts like a detergent to break down fat in the intestine into tiny globules that can be dissolved and suspended in water; the tiny globules can then pass through the walls of the small intestine into the bloodstream. The bile salts are also absorbed through the walls of the intestine but are returned to the liver to form new bile. The yellow-green or golden color of bile is due to the pigments bilirubin and biliverdin.

Bilirubin is a yellow pigment derived from decomposed red blood cells. Biliverdin is a green pigment derived from conversion of bilirubin by a chemical reaction. These pigments are also responsible for some of the color of body wastes.

Bile is produced continuously in the liver and passes through ducts to be stored in the gallbladder until mealtime, at which time it is emptied into the duodenum. Digestive disturbances result if the flow of bile is stopped or reduced, either because of a liver disorder or because a duct has been blocked by inflammation or a gallstone (a solid mass of material usually composed of calcium, cholesterol, bilirubin, or a combination thereof) formed in the gallbladder. Any of these conditions can also cause jaundice, in which the pigments bilirubin and biliverdin accumulate in the blood. Jaundice, although not a disease in itself, shows up as yellow staining of the skin, eyes, and body fluids.

Cholecystitis

Cholecystitis is an inflammation of the gallbladder. The gallbladder is a small, pear-shaped organ that stores the bile produced by the liver and releases it as needed to help digest foods—particularly fats—in the small intestine. Cholecystitis may be either acute (sudden and severe) or chronic (recurring but less severe).

Acute cholecystitis

In about 90 percent of cases, acute cholecystitis results when the outlet of the gallbladder or the duct leading from it is plugged by a gallstone. A gallstone is formed in the gallbladder from cholesterol, calcium, bile pigments, or a combination of these substances. Unless the stone becomes dislodged, inflammation and pressure build up behind it. In severe cases, the swollen gallbladder may not receive enough blood, resulting in tissue death. The gallbladder may become gangrenous or perforated, causing bile to spill into the abdominal cavity. An abscess (a collection of pus within a cavity) usually forms, and bacteria may colonize the region. Occasionally, the resulting leakage of infected bile causes peritonitis (an inflammation of the lining of the abdominal cavity). However, not all gallbladder attacks progress to this extreme; they may subside only to recur later. Cholecystitis can also result from a blockage caused by enlargement of the veins in the common bile duct, which the gallbladder shares with the liver.

Acute cholecystitis often begins after a meal rich in fats, such as one containing fried foods, chocolate, or cream. The individual may awaken in the middle of the night with indigestion, gas, and a sharp pain in the upper right quarter of the abdomen, which is often hard and sensitive to the touch. Pain may also be felt in the middle of the abdomen and may spread to the tip of the right shoulder blade. The pain is crampy and severe. Vomiting is likely and provides some relief. If fever is present, infection of the gallbladder or bile duct is likely. If jaundice (yellowing of the skin, caused by bile pigment in the blood) is present, the symptoms are probably due to blockage of the common bile duct by a gallstone or tumor.

Nuclear medicine scanning confirms the diagnosis of cholecystitis. In this procedure, a radioactive material is administered, and its distribution in the affected area is recorded on X-ray film. X-ray examination and ultrasonography, a technique that uses sound waves to create images of internal structures, may also be used to confirm the diagnosis and to locate gallstones.

Treatment of an acute attack may include rest, intravenous feeding, painkilling drugs, and antibiotics. Because attacks are likely to recur, however, the usual solution is surgical removal of the gallbladder. This is often done immediately. Removal of the gallbladder does not hinder the digestive process, since the liver can compensate for the lost organ.

The mere presence of gallstones found incidentally during tests for other problems does not always mean that surgery is necessary, however. In many cases, gallstones can be present for life without ever causing acute cholecystitis.

The gallbladder can now be removed without the standard incision. Instead a periscope-like instrument called a laparoscope is inserted through a puncture in the abdominal wall. After the laparoscope is inserted, a laser is used to free the gallbladder from its bed underneath the liver. The gallbladder is then removed through the puncture by suction. Laparoscopy has shortened hospital stays and decreased complications from surgery. In addition, instead of having a large scar, the patient usually has only four small puncture marks. This procedure is not for everyone with gallbladder problems, however. Individuals who have had numerous abdominal surgeries are usually not candidates for the procedure. Furthermore, if the attempted laparoscope surgery proves to be unsuccessful, the standard incision may need to be made anyway.

Nonsurgical methods for removing gallstones, including drug and chemical therapy and lithotripsy (the use of shock waves to shatter the stones), have been tried with varying degrees of success. The criteria for using these methods, however, is very strict; surgical removal of the gallbladder is still the method of choice in most cases.

Chronic cholecystitis

Chronic cholecystitis is a continued inflammation of the gallbladder, with repeated attacks over time that are similar to, but milder than, those of acute cholecystitis. Gallstones are usually present; whether they develop before or after the emergence of the disease is unknown. The causes of chronic cholecystitis are not entirely understood, although occasionally bacterial infection is the reason. Diet, heredity, and hormones also appear to be involved, and chronic cholecystitis is more likely to affect women than men.

The pains of chronic cholecystitis commonly appear over the pit of the stomach and in the upper right quarter of the abdomen. They may range in intensity from mild to unbearable. The pains are crampy and usually come on suddenly, but they may be separated by pain-free intervals of 15 minutes to an hour. The pains may disappear after several minutes or continue for several hours; the average attack lasts about an hour. Although the pains may appear together with nausea, gas, and belching and may occur after eating fatty foods, these indications may not be directly related to the disease.

Diagnosis of chronic cholecystitis is based on the symptoms and can be confirmed by the same studies used for diagnosis of acute cholecystitis—nuclear medicine scanning and ultrasonography. The doctor must make a careful investigation of other possible causes of the symptoms, including peptic ulcer (which occurs in the stomach or in the beginning of the small intestine), inflammation of the pancreas, and bowel disease.

The ideal way to treat chronic cholecystitis is to remove the gallbladder, together with any gallstones in the duct leading from the liver to the duodenum (the first part of the small intestine). If it is not clear that the symptoms are caused by gallbladder inflammation, or if the patient cannot withstand an operation, other methods are used. These include a low-fat diet, weight reduction, and use of medications.

As with acute cholecystitis, the use of medication, chemicals, or lithotripsy (shock waves that shatter stones) to get rid of the stones has very strict criteria, and in most cases, surgical removal of the gallbladder is still the treatment method of choice.

Cirrhosis

Cirrhosis is a disease in which the cells throughout the liver are progressively destroyed. The liver tissue is replaced by areas with normal new cells as well as scar tissue, which alters the structure of the organ. The flow of blood and lymph through the damaged liver is much less efficient, and eventually the liver fails.

Causes
Cirrhosis represents an attempt by the liver to rebuild itself and continue despite injury. The injury may be a sudden and massive infection, as in acute hepatitis, or it may occur in a less dramatic manner over a period of months or years, as in chronic active hepatitis or obstruction of the bile ducts within the liver. The process of obstruction starts with inflammation and progresses to scarring and then closure of the ducts. A similar condition is caused by obstruction of the external bile ducts by a stone, scar, inborn defect, or tumor. The damage can also be caused slowly and steadily, by alcohol abuse, which is by far the most common cause of cirrhosis. Other causes include the following:

• Use of certain medications
• Inborn errors in physical or chemical processes of the body
• Syphilis
• Passive liver congestion, due to inability of the heart to accept a normal flow of blood from the liver or to obstruction of one of the drainage systems of the liver

Symptoms

Frequently, because it imitates many other diseases, cirrhosis is not suspected until it is well advanced. Symptoms include general weakness, a vague feeling of being unwell, loss of appetite, loss of weight, and a loss of interest in sex. There may be a dull abdominal ache, nausea, constipation, or diarrhea. In a malnourished patient, the tongue may be inflamed.

Many symptoms of cirrhosis are the result of high blood pressure in the portal vein, which brings blood from the intestinal area to the liver. In cirrhosis, the liver cannot handle a normal flow of blood, so the pressure in the portal vein rises. One result is that fluid from the blood is lost into the abdominal cavity. The fluid may accumulate and press against the diaphragm (the muscular wall separating the abdominal and chest cavities) and interfere with breathing. Collateral blood vessels form to carry away the excess blood into the general circulation. There may be bleeding in the esophagus or stomach when these smaller collateral vessels burst under pressure. The patient may vomit blood. Serious, life-threatening hemorrhage may occur.

The liver may be enlarged and firm or, in advanced cases, shrunken. Other symptoms include an enlarged spleen, mottled redness of the mound at the base of the thumb, "spider veins" on the skin of the upper body, loss of hair from the chest and the pubic area, diminished size of the testes, and tingling sensations in the skin of the hands and feet.

Diagnosis

A liver biopsy is used to diagnose cirrhosis of the liver. A hollow needle is inserted through the skin and into the liver itself to obtain a tissue sample for analysis. Examination of tissue from a diseased liver reveals destruction of cells and scarring. Other diagnostic procedures include nuclear medicine scanning, in which radioactive material is administered and its distribution to the liver is recorded on X-ray film. X-ray pictures are taken of the gallbladder and of bile ducts both inside the liver and leading from it. Important clues that may be found in blood and urine tests include the presence of high levels of bile pigments in the blood, a low red blood cell count (anemia), vitamin and mineral deficiencies, and protein in the urine.

Treatment

Treatment is aimed first at removing the cause of the original injury. For example, an alcoholic patient is told to stop drinking and is placed on a well-balanced diet. Often, thiamin (vitamin B_1) and folate supplements are also given. If a stone is obstructing an external bile duct, it can be removed. Fluids and salt are usually restricted, to prevent fluid buildup. Liver transplantation is sometimes considered.

Good care includes getting plenty of rest and avoiding infection, which places stress on the liver. Avoidance of alcohol intake is paramount in the treatment of cirrhosis and most other liver diseases. A physician should be consulted before any medication, including over-the-counter preparations, is taken.

Prevention

Many of the various causes of cirrhosis of the liver cannot be predicted and guarded against, but the major one can be. Drinking moderately or not at all is the best way to reduce the risk of developing cirrhosis.

Colostomy

Colostomy is the creation of a stoma (opening) in the wall of the abdomen to which an opening in the colon is attached. Thereafter, the contents of the colon are eliminated through the stoma instead of through the rectum and anus.

The opening may be permanent (as in some operations for cancer of the rectum), or it may be temporary (as in treatment of severe diverticular disease or Hirschsprung disease).

Correction of Hirschsprung disease

In Hirschsprung disease, an inherited disorder of newborns, the last portion of the bowel lacks specialized nerves and cannot function normally. The healthy portion of the bowel above this segment is connected to a stoma. Elimination takes place via this route for several months until the baby is strong enough for a second surgical procedure, in which the defective portion of the bowel is removed and the healthy portion is connected to the anus, permitting normal bowel movements.

Permanent colostomy

Having a permanent colostomy does not prevent a person from leading a normal life. The patient is taught how to empty the colon once a day by using irri-

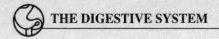

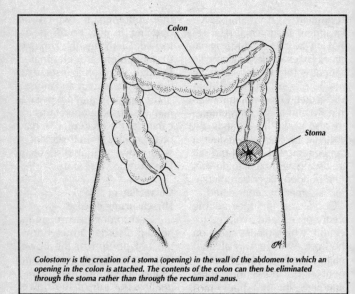

Colostomy is the creation of a stoma (opening) in the wall of the abdomen to which an opening in the colon is attached. The contents of the colon can then be eliminated through the stoma rather than through the rectum and anus.

gations (enemas) and a special collecting device. By manipulating the diet, it becomes possible to anticipate bowel movements. At first, patients wear a pouch over the stoma to collect any leakage from the colon. An adhesive is used to form a tight seal around the opening of the pouch and the stoma, and a deodorant in the pouch controls odor. After a while, many patients with so-called dry colostomies need only wear a stoma cap or a small gauze patch over the stoma to absorb mucous secre-

tions. Physical activities can be resumed, with or without a pouch, including swimming, other noncontact sports, and sexual relations. The only exceptions are heavy lifting, which could cause a hernia through the weakened abdominal muscles, and any activity that could injure the stoma or abdomen.

To avoid infection of the stoma and irritation of the skin around it, the patient needs to wash the surrounding skin area with mild soap and water each day and then rinse and dry it.

Special adhesive materials that protect and soothe the skin have become available. These products are applied after cleaning the skin.

Support, encouragement, and practical advice from those who have undergone the operation are available through local chapters and the national headquarters of the United Ostomy Association.

Crohn disease

Crohn disease (also known as *regional enteritis* and *ileitis*) is characterized by inflammation of a section or sections of any part of the digestive tract—most often, the ileum (the last third of the small intestine). The disease begins as patches of tiny ulcers in the innermost lining of the intestine, with swelling of nearby tissues. The inflammation eventually extends through all layers of the intestine, which becomes thickened, hard, and brittle. Deepening ulcers, scarring, and swelling may obstruct the intestinal tract.

Causes

The cause of Crohn disease is unknown. However, research indicates that infection, immune disorders, or an inherited defect may play a part. There is some evidence of an increased incidence of Crohn disease in Jews; black people are least likely to have the disease. The disease usually begins between the ages of 15 and 35, but can occur at any age.

Symptoms

Symptoms usually develop gradually, with spells of diarrhea (four to six stools a day, frequently bloody), low fever, weight loss, loss of appetite, general weakness, and steady or colicky pains in the abdomen, commonly on the right side. Milk, milk products, and coarse foods may make symptoms worse.

Occasionally an acute (sudden and severe) case resembles appendicitis, with sharp pain in the lower right portion of the abdomen, cramping, nausea, fever, and diarrhea. There may or may not be bloody stools. An acute case can also resemble infectious diarrhea.

Diagnosis

While probing the abdomen and pelvis, the doctor may detect a tender mass of thickened or matted loops of intestine. The chronic form of the disease can occasionally be mistaken for other problems, such as irritable bowel syndrome. However, an X ray of the small intestine taken after administration of the contrast medium barium may reveal the characteristic pattern of narrowed portions of the bowel. The physician may use a proctosigmoidoscope (a lighted, hollow instrument that is inserted through the anus) to inspect the lower intestinal lining for patchy areas of inflammation or to perform a biopsy (obtain a sample of tissue from the lining for microscopic examination).

The physician may also use a colonoscope to study the lining of the colon and the last several inches of the ileum.

Complications

Complications include abscesses (pus-filled cavities) and fistulas. Fistulas are abnormal connecting channels that originate from inflamed portions of the bowel and commonly extend into and around adjacent tissue. In the anorectal area, they may sometimes be seen as openings in the skin. They can also extend from one section of the bowel to another, from the bowel to the bladder or vagina, and from the bowel to the abdominal wall. Fistulas are frequently infected, and they discharge pus.

Perforation of the intestine can also occur, leading to peritonitis (inflammation of the lining of the abdominal cavity). This is marked by severe abdominal pain and rigidity of the abdomen, and is most often a surgical emergency. On occasion, a small perforation may become walled off, creating an abscess.

Malnutrition is a very common complication of Crohn disease, because areas of inflamed intestine cannot properly absorb nutrients. The risk of cancer of the colon and rectum is also increased. Arthritis, eye disorders, kidney stones, and certain skin disorders may also accompany this illness.

Treatment

At present, there is no cure for Crohn disease. Surgery is sometimes necessary to remove an entire section of diseased bowel, drain an abscess, or eliminate a fistula. This relieves the condition for a temporary period, but symptoms almost always recur, and another operation may be necessary.

Treatment of this disease is directed at making the patient as comfortable and functional as possible by helping to reduce the severity of his or her symptoms.

A diet rich in calories and vitamins with adequate protein is desirable to compensate for the patient's poor absorption of nutrients from the intestines. Individuals with severely inflamed or obstructed bowels may be placed temporarily on intravenous feeding or a special diet. Patients with anemia may need supplements of vitamins and minerals (such as iron, folate, and vitamin B_{12}) and sometimes blood transfusions; those patients with severe diarrhea or dehydration (severe loss of body fluids) may need intravenous fluids.

Cramps and diarrhea are frequently controlled by various medications that are designed to relax the bowel wall, while preparations such as psyllium may help to firm stools.

Antibiotics are used on a short-term basis to treat abscesses and infected fistulas. Sulfa–salicylate combination drugs may be used on a long-term basis to curb inflammation and prevent acute episodes, particularly in disease involving the large intestine. The steroid drug prednisone is a mainstay in treating flare-ups of symptoms. Newer salicylate (aspirin-like) drugs, either in enema or oral form, are also quite effective in relieving symptoms.

Diverticulosis and diverticulitis

Diverticulosis is the occurrence of diverticula (little pouches) that form when the inner lining of the large intestine is forced, under pressure, through weak spots in the muscular outer layer of the colon. Diverticulosis may be present in about one third of people over the age of 60 in the United States, and both its incidence and the frequency of complications increase with age. Diverticulitis is inflammation or infection of the diverticula.

Causes

One theory about the cause of diverticulosis is that abnormal movement of the colon (possibly because of too little bulk in the diet) produces intense pressure, which forces the intestinal lining through weak spots in the muscular layer.

Most people with simple diverticulosis have no discernable symptoms. Occasionally, however, a pouch next to a blood vessel may ulcerate, causing it to bleed. If the vessel is an artery, severe bleeding can result, which can become visible as bleeding from the anus. Shock and even death may re-

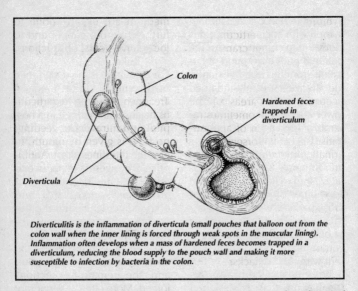

Colon

Hardened feces trapped in diverticulum

Diverticula

Diverticulitis is the inflammation of diverticula (small pouches that balloon out from the colon wall when the inner lining is forced through weak spots in the muscular lining). Inflammation often develops when a mass of hardened feces becomes trapped in a diverticulum, reducing the blood supply to the pouch wall and making it more susceptible to infection by bacteria in the colon.

sult if the condition is not promptly given medical attention.

It has been estimated that about one fifth to one fourth of those who have diverticulosis will suffer from diverticulitis. Diverticulitis develops when a mass of hardened waste matter (called a fecalith) forms in a pouch and reduces the blood supply to the thin walls of the pouch (by means of pressure against the wall), making them more susceptible to infection by the bacteria of the colon. The inflammation that follows can lead to perforation, formation of

an abscess (an enclosed sac of pus around the perforation), or peritonitis (infection of the lining of the abdominal cavity). Not infrequently, the inflamed section of bowel becomes attached to the urinary bladder or vagina, burrowing out from the colon to create a fistula (abnormal channel), which leaks infectious material into the other organ.

Repeated inflammation can cause thickening of the wall of the colon. As a result, narrowing the colon can cause partial or sometimes total obstruction of the colon.

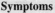
Symptoms

Symptoms of diverticulitis include intermittent crampy abdominal pains and tenderness, usually on the lower left side of the abdomen. Pain can also occur in other areas of the lower abdomen, sometimes resembling the pain of appendicitis. Pain that worsens during urination may indicate that the inflamed colon has become attached to the bladder. Stool (feces) or air in the urine may indicate a colon-to-bladder fistula. Constipation or constipation alternating with diarrhea is common. Fever is usually present with acute attacks.

Diagnosis

The diagnosis of diverticulitis usually is made if there is a history of pain in the left lower section of the abdomen, accompanied by fever and a change in bowel habits. A physical examination may reveal a mass in that area, along with extreme tenderness. After the acute episode has subsided, the doctor may insert a proctosigmoidoscope (a lighted, tubelike instrument) through the anus and into the lower part of the colon to see if there is any evidence of cancer that might be causing the symptoms. X-ray examinations with a contrast medium are usually done to further rule out cancer and to locate diverticula, obstructions, and fistulas.

Treatment

Treatment of severe diverticulitis begins with bed rest in a hospital and intravenous feeding; no food is given by mouth, to give the intestines a rest. Antibiotics are given if there is evidence of infection. (Less severe cases can be treated at home—with bed rest, fluids, and antibiotics.) If peritonitis develops, it may be necessary to operate. The inflamed section of the colon may simply be cut out, and the remaining sections joined. More often, a temporary colostomy (a surgically created opening in the abdominal wall, which allows the colon to empty to the outside of the body) is necessary. Later, after all inflammation and infection have subsided, the redirected portion of the colon is reconnected to the remaining portion of the colon or to the rectum.

Prevention

Choosing a diet with plenty of bulk may help prevent diverticulosis. People who have diverticulosis should eat a relatively high-fiber diet. Food supplements, such as psyllium, that serve to increase bulk may be recommended to move the stool through the colon at a normal rate.

Food poisoning

The term *food poisoning* generally refers to an illness caused by the ingestion of food that is either poisonous itself (such as certain kinds of wild mushrooms) or that has been contaminated, usually by bacteria or their toxic by-products.

Many of the symptoms commonly associated with food poisoning—nausea, vomiting, and diarrhea—are unpleasant but not generally life-threatening and usually subside within a relatively short period of time without medical treatment. However, for some groups—particularly the very old, the very young, and the seriously ill—food poisoning can be extremely serious, and some forms, such as botulism and mushroom poisoning, are potentially fatal for anyone.

In general, bacterial food poisoning can be prevented by careful observance of proper procedures in food processing and preparation. Special attention should be given to hand washing by food handlers, prompt refrigeration of food, and cleanliness in food preparation areas.

Botulism

The *Clostridium botulinum* bacterium produces a toxin which, when ingested, prevents the transmission of nerve impulses to muscle. Nausea, vomiting, and abdominal cramps are common. The effects on the nervous system begin in the head, causing double or blurred vision and difficulty in swallowing, and then proceed downward as paralysis of the arms, the muscles that aid in breathing, and eventually the legs. These symptoms usually appear 4 to 36 hours after ingestion of the toxin, but can be delayed as long as eight days.

The foods most commonly implicated in botulism are home-canned preparations. Also, honey should not be given to infants because it has been reported as a source of fatal botulism in that age group. The best way to prevent botulism is to strictly follow established guidelines when canning foods at home. Contaminated foods sometimes have a foul odor, but this warning is not always present.

With the availability of *Botulinum* antitoxin, fewer than 10 percent of cases are now fatal. However, suspicion of botulism should still be considered a medical emergency.

Salmonellosis

Salmonellosis is any number of diseases caused by *Salmonella* bacteria. One of those diseases is typhoid fever, which fortunately is now uncommon in the United States. A very common form of salmonellosis is *Salmonella* gastroenteritis.

The foods that most commonly harbor *Salmonella* bacteria are meat, poultry, milk, and eggs. *Salmonella* bacteria are frequently transmitted by contact with human or animal fecal material or by eating food contaminated with such material. The symptoms of *Salmonella* gastroenteritis include nausea, abdominal cramps, and diarrhea. In severe cases, mucus and blood are present in the stools.

The symptoms of salmonellosis usually appear 12 to 24 hours after ingestion of contaminated food. Most cases occur in children during the summer and early fall. The illness is generally mild, usually lasting two to five days. However, salmonellosis can be fatal for very young infants, seriously ill patients, and the elderly.

Treatment of most Salmonella infections involves replacing the fluids lost from diarrhea. If fluid loss is severe, hospitalization and intravenous fluid supplementation may be necessary. Use of antibiotics is reserved for patients with severe symptoms because, if used indiscriminately, such drugs can actually prolong the illness. Antidiarrheal medications can also prolong the illness and should be used only to control the most severe symptoms. Laboratory analysis of stool or blood samples may be necessary to establish the diagnosis and prescribe the appropriate treatment. Cultures of the stool should also be performed after the illness has passed to confirm that the bacteria are not still being shed, creating the potential for spread of infection.

Staphylococcal gastroenteritis

Gastroenteritis caused by *Staphylococcus aureus* bacteria is a very common form of food poisoning. Foods that are cooked at low temperatures and then allowed to cool at room temperature for long periods of time are most frequently the source. (Creamy foods and dressings made with mayonnaise are often responsible for harboring the bacteria.)

343

The symptoms—excessive salivation, nausea, diarrhea, abdominal cramps, and vomiting—usually occur within two to four hours after eating the contaminated food. The illness usually lasts less than 24 hours and requires no treatment in otherwise healthy individuals. Antibiotics and antidiarrheal medications can, in fact, prolong the illness. In elderly or ill people, hospitalization and intravenous fluid replacement may be necessary. Symptoms of dehydration, such as dryness of the mouth and light-headedness, should receive prompt medical attention.

Other bacterial causes

Clostridium perfringens is a bacterium commonly found in raw meat and poultry. Its growth in foods is encouraged by slow cooking at low temperatures. Symptoms of infection—abdominal cramps, nausea, and diarrhea—usually appear about 8 to 12 hours after ingestion of contaminated food, but can be delayed as long as 24 hours. The illness generally lasts less than one day and requires no treatment other than getting plenty of fluids.

Infection with the *Vibrio parahaemolyticus* bacteria is most often associated with ingestion of raw or improperly refrigerated seafood. This illness usually occurs during the warmer months and is most common in the coastal regions of the United States. The primary symptom—severe, watery, occasionally blood-tinged diarrhea—generally occurs 12 to 24 hours after eating the contaminated food. The illness rarely lasts more than two days. In severe cases, antibiotics may be necessary.

Bacillus cereus infection is commonly associated with rice products, particularly fried rice and unrefrigerated boiled rice. The primary symptoms—typically nausea and vomiting—are usually mild.

Mushroom poisoning

Do not consume wild mushrooms. It is all but impossible for anyone but an expert to discriminate nontoxic mushrooms from the more than 50 toxic varieties of mushrooms.

Mushroom poisoning usually begins 6 to 24 hours after ingestion of the mushrooms. Starting with severe abdominal cramps, nausea, vomiting, and diarrhea, the illness rapidly progresses to involve the liver, kidneys, and heart. Mushroom poisoning has proven to be fatal.

Gallstones

Gallstones are hardened masses that consist mainly of cholesterol, blood, bile (fluid produced in the liver and stored in the gallbladder), calcium, and other substances. The stones form in the gallbladder or in the bile duct leading into the small intestine.

Causes

When bile contains excessive amounts of cholesterol, the unnecessary cholesterol separates from the solution and forms stonelike masses. Unfortunately, since the body itself produces cholesterol, formation of these types of stones cannot always be prevented merely by controlling cholesterol intake in the diet.

Pregnancy, obesity, diabetes, liver disease, and certain forms of anemia can increase the risk of gallstones. For some reason, overweight people who frequently lose and gain large amounts of weight seem more susceptible to gallstones, as do women who have had two or more children.

Although the reasons are unclear, twice as many women as men over age 40 develop gallstones. Gallstones do not commonly occur in young people.

Symptoms

By themselves, gallstones often produce no signs of disease. About half the people with gallstones have no visible symptoms. Symptoms that do appear are usually chronic (long-term) in nature, including discomfort and pain in the upper abdomen, indigestion, nausea, and intolerance of fatty foods. Sometimes the gallstones may pass through the bile duct into the intestines to be excreted naturally.

However, symptoms can occur when a stone that had been floating in the gallbladder becomes trapped inside the bile duct. In an acute gallbladder attack, a sharp pain (often on the right side of the upper abdomen) may travel to the back and under the right shoulder blade. Frequently, the pain develops suddenly after a meal and leads to fever, chills, vomiting, and possibly jaundice (yellowing of the skin and whites of the eyes caused by the presence of excess bile pigment in the bloodstream).

Complications

Serious complications of liver damage can develop if gallstones become lodged between the gallbladder and small intestine and block the flow of bile.

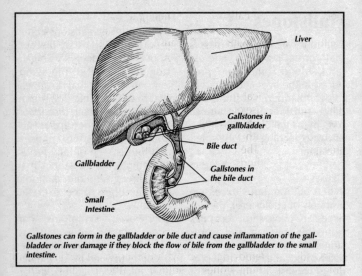

Gallstones can form in the gallbladder or bile duct and cause inflammation of the gallbladder or liver damage if they block the flow of bile from the gallbladder to the small intestine.

When gallstones remain in the gallbladder, the organ may become inflamed. Patients with this condition, called chronic cholecystitis, may appear to have few or no symptoms. However, in most cases, repeated attacks of pain occur.

Diagnosis
Gallstones that cause no symptoms can be detected by an X-ray study of the gallbladder, called a cholecystogram. A cholecystogram is performed after the patient has swallowed a tablet containing dye that outlines the gallbladder and any stones that may be present.

Nowadays, most physicians prefer to use ultrasound (a technique that uses sound waves to create images of internal structures). Some studies using radioactive isotopes have been developed to differentiate between acute and chronic cholecystitis.

Treatment
For acute gallbladder attacks due to gallstones with severe and prolonged symptoms, doctors generally recommend a cholecystectomy (surgical removal of the gallbladder). This treatment is one of the most common forms of abdominal

surgery. A technique called laparoscopy can be used to remove the gallbladder without a standard surgical incision.

Other nonsurgical methods for removing gallstones, including drug and chemical therapy and lithotripsy (the use of shock waves to shatter the stones), have been tried with varying degrees of success. The criteria for using these methods, however, is very strict; surgical removal of the gallbladder is still the method of choice in most cases.

Since the gallbladder is not necessary to maintain life, some doctors suggest removing a gallbladder containing stones even if they are not causing any obvious symptoms.

Gastroenteritis

Gastroenteritis is an inflammation of the lining of the stomach and the intestines.

Causes

Gastroenteritis can be caused by bacteria or viruses; by allergic reactions to certain foods or drinks; by infectious diseases, such as typhoid fever and influenza; by food poisoning; by overconsumption of alcohol; or by certain drugs.

Symptoms

Symptoms include headache, nausea, vomiting, diarrhea, and gas pains in the stomach and the intestines. Often, the individual will feel that gas is "caught" in certain portions of the intestine. On occasion, cramps may produce severe pain.

Diagnosis

The first task in treating gastroenteritis is to identify the cause or causes of the inflammation. Blood tests and cultures for viruses or bacteria may be done. If the problem is caused by an allergic reaction, the source of the reaction can sometimes be identified by allergy tests.

Treatment

Antibiotics can be used to treat bacterial infections. A variety of medicines (many of them nonprescription) can ease the effects of stomach cramps and gas pains. Diarrhea may necessitate replacement of lost fluids. Elderly or extremely ill individuals may have to be hospitalized for intravenous replacement of fluids.

Prevention

Maintaining a clean kitchen, eating in restaurants where the

347

kitchens are kept clean, washing fresh foods thoroughly, and cooking foods carefully are all safeguards against bacterial and viral infections. Identification of allergy-causing foods and moderation in alcohol consumption can also help prevent gastroenteritis.

Hemorrhoids

Hemorrhoids are enlarged veins inside or just outside the anal canal, which is the opening at the end of the large intestine. As the veins swell, they can cause severe inflammation and discomfort.

Causes

In some cases, hemorrhoids are the result of poor toilet habits. Habitual postponement of bowel movements can lead to loss of rectal function and undesirable straining during elimination.

Straining puts increased pressure on the veins and slows the flow of blood, thereby contributing to swelling and inflammation of veins. If bowel movements are postponed, the stools retained in the bowels may lose moisture. When feces becomes dry and hard, the added strain of constipation favors the development of hemorrhoids.

Another source of hemorrhoid irritation comes from pressure on the veins due to diseases of the liver or heart or from a tumor. Pregnancy may also contribute to the development of hemorrhoids, because the enlarged uterus increases pressure on the veins. Moreover, prolonged pressure from pushing during labor and delivery can also lead to hemorrhoids.

Diet plays a major role in the development of hemorrhoids as well. A diet containing a high proportion of refined foods rather than foods with natural roughage increases the likelihood of constipation and, therefore, the likelihood of hemorrhoids.

Hemorrhoids seem to be more prevalent in some families. However, this tendency has been attributed to similar dietary and personal habits rather than heredity.

Symptoms

Hemorrhoids may take years to develop and almost always cause irritating symptoms. The first signs of hemorrhoids include itching and discomfort during and after bowel movements. Continued straining dur-

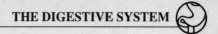

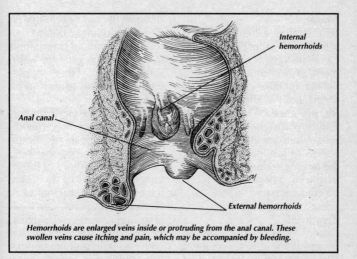

Internal hemorrhoids

Anal canal

External hemorrhoids

Hemorrhoids are enlarged veins inside or protruding from the anal canal. These swollen veins cause itching and pain, which may be accompanied by bleeding.

ing elimination will eventually produce slight swelling of the lining of the anal canal. This swelling may not be noticed until hard stools scrape the anal lining and cause bleeding—an early clue that a hemorrhoid has developed.

With prolonged straining, a portion of the anal canal may jut out of the anus during a bowel movement. As long as the elastic connective tissue is still strong enough to pull the hemorrhoid back into the anal canal unassisted, the individual may not notice the growing problem. However, with persistent pressure, the protruding tissue may remain outside the anus after a bowel movement and need to be manually returned to the anal canal. Once outside the anal canal, the hemorrhoid creates a dull aching sensation or ulcerates and bleeds.

A more involved problem develops when the hemorrhoid is difficult or impossible to return within the anal canal, and permanent swelling at the anal opening interferes with elimination. The patient may then postpone bowel movements in an effort to avoid pain. Instead of helping, this avoidance of bowel movements intensifies the problem because it leads to constipation.

Diagnosis

To diagnose a hemorrhoid, a physician inspects the anal canal, often with special instruments. An anoscope (a short, lighted, tubelike instrument) inserted into the anus can reveal the presence of hemorrhoids. The proctosigmoidoscope, a longer instrument that provides a view of the lower portion of the large intestine, may be used to rule out other causes of rectal bleeding or pain.

Treatment

Painful hemorrhoids can be treated at home by taking warm sitz baths (sitting in a tub of warm water). Over-the-counter preparations cannot cure hemorrhoids, but they can help relieve itching and swelling. Nonirritating laxatives may be useful in softening stools and easing bowel movements. Should symptoms worsen after application of any remedy, its use should be suspended and a doctor consulted. Chemicals in these preparations may produce an allergic reaction.

In the early stages of hemorrhoid development, adjustment of personal habits may prevent progression of the condition. A bowel movement should never be delayed once the urge is felt. During bowel movements, straining should be avoided. A diet including plenty of roughage—natural grains, fresh fruits, and vegetables—also softens stools. Fiber supplements have also proven to be quite helpful.

For severe cases of hemorrhoids, a doctor may recommend a surgical procedure called hemorrhoidectomy to remove dilated portions of the affected veins and to tie off the remaining parts of the vein. Newer procedures, such as cryosurgery and laser surgery, remove the hemorrhoid, but with less pain and fewer postoperative complications. Laser surgery uses an intensified beam of light to burn off the hemorrhoid. With cryosurgery, the hemorrhoid is frozen with an extremely cold probe; the frozen tissue dies, and the hemorrhoid falls off within several days. Many physicians can perform cryosurgery in their offices in a matter of minutes. Frequently, the only postoperative complaint is a slight watery discharge from the anal canal for a few days after the procedure.

Another technique used to eliminate hemorrhoids is rubber-band ligation. With this procedure, which can be performed in the physician's office, the blood supply of the hemorrhoid is cut off by tying a rubber band around the swollen tissue. The hemorrhoid usually drops off within three to nine days. Unfortunately, as is the case with the nonsurgical procedures, this procedure is not always suitable for all patients. As a result, it is often done only to remedy internal hemorrhoids.

Recurrence of hemorrhoids after any type of treatment is not uncommon.

Hiatal hernia

A hernia is a protrusion of a body part through the structures that surround it. A hiatal hernia (also referred to as a hiatus or diaphragmatic hernia) occurs when a portion of the stomach protrudes above the diaphragm (the muscular wall separating the chest and abdominal cavities) into the chest.

Sliding hiatal hernia
Normally, the esophagus (the passageway from the throat to the stomach) passes through a tight muscular collar, called a hiatus, that prevents the stomach from squeezing up into the chest cavity. However, if the collar is too large or if it relaxes, a sliding hiatal hernia may occur. Pressure in the abdomi-

nal cavity (such as that caused by obesity, pregnancy, tight clothing, bending or other changes in position, coughing, or straining) causes the top part of the stomach to herniate (slide through the opening) along with the gastroesophageal junction (the junction of the stomach and the esophagus). This condition is very common but occurs more frequently with women and older people. It may be hard to diagnose, since often there are no visible symptoms. Surgical treatment is recommended in only the most severe cases of hiatal hernia.

Until recently it was believed that the mere presence of a sliding hiatal hernia causes regurgitation (backward flow) of food and harsh stomach acid into the esophagus, which produces the burning sensation of heartburn. Current thinking, however, is that regurgitation and heartburn are the result of functional problems of the esophageal sphincter (band of muscle fibers between the stomach and the esophagus).

Paraesophageal hiatal hernia
A relatively uncommon but quite dangerous type of hiatal hernia is the paraesophageal, or rolling, hiatal hernia. In this type, the gastroesophageal

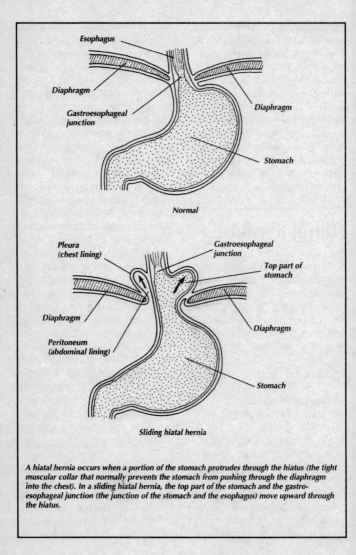

Esophagus

Diaphragm

Gastroesophageal junction

Diaphragm

Stomach

Normal

Pleura (chest lining)

Gastroesophageal junction

Top part of stomach

Diaphragm

Diaphragm

Peritoneum (abdominal lining)

Stomach

Sliding hiatal hernia

A hiatal hernia occurs when a portion of the stomach protrudes through the hiatus (the tight muscular collar that normally prevents the stomach from pushing through the diaphragm into the chest). In a sliding hiatal hernia, the top part of the stomach and the gastro-esophageal junction (the junction of the stomach and the esophagus) move upward through the hiatus.

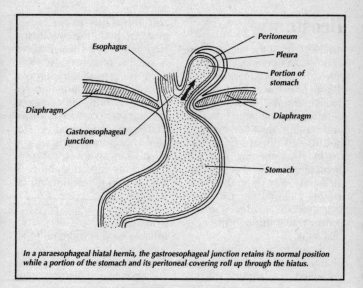

In a paraesophageal hiatal hernia, the gastroesophageal junction retains its normal position while a portion of the stomach and its peritoneal covering roll up through the hiatus.

junction retains its normal position while a portion of the stomach and part of its peritoneum (covering membrane) rolls up through the opening in the diaphragm, alongside the junction. The danger is that the herniated section may become trapped in the chest with its blood supply choked off, thereby causing death of stomach tissue. Bleeding is also a common complication.

Although dangerous, this condition may have no visible symptoms and is usually found accidentally on an X ray taken for another purpose. The only common symptom of this condition is a sense of fullness in the chest after eating.

Because of the potential complications of the paraesophageal hernia, some authorities recommend surgery, even in the absence of symptoms. Surgery for the paraesophageal hernia involves entering the abdomen and pushing the herniated portion of the stomach back into its proper position while removing the sac of peritoneum around it. After this, the muscular collar of the diaphragm is tightened with stitches.

Ileostomy

An ileostomy is the surgical creation of an opening, or stoma, through the abdomen into the ileum (the lower part of the small intestine). An ileostomy is performed if the large intestine and rectum must be removed because of disease or abnormality. The opening into the small intestine then becomes an artificial anus through which waste material is expelled, since waste matter can no longer travel through the normal anus.

The waste matter that is discharged through the stoma is collected in a bag that the patient wears continuously. Because this waste matter does not pass through the large intestine, where water is absorbed from the waste matter, the material excreted through the stoma is watery. Patients learn to care for their stomas in the hospital after surgery.

Irritable bowel syndrome

Irritable bowel syndrome, also called *spastic colon* and *mucous colitis*, is a collection of symptoms caused by irritability and irregularity in the movement of both the small and large intestines. The syndrome is usually influenced by emotions. Feelings of nervousness, anxiety, guilt, depression, or anger may bring on or aggravate this very common disorder. Coffee, raw fruits and vegetables, hormones, drugs, and overuse of laxatives can promote it, as can an inability of the body to digest the natural sugar in milk.

Symptoms

Irritable bowel syndrome is not a disease, but a collection of symptoms that includes both constipation and diarrhea, often alternating and sometimes accompanied by abdominal cramps and straining during elimination. Stools may be loose or compacted and may include mucus, which is produced by the bowel lining in greater than usual amounts as a response to irritation. Gas, bloating, nausea, headache, and fatigue may accompany the other symptoms of irritable bowel syndrome.

There are two main types of irritable bowel syndrome. The first type, spastic colon, is marked by cramps or a dull, aching pain in the abdomen, usually the lower part. The discomfort often begins at mealtime and may disappear after a bowel movement. The second type of irritable bowel syndrome is characterized by painless diarrhea, especially an urgent need for a bowel movement on awakening or during or right after a meal.

Diagnosis

If a patient appears to have irritable bowel syndrome, the doctor will initially want to rule out diseases that can have similar symptoms. The patient may be requested to bring in a stool specimen to be examined for traces of blood and microorganisms. The colon may be X-rayed after a barium enema. The doctor may examine the lower portion of the colon with a proctosigmoidoscope (a lighted tubelike instrument inserted through the anus) to check for more serious disorders, such as ulcerative colitis.

Treatment

If no organic disease is found, the doctor will reassure the patient and discuss ways in which the symptoms can be relieved. There may be methods by which the patient can reduce the anxiety or depression that may be causing the syndrome. The doctor may prescribe a tranquilizer, sedative,

antidepressant, or antispasmodic medication. Long walks, bike rides, or other exercise may help to relax the person while promoting better bowel action.

If constipation is a problem, the doctor will advise the patient to add bulk (such as whole bran) to the diet and to stop depending on laxatives. If diarrhea is present, avoiding laxative foods, such as prunes, may help.

Patients bothered by gas will be warned against foods such as cabbage and beans. Milk may be barred from the diet. Most people, with the general exception of those of northwestern European origin, lose some or all of the ability to digest lactose, the natural sugar in milk, by the time they are 20 years old. A test for this is an oral dose of lactose. If it results in diarrhea and bloating, it is a good indication that the symptoms of irritable bowel syndrome could have been caused by drinking milk.

If irritable bowel syndrome continues despite treatment, it is important to remember that it is not dangerous. However, to be on the safe side, regular medical checkups should be scheduled, especially if the patient is over 40 years of age.

Jaundice

Jaundice is a yellowish discoloration of the skin, the whites of the eyes, the mucous membranes, and other tissues of the body caused by the accumulation of the bile pigment bilirubin in the blood.

Bilirubin consists primarily of the hemoglobin (a pigment that carries oxygen) of used red blood cells and is found in bile, a yellow-green fluid that aids in digestion by breaking down fat. Bile is secreted by the liver, stored in the gallbladder, and discharged into the small intestine when it is needed for digestion.

Causes

In many cases, jaundice occurs when an obstruction prevents bile from being discharged into the small intestine. The obstruction may be caused by gallstones, tumors, or parasites in the bile ducts. Jaundice may also be a sign of hepatitis, in which the inflamed or damaged liver cannot process the bilirubin it receives. Occasionally, jaundice appears if red blood cells are destroyed too rapidly and the liver cannot accommodate the excess pigment. Jaundice is also associated with many other diseases in which the functioning of the liver is disrupted, including various forms of cancer and certain viral and parasitic infections. More than 50 percent of full-term newborn infants and 80 percent of premature newborn infants show signs of jaundice by the third day after birth. In most of these cases, the condition is nothing to worry about and disappears in about a week or so.

Symptoms

Usually when jaundice occurs, the liver has become enlarged and is functioning less than optimally. Bowel movements may be clay-colored, and urine can vary in hue from light yellow to brownish green. Jaundiced skin ranges in color from lemon yellow to olive green.

Diagnosis

Routine blood testing will determine the origin of some cases of jaundice, but usually it is necessary to examine the bile ducts using ultrasound, in which sound waves are used to create images of internal structures, and computed tomography, a special X-ray technique that provides cross-sectional pictures of an area. Endoscopic retrograde cholangiopancreatography (ERCP) is a technique used to identify gallstones, inflammatory disease of the pancreas, or obstruction of the bile ducts. This is accomplished by threading an endoscope (a flexible, lighted, tubelike instrument) through the mouth, down the esophagus, through the stomach, and into the duodenum (the first part of the small intestine). A small flexible tube is then inserted into the opening of the bile duct, and a contrast medium is infused. X rays are immediately taken. Bile samples for testing can also be obtained in this manner. During this procedure, the patient is sedated but is not under general anesthesia. Usually the individual goes home the same day or the following day, depending on the underlying condition.

Treatment
Surgery may be necessary if an obstruction is present. Otherwise, treatment depends on the underlying condition.

Occult blood

Occult blood is blood that is present in an amount so small that it is detectable only with a chemical test or microscopic examination. This term is generally used to refer to blood in the stools that indicates bleeding along the gastrointestinal tract.

Symptoms
Often, the only symptom of occult bleeding is fatigue due to loss of oxygen-carrying red blood cells. A significant amount of blood can be passed in one stool with no visible indication that blood is present.

Diagnosis
Occult bleeding is not always constant, so tests are typically performed on stool samples obtained on three separate occasions if a problem is suspected. The patient must not eat red meat for three days before the samples are obtained; even cooked blood from meat can cause a positive test result. Aspirin can also cause minute amounts of blood to appear in the stools and should not be taken for at least several days before testing. Tests for occult blood are commonly done as a screening examination for colon cancer and polyps. These tests are highly effective in early diagnosis of these conditions.

Pancreatitis

The pancreas has many functions. The endocrine portion of

357

the pancreas secretes hormones directly into the bloodstream, such as the hormones insulin and glucagon, which are critical to the processing of glucose (the form of sugar used by the body for energy). The exocrine portion of the pancreas secretes digestive enzymes (proteins that promote chemical reactions), such as amylase, which aids in the breakdown of starches, and lipase, which aids in the breakdown of fats. Pancreatitis is an inflammation of the pancreas.

Causes

Pancreatitis commonly results from an obstruction of the pancreatic ducts, which convey enzymes to the small intestine. Why these blockages occur is often hard to determine; however, most cases of pancreatitis are related to gallbladder disease or alcoholism. Acute attacks are frequently associated with gallstones or alcoholic binges. If hereditary factors are involved, the disease may begin in childhood, as early as eight or ten years of age. Direct blows to the abdomen or injury during an operation may also lead to pancreatitis. Mumps and other viral infections, tumors, and the use of certain drugs, including steroids, thiazide diuretics, and oral contraceptives, have all been associated with pancreatitis.

Symptoms

The disease is characterized by the sudden onset of steady, severe, piercing, upper abdominal pain (frequently radiating to the middle portion of the back) accompanied by nausea and persistent vomiting. Eating—or even the sight of food—may bring on the pain or make it worse. Vomiting provides no relief, a feature that distinguishes pancreatitis from some stomach or intestinal disorders. Fever, shock (circulatory collapse), jaundice (yellowish discoloration of the skin and whites of the eyes), dehydration (excessive fluid loss), bleeding, and infection may occur in severe attacks of pancreatitis.

Diagnosis

The existence and degree of inflammation in the pancreas may be hard to determine, not only because of the hidden position and dual purpose of the gland, but also because the symptoms are easily confused with those of other abdominal disorders. Blood and urine tests, as well as microscopic tissue examination, may be inconclusive, but can at least be helpful in excluding other abdominal disorders.

A special X-ray study, endoscopic retrograde cholangiopancreatography (ERCP), may be used to inspect the pancreatic ducts. The technique is performed by inserting an endoscope (a flexible, lighted, tubelike instrument) through the mouth and stomach into the duodenum (the first part of the small intestine). In the duodenum is the opening to the common bile and main pancreatic ducts. A special device is inserted through this opening, and X-ray contrast material is injected. Obstructions, tumors, and characteristic ductal patterns associated with chronic pancreatitis can be seen on the X-ray films.

Treatment

The patient is usually hospitalized for 3 to 14 days for a mild to severe acute attack of pancreatitis. Correction of an underlying problem (for example, removal of gallstones) improves the chances for complete recovery.

Initial treatment is aimed at relieving the pain and reducing stomach secretions, which can stimulate the pancreas. To allow the pancreas to rest, eating and drinking are replaced by intravenous feeding. Antacids are also frequently given.

During convalescence, a low-fat, high-protein diet should be followed, and antacids may be prescribed. If the disease is chronic, it may be necessary to use pancreatic extracts to supplement the insufficient quantities of enzymes secreted by the diseased pancreas. This helps to normalize digestion and thereby maintain adequate nutritional status.

After an acute episode of pancreatitis, tissue debris, blood, and pancreatic enzymes may form a pseudocyst (an internal space filled with a collection of material but not within a sac). Rupture or enlargement of a pseudocyst can be a very serious or even fatal event. If a pseudocyst does not clear up spontaneously, surgery is necessary to drain it.

Chronic pancreatitis is an indication of continued degenerative tissue damage, which may impair pancreatic function. In some cases of chronic pancreatitis, surgical exploration might be used to locate a previously unidentified blockage or to remove diseased tissue; however, surgery is unlikely to help the patient who continues to drink excessive amounts of alcohol. Recently, procedures to remove stones or otherwise relieve obstruction have been successfully performed through a gastroscope thus eliminating the need for surgery.

Periodontal disease

Periodontal disease (also known as periodontitis) is a progressive deterioration of the gums, bones, and other tissues around the teeth.

Causes

One theory is that periodontal disease begins with an accumulation of bacteria and food particles within the tissues surrounding the teeth. These bacteria emit toxins (poisons) that cause gum tissue to swell, bleed, and deteriorate.

Stages of periodontitis

Gingivitis (inflammation of the gums) is the first stage of periodontitis. The second stage results when the soft tissues become separated from the bone and teeth, leading to "pocket" formation. Pockets of

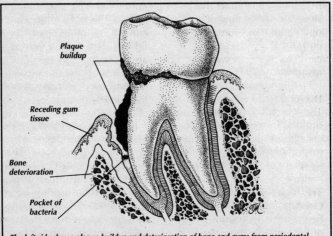

Plaque buildup

Receding gum tissue

Bone deterioration

Pocket of bacteria

The left side shows plaque buildup and deterioration of bone and gums from periodontal disease; the right side shows healthy tooth, bone, and gums.

bacteria and pus accumulate around the teeth, leading to weakening of the tissues holding the teeth in their sockets and destruction of the bone supporting the teeth. As the disease advances, teeth become loose and fall out. They may also move out of alignment with one another, causing problems with chewing.

Symptoms

In the early stage of periodontal disease, gums become sore, red, and slightly swollen. They may be sensitive to the touch and may bleed when brushed or flossed. The presence of pus in the gums around the teeth signals the beginning of the second stage. If pus remains in the gum tissue without draining, extreme pain and swelling can result.

Diagnosis

The diagnosis of periodontal disease is based on the presence of swollen gums and deposits of plaque around the teeth.

Treatment and prevention

Once periodontal disease has been detected, continued care of the mouth at home can help prevent extension of disease and can reduce gum problems.

Oral hygiene to prevent gum disease is the same as treatment to prevent tooth decay. Ideally, the mouth should be cleaned after every meal. At the least, a thorough cleansing at bedtime is necessary to reduce the risk of gum disease.

Dentists suggest brushing with a soft-bristled toothbrush. Gentle movements within the crevices dislodge decay-causing material, and firm strokes over the teeth remove plaque. Flossing is recommended to clear plaque from between teeth. After brushing and flossing, vigorously rinsing the mouth with mouthwash containing an antimicrobial agent (a substance that kills bacteria) can also help eliminate bacterial growth, but mouthwash alone cannot prevent plaque formation. For self-checking, a dental mirror provides a view of the teeth and gums in the back of the mouth.

In advanced cases, a dentist may scrape the affected tissue pockets and apply antiseptics every few months in an effort to kill the bacteria. Should this procedure fail to check the spread of the disease, surgery by a periodontist (gum specialist) may be needed to remove deep pockets in the gums. Once the bacteria have been eliminated, good oral hygiene should control the disease.

Peritonitis

Peritonitis is a term used to describe an inflammation or infection of the peritoneum, the thin, double-layered membrane that lines the abdominal cavity and covers the abdominal organs.

Causes
Peritonitis occurs when the peritoneum is invaded by bacteria or irritated by toxins (poisons), bile (a substance produced by the liver and stored in the gallbladder), blood, or urine. Because the peritoneum is well sealed, it can be infiltrated only when one of the hollow organs of the abdomen ruptures; when a solid organ is somehow damaged, causing it to leak; or when there is a penetrating injury from the outside. (If the colon is perforated, feces, which contain bacteria and toxins, are discharged, causing bacterial peritonitis.)

Symptoms
A main symptom of peritonitis is severe pain that intensifies with any movement and often forces the person to lie very still with the legs drawn up. The abdominal area becomes very tender and rigid; commonly there is vomiting, fever, and dehydration (excessive loss of body fluids). When the peritoneum is inflamed, fluid begins to leak out of the blood vessels into the peritoneum. If this condition is not corrected, it may lead to shock (failure of the circulatory system). Swelling of the abdomen is a sign that the intestines have become paralyzed and bloated with air or that a large amount of fluid is accumulating.

Treatment
These symptoms of peritonitis call for immediate medical care, including intravenous administration of antibiotics to fight infection. Intravenous fluids are also given to replace lost fluids. In addition, a tube is usually inserted through the nose and into the stomach to relieve bloating and remove pooled fluids. After the patient's condition has stabilized, surgery is performed to remove or repair the cause of peritonitis.

Pyloric stenosis

Pyloric stenosis is a constriction (narrowing) of the passage between the stomach and the small intestine. The stomach has two openings—one at the top, where it joins with the esophagus (food tube), and one at the bottom, where it joins with the small intestine. The lower opening is called the pylorus.

Causes

Pyloric stenosis, or gastric outlet obstruction, can be caused by many conditions, including cancer, spasm, a nearby ulcer in the part of the intestine directly below the pyloric opening, gastritis (inflammation of the stomach), and enlargement of the pyloric sphincter (the muscle that rings the pyloric opening and controls its movement).

Symptoms

In the case of congenital (present at birth) pyloric stenosis, ten days to three weeks after birth the infant will experience regurgitation ("spitting up" of part of the stomach's contents), projectile vomiting (vomiting with great force), weight loss, and dehydration (excessive loss of body fluids) without appetite loss.

Adults that have pyloric stenosis experience discomfort in the upper and middle portions of the abdomen, pain, bloating of the abdominal area, nausea, vomiting, and weight loss.

Treatment

In most mild cases of temporary pyloric stenosis, such as that caused by an ulcer, the condition can be treated by offering only small meals or intravenous feeding, restoring normal fluid levels, and administering antacid drugs (drugs that help block the production of stomach acid).

In severe cases, a pyloromyotomy (a lengthwise incision into the pyloric muscle) may be indicated. A portion of the pyloric sphincter may also have to be removed.

Tooth decay

Tooth decay (dental cavities, or caries) is the gradual process of destruction and mineral loss that affects the enamel (outer layer) and dentin (the bony second layer) of a portion of a tooth, causing it to become soft, discolored, and porous.

Causes

A combination of factors causes tooth decay. A substance called plaque, made up of sugars, starches, bacteria, and proteins, builds up on dental surfaces, especially near the gums and in

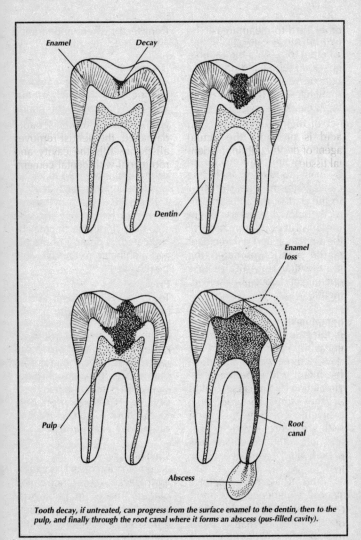

Tooth decay, if untreated, can progress from the surface enamel to the dentin, then to the pulp, and finally through the root canal where it forms an abscess (pus-filled cavity).

other hard-to-clean areas. The plaque prevents the saliva from performing its natural protective function. The bacteria in the plaque feed on the sugars and starches that cling to the teeth and produce acid as a by-product of their metabolism. That acid is probably the actual agent of destruction in the dental tissue.

Symptoms
When the cavity has progressed into the dentin or the surface of an exposed root, the tooth becomes sensitive to touch and rapid temperature changes. Sweet foods can cause pain as dissolved sugar enters the cavity. Bacteria may pass through tiny channels in the dentin and inflame the pulp, which contains blood vessels and nerve tissue, producing a toothache.

Diagnosis
The cavity reveals itself to the examining dentist as a darkened area or as an area of softness when probed with a sharp instrument. An X ray is also helpful in locating and identifying cavities.

Treatment
Cavities are treated by drilling out the decayed material and replacing it with a filling. In front teeth, where appearance is important, the filling may be porcelain or a plastic resin (which is also used to fill pits and tiny cracks in the enamel). In other teeth, the filling is usually silver-colored or an alloy of gold. When a tooth is badly damaged, the dentist removes all decay, fills the cavity and root canal with dental cement, then grinds and tapers the outer surface and covers it with what is known as a gold crown. On teeth toward the front, the gold crown is sometimes overlaid with porcelain to provide a natural appearance.

Prevention
To prevent decay, teeth should be cleaned daily with a soft-bristled brush, preferably after each meal, to remove food particles and plaque. Equally important is the use of dental floss to remove debris between the teeth. Avoiding sweet, sticky foods, or at least rinsing or brushing shortly after eating them, may also aid in the prevention of tooth decay.

A child's teeth will be more resistant to decay if the child drinks water containing the proper amount of fluoride in the first 12 years of life, which is the critical period when the teeth are developing.

If the water supply is not fluoridated, a vitamin supplement containing fluoride can be taken daily. In addition, fluoride treatments are often a routine part of a child's dental examination. Adults and children alike can benefit by using a toothpaste or mouthwash that contains fluoride.

Traveler's diarrhea

Of all the illnesses likely to afflict travelers to foreign countries, the most common is "traveler's diarrhea." This disorder, an intestinal infection caused by microorganisms to which the traveler is unaccustomed, is characterized by loose, watery stools often accompanied by nausea and abdominal cramps.

Causes

The organism most commonly responsible is *Escherichia coli (E. coli).* This bacterium is a normal inhabitant of the intestines, but in some areas of the world it has evolved into a strain called *enterotoxigenic* (poisonous to the intestines) *E. coli,* or *ETEC,* which can cause moderate to severe diarrhea. Other organisms that can cause traveler's diarrhea include *Campylobacter, Salmonella,* and *Shigella* bacteria; parasitic protozoa (one-celled organisms), such as *Entamoeba histolytica* (the cause of amebic dysentery) and *Giardia lamblia*; and a number of viruses.

Symptoms

The major symptom of the illness is, of course, diarrhea, which can range in intensity from mild (three to four loose, watery stools per day) to severe (10 to 20 bloody stools per day). The severity of traveler's diarrhea is largely dependent on the type of organism that is causing the infection and the health status of the individual. Traveler's diarrhea caused by bacteria usually begins a few days after the beginning of the trip and may last for several days to a few weeks if not properly treated. *Campylobacter* and *Shigella* infections commonly are marked by severe, bloody diarrhea. The diarrhea caused by *Giardia* organisms is usually characterized by abundant stools (rarely blood-tinged) and can be associated with other symptoms, such as fever, weight loss, and weakness. Traveler's diarrhea caused by protozoa can be mild or very severe, with involvement of other organs, such as the liver.

Diagnosis

Knowledge of which foreign countries have been visited recently will help the doctor in making a preliminary diagnosis. Because it is very difficult to differentiate among the various infectious causes of diarrhea, laboratory studies, such as stool cultures and blood tests, are often needed. Parasitic diarrhea is especially difficult to diagnose; occasionally, multiple cultures are necessary, as well as proctosigmoidoscopy (visual examination of the rectum and lower portion of the large intestine with a special instrument).

Treatment

Mild cases of traveler's diarrhea usually clear up without treatment in a few days. Diarrhea that lasts for more than several days or that is associated with persistent fever or with the presence of blood, pus, or mucus in the stools calls for immediate medical attention.

Prevention

Much has been written in recent years about prevention of traveler's diarrhea by taking medication before and during the trip. It must be remembered that all medications have potential side effects and that the indiscriminate use of antibiotics and antidiarrheal medications can be dangerous. Except in special circumstances (for example, a person with severe health problems, for whom an episode of severe diarrhea could be catastrophic), routine preventive treatment with antibiotics is not recommended.

Because there are no vaccines or universally effective prophylactic drugs to use against traveler's diarrhea, caution should be exercised when eating or drinking in many foreign countries. Avoid unboiled water (and ice made from unboiled water). Be careful of water that you use to brush your teeth, too. Do not assume that bottled water that is available locally is safe. Lettuce and other fresh vegetables are common food culprits. Fruit with intact skin is usually safe if you wash it with uncontaminated water and peel it yourself before eating. Beer, wine, and carbonated beverages are usually safe, but it must be remembered that the addition of alcoholic beverages to water does not kill infectious organisms. Food obtained from local street vendors should always be avoided.

Ulcer

An ulcer is an erosion (open sore) on the surface of an organ or tissue. Ulcers most commonly erupt in the esophagus, stomach, and duodenum, in which case they are known as *peptic ulcers*.

Causes

Research suggests that both duodenal and gastric ulcers may be caused by infection with the organism *Helicobacter pylori*. In addition, aspirin, caffeine, and nonsteroidal anti-inflammatory drugs (such as ibuprofen) may also contribute to the development of ulcers.

Heredity plays an important role in contributing to ulcers. People who have a family history of ulcers seem to have a greater likelihood of acquiring the condition, as do people with type O blood. In addition, liver disease, rheumatoid arthritis, and emphysema are among the conditions that may increase vulnerability to ulcers.

Symptoms

Ulcers can produce mild symptoms resembling heartburn or severe pain radiating throughout the upper portion of the body. The most common discomfort of ulcers is a burning sensation in the abdomen above the navel that may feel like hunger pangs. Pain comes about 30 to 120 minutes after eating or in the middle of the night when the stomach is empty. At this time, the acidic stomach juices are more apt to irritate the unprotected nerve endings in the exposed ulcer. Usually, pain subsides after eating or drinking something or taking an antacid to neutralize stomach acid.

Some people experience nausea, vomiting, and constipation. Blood in the feces (discoloring them black), blood in the vomit, extreme weakness, fainting, and excessive thirst are all signs of internal bleeding and may appear in more advanced cases.

While ulcers are not usually life-threatening, they can cause serious damage if left untreated. Ulcers may erode nearby blood vessels and cause internal seepage of blood or hemorrhage (massive internal bleeding). A perforated ulcer may penetrate an adjoining organ, causing infection.

Diagnosis

Physicians diagnose peptic ulcers primarily on the basis of an X-ray examination after the patient has swallowed a special

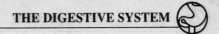

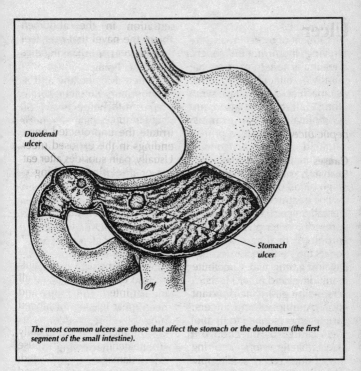

Duodenal ulcer

Stomach ulcer

The most common ulcers are those that affect the stomach or the duodenum (the first segment of the small intestine).

chalky substance called *barium*. The barium makes the digestive tract visible on X-ray film, allowing the doctor to view any abnormalities.

A second diagnostic technique is called an *upper GI endoscopy* (also called *gastroscopy*). The doctor inserts an endoscope (a flexible, lighted, tubelike instrument) through the mouth and down the esophagus to directly view the lining of the esophagus, stomach, and duodenum. An endoscopic examination and a biopsy (removal of a tissue sample for analysis) are necessary to confirm that an apparent ulcer is not actually a cancerous growth. *Helicobacter pylori* can be diagnosed with endoscopic biopsy or though a blood or breath test.

Treatment

Treatment of ulcers involves relieving the irritation so that healing is able to progress naturally. Antacids counteract stomach acid and relieve symptoms, but they can also cause complications. For example, sodium bicarbonate, a primary antacid ingredient, contains large amounts of sodium, which can aggravate kidney disease or high blood pressure.

For treatment of more problematic ulcers, a physician may prescribe other preparations to promote healing. Sucralfate coats the stomach, protecting it against gastric acid. Cimetidine, ranitidine, and other H_2 blockers inhibit gastric acid production. Antibiotics and antacids are often prescribed to treat ulcers caused by infection with *Helicobacter pylori*.

Although recent studies have shown that a bland diet is not necessary for ulcer management, such a diet is sometimes recommended until the acute symptoms disappear. Thereafter, many doctors suggest avoiding only those foods known to cause stomach distress.

Most ulcers heal within two to six weeks after treatment begins. To prevent recurrence, patients should continue to refrain from use of cigarettes, caffeine, alcohol, and other substances that stimulate stomach acid production or irritate the digestive tract lining.

When drug therapy and diet cannot cure an ulcer, surgical repair may be necessary. Surgery is appropriate for repeated ulcers that recur or are life-threatening, such as perforated ulcers. Sometimes, surgeons remove a portion of the stomach and parts of the vagus nerve (which controls digestive secretions) to reduce stomach acid production. Usually, ulcers do not reappear after surgery.

Recently, endoscopic cautery (burning of tissue through an endoscope), direct injection of medications, and lasers have been quite successful in stopping bleeding, reducing the size of lesions, and correcting strictures (narrowing of the ducts due to scar formation). These procedures have spared many individuals from surgery.

Ulcerative colitis

Ulcerative colitis is a chronic inflammatory disease of the large intestine characterized by bloody diarrhea and the development of erosions (open sores) on the lining of the colon.

Causes

Although there is a familial tendency to develop ulcerative colitis, the cause of the disorder is unknown. Any age group may be affected, but it tends to begin in people between the ages of 15 and 40.

Among possible contributing factors are infection, immunologic derangement (a breakdown in the body's defense system), lack of protective elements in the bowel wall, nervous or psychological disturbances, and alterations in the connective tissue in the colon.

Symptoms

The first sign of ulcerative colitis is usually a series of attacks of bloody diarrhea. The attacks can vary in intensity and duration and are usually interspersed with periods of normal bowel movements. The attacks may be severe, with sudden violent diarrhea, high fever, symptoms of abdominal inflammation, and bacterial invasions. Often, an attack will be preceded by mild lower abdominal cramps and the appearance of blood or mucus in the feces.

If ulceration is confined to the rectum and the terminal portion of the colon, the bowel movements may be normal or bloody, with discharges of mucus containing red and white blood cells between stools. If the disorder extends to other portions of the colon, stools become looser and more frequent, and the patient suffers severe cramps, watery stools, fever, anemia, and loss of appetite.

Complications

If the condition persists in this severe form, hemorrhage (internal bleeding) is the most common complication. In toxic megacolon, a serious complication, the colon loses muscle tone and dilates almost completely, resulting in perforations of the organ. The risk of colon cancer and cancer of the bile ducts increases in patients with ulcerative colitis.

Diagnosis

Ulcerative colitis is diagnosed by medical history, physical examination, and colonoscopy (in which a lighted, flexible, tubelike instrument is inserted through the anus and into the colon for a visual examination of the interior).

Treatment

Treatment for milder cases of ulcerative colitis consists of a diet low in milk, milk products, nuts, kernels, and seeds and the prescription of antidiarrheal

THE KIDNEYS AND URINARY SYSTEM

The urinary system includes those organs of the body that produce and eliminate urine (a combination of water and waste products that passes out of the body as fluid). By controlling urine flow, the system maintains proper water balance in the body. Individual parts of the urinary system monitor the concentration of salts and other necessary nutrients.

Functions of organs

The organs most responsible for the control of the balance of chemicals and water in the blood are the two kidneys. The kidneys are bean-shaped structures located in back of the abdomen. Their chief functions are to filter wastes from the blood and to ensure reabsorption of essential chemicals back into the bloodstream. The kidneys also play a major role in blood pressure regulation, and they influence the production of red blood cells. In the kidneys, waste products combine with water and salts to form urine.

Urine passes from each kidney into the bladder through tubes called *ureters*. The bladder stores the urine until elimination.

A sphincter muscle around the exit from the bladder prevents urine from escaping. When the bladder is about half full, the body feels an urge to urinate. At this time, the muscle can be relaxed voluntarily to release the urine and empty the bladder during the elimination process.

The urethra is a tube that transports urine from the bladder to the exterior of the body. The female urethra is about an inch and a half long and is enclosed within the body.

The male urethra passes through the penis and is approximately eight inches long. For the male, the urethra serves the dual function of transporting urine and semen (the fluid from the male reproductive organs). Semen is released during sexual intercourse, at which time urine is blocked from leaving the bladder.

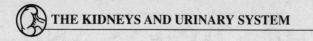

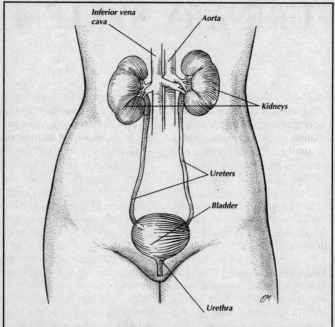

The role of the urinary system (the female urinary tract is shown here) is to cleanse the blood. Arterial blood is filtered through the kidneys and returned to the circulation. Waste products, plus excess water, are sent through the ureters to the bladder, to be excreted as urine.

Disorders

Changes in urine and urinary habits that do not seem to have an obvious cause may be symptoms of disease.

Some symptoms that require medical attention are changes in frequency, timing, and control of urination; changes in the quantity and color of urine; and the presence of pain accompanying urination. A doctor should be contacted if any of the following symptoms is noted: extreme pain while urinating, blood in the urine, a noticeable increase or decrease in frequency of urination (a symptom of kidney failure), marked changes in the color of the urine, or cloudiness in the urine accompanied by pain or fever.

Changes in urine or urinary habits may be caused by a variety of disorders involving the kidneys, urinary tract, bladder, and prostate (a gland that surrounds the male urethra).

Increased frequency of urination may be caused by inflammation of the kidneys, bladder, or urethra; diabetes mellitus (a disorder of carbohydrate metabolism); or an enlarged prostate gland.

A change in timing of urination, usually in the form of very frequent nighttime awakenings accompanied by the urge to urinate (called nocturia), is often coupled with painful urination, a weak stream, or difficulty in starting urination. These may be symptoms of an enlarged prostate gland or an inflammatory or infectious disease within the urinary tract, as well as tumors or other disorders that result in increased pressure on the bladder.

Difficulty in controlling, starting, and maintaining the flow of urine may also be symptoms of an inflammation of the prostate gland. Inability to hold back urine is a common problem of elderly people, as their control of the sphincter muscle of the bladder weakens. Also affected by this problem are women who are in the late stages of pregnancy, when the enlarged uterus continuously presses on the bladder.

Changes in the quantity of urine normally produced can also be an indication of disease. Producing an excessive amount of urine (called polyuria) may be a symptom of kidney disease, diabetes, or glandular disorders. Decreased production of urine may indicate the presence of dehydration, internal hemorrhaging, or acute renal failure.

Slight changes in the color and clarity of the urine from day to day are normal, but strikingly obvious color changes and extreme cloudiness may signal infection, tumors, kidney stones, prostate problems, or other abnormalities in the urinary tract.

Pain while urinating, most commonly in the form of a burning sensation felt along the urethra, may be a sign of a lower urinary tract infection. Excruciating pain across the abdomen or the back may signal the presence of kidney stones.

Treatment of urinary problems usually involves treating an underlying cause, which can range from a mild infection to a very serious disease. An accurate diagnosis by a physician is the first step to proper treatment of these disorders.

Cystitis

Cystitis is an inflammation of the bladder; the term, however, is commonly used to mean bladder infection.

Causes

Cystitis is usually caused by bacteria that have invaded the urethra and entered the bladder. Women are more susceptible than men because their urethras are shorter (approximately one and a half inches long, compared with about eight inches in men), thus presenting less distance for the bacteria to travel. Also, in women, the anus and the external openings of the urethra and the vagina are so close together that bacteria can easily migrate from one to another. The bacteria that are almost always responsible for cystitis are types that normally live harmlessly in the human intestine.

Obstruction is also a common cause of urinary tract infection. When obstruction occurs, the bladder may not empty properly. The urine remaining in the bladder can then create a breeding ground for bacteria to multiply. Causes of obstruction include tumors, kidney stones, and an enlarged prostate gland.

The urethral lining may have a defect that allows bacteria to enter the urinary tract. For example, frequent intercourse may traumatize the urethra, disrupting its lining and making it more susceptible to infection.

Cystitis in men is uncommon. When it does occur, the usual cause is an infection that has spread from an inflamed prostate gland or that has developed in the bladder because of an enlarged prostate.

Urethritis, an infection or inflammation of the urethra, often sets the stage for the development of cystitis. Urethritis occurs in both men and women and is usually acquired through sexual intercourse with an infected individual. Gonorrheal and nongonococcal urethritis are the two most common types.

Symptoms

The symptoms of cystitis include a painful sensation or burning on urination, a frequent and often urgent need to urinate (sometimes causing awakening during the night), and occasionally, low-back pain. These symptoms, along with bloody urine, indicate hemorrhagic cystitis, which is relatively common in women. Although quite frightening, this is most often a minor and easily treatable condition. However, repeated episodes or persistent bleeding, whether it's visible or microscopic, requires further investigation. In men, however, bloody urine is not usually attributable to hemorrhagic cystitis and demands immediate investigation.

With the exception of visibly bloody urine, all of the symptoms mentioned can be present in urethritis, which is also commonly accompanied by a discharge. High fever, chills, and back pain (usually one-sided), with or without any other symptoms, usually indicate pyelonephritis (kidney infection), which demands immediate attention of a doctor.

Diagnosis

The diagnosis of urinary infection rests on the urinalysis and urine culture results. The presence of moderate to large numbers of white blood cells, along with at least 100,000 colonies of any one type of bacteria in a culture, provides conclusive evidence of infection.

Not infrequently, it is difficult to determine which part of the

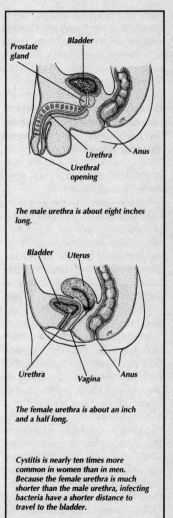

The male urethra is about eight inches long.

The female urethra is about an inch and a half long.

Cystitis is nearly ten times more common in women than in men. Because the female urethra is much shorter than the male urethra, infecting bacteria have a shorter distance to travel to the bladder.

urinary tract is infected, or if there is infection at all. In women, some white blood cells and bacteria are usually present at the opening of the urethra. Therefore, in order to keep the urine specimen free of these contaminants, a midstream specimen is usually requested. The first spurt of urine is thought to wash away the urethral contaminants, and the rest of the urine sample is then normally uncontaminated.

For the vast majority of cases of simple cystitis, this procedure is adequate; however, if a question exists as to the validity of the specimen or if for some reason the specimen must be absolutely free of contaminants, a catheter (thin, flexible tube) may be inserted into the bladder through the urethra.

In women, this is an easy procedure and eliminates vaginal and anal contaminants. If the catheter-obtained specimen is free of pus and bacteria, the symptoms are the result of another condition—commonly vaginitis or urethritis. In a man, the procedure is somewhat more difficult and often not necessary. If prostatitis is the suspected cause of the infection, the physician can insert a gloved finger into the anus and feel the gland directly. A specimen of prostatic fluid is usually obtained (by massaging the gland at the time of examination) through the urethra for culture.

In difficult chronic cases of cystitis in both men and women, in which the cause of recurring infection may be an obstruction or a drainage problem, special X-ray studies are necessary; contrast material is placed in the bladder by means of a catheter, and X-ray pictures are taken of the bladder and the urethra during urination. With such studies, narrowing of a portion of the urethra, the presence of kidney stones, and incomplete emptying of the bladder (which promotes cystitis) can be detected. The bladder can also be examined through cystoscopy (examination by means of a flexible, lighted, tubelike instrument called a *cystoscope*, which is inserted through the urethra). These procedures are preceded by an intravenous pyelogram, in which contrast material injected through a vein is eliminated by the kidneys, providing an X-ray picture of the kidneys, ureters, and bladder.

Treatment
Treatment of first-time cystitis is usually by means of antibiotics

taken by mouth. Occasionally, large single doses of drugs are used. Recurrences may be treated in the same way if they are due to a different organism. If the same organism is causing the trouble, the condition may require larger doses of medication or long-term treatment. (Daily doses of medications may be necessary for six months or more.) It is important that dosage instructions be followed exactly, because a person is vulnerable to a new infection or reinfection if the entire course of recommended drug therapy is not completed.

Some individuals are prone to repeated episodes of cystitis or upper urinary tract infections. If there is an anatomic defect, such as a narrowed urethra, dilation (enlarging) may be needed. If stones are present, they may have to be removed. If an infected prostate is the source of infection, antibiotics are usually tried first; surgery is a last resort. If no obvious cause of recurrent cystitis is found, low doses of antibiotics may be prescribed for long periods of time (this is called prophylactic, or preventive, therapy).

Prevention
Women may be able to guard against recurrent cystitis by front-to-back wiping with toilet tissue and by cleansing with soap and water after each bowel movement. They should also try to urinate immediately after sexual intercourse to wash away infecting bacteria that might enter the urethra. Loose, absorbent underclothes allow evaporation and absorption of body fluids and thus help prevent infection. Both men and women should drink plenty of fluids and urinate frequently, completely emptying the bladder each time.

Dialysis

Dialysis is the removal of wastes and other undesirable substances from the blood by means of a special membrane that is selective in what it allows to cross. In the healthy body, this task is performed by the kidneys.

Hemodialysis
In a patient suffering from temporary or permanent kidney failure, cleansing of the blood can be done with an artificial kidney machine; this is known as *hemodialysis*. Two plastic tubes, one connected to an artery and one to a vein, are implanted in the patient's arm or

leg. During dialysis, which can take three to five hours per treatment, blood from the artery tube enters the machine and comes into contact with a thin membrane. Wastes from the blood pass through the membrane into circulating fluid on the other side of the membrane. The blood cells themselves cannot cross the membrane. The cleaned blood is then piped back into the patient through the vein tube.

Peritoneal dialysis

In peritoneal dialysis, the patient's own peritoneum (lining of the abdominal cavity) is used as the dialysis membrane. A sterile plastic catheter (tube) is passed into the abdominal cavity, and a solution of glucose (a form of sugar) and mineral salts is periodically injected into and withdrawn from the cavity. The fluid comes into contact with delicate blood vessels in the peritoneum.

Because of the difference in concentration of certain chemical elements in the blood and the dialysis solution, wastes from the blood are forced through the membrane of the peritoneal wall. The dialysis liquid is periodically withdrawn and replaced with a fresh solution.

Continuous ambulatory peritoneal dialysis

A new method called continuous ambulatory peritoneal dialysis has greatly lowered the cost of dialysis and made the procedure more convenient. It can be done at home by the patient without the complex equipment and the skilled supervision that has made machine dialysis so expensive. A tube is surgically implanted in the patient, just below the navel. About every four to five hours and just before bedtime, the patient drains out the old fluid and empties a bag of fresh dialysis fluid into the abdominal cavity through a tube. The fluid remains in the cavity, soaking up wastes from the blood, while the patient sleeps or goes about his or her usual daily activities. The procedure enables the patient to be independent and mobile.

Glomerulo-nephritis

Each kidney contains more than a million filtering units called *nephrons,* in which wastes are drawn from the blood to form urine. In each nephron is a network of capillaries (tiny blood

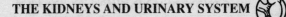
vessels) called a *glomerulus*. Glomerulonephritis is an inflammation of the glomeruli (the plural of glomerulus), which interferes with the normal operation of the kidney.

Causes

Glomerulonephritis can be caused by an infection in the kidneys, but most often it is due to an allergic reaction or immune response to infections in other parts of the body. Although many different kinds of infections can lead to glomerulonephritis, including pneumonia, bacterial infection of the heart, syphilis, malaria, hepatitis, and measles, the most common cause is infection of the throat, tonsils, or skin by certain types of *Streptococcus* bacteria. The body's immune response to the infection occurs as an inflammation of the capillaries in the glomeruli. The capillaries become congested and surrounded by blood cells and pus.

Fluid builds up in surrounding tissues, sometimes causing the kidneys to enlarge. Protein, which should remain in the blood, is discharged into the urine through the diseased glomeruli, and there is edema (fluid buildup) in body tissues. These two signs—edema and the presence of albumin (a type of protein) in the urine—are the chief indicators of the disease.

If the disease continues to progress, the tiny arteries in the kidneys become thickened and scarred so that some can no longer carry blood. The parts of the kidneys that they serve shrink. The eventual result of this process may be total kidney failure. The disease affects both kidneys.

Symptoms

Symptoms of glomerulonephritis usually begin one to three weeks after an initial infection, such as strep throat. The patient has headaches, a mild fever, a puffy face, pain in the area between the ribs and the hips, and decreased urine output. The urine may be bloody, smoky, or coffee-colored. Shortness of breath may occur, together with increased heartbeat and a rise in blood pressure. Detection of protein and red blood cells in the urine confirms the diagnosis.

Treatment

Treatment includes antibiotics, if streptoccoccal organisms are still present. Rest and symptomatic treatment are necessary for at least a week after tests of blood, blood pressure, and the urine indicate that the kidneys are back to normal.

Sodium and protein may be restricted or even forbidden for a time. Fluids are restricted until the output of urine returns to normal. Any infection is treated promptly with antibiotics. The overwhelming majority of patients with glomerulonephritis due to streptococcal infection recover fully.

Guarding against infection, injury, and fatigue can help prevent flare-ups of the disease. Intake of protein may have to be limited, depending on how well the kidneys are working. A return to normal activity is desirable, but strenuous exercise should be avoided.

If the disease is still present after one to two years, it may be considered chronic. This occurs in 5 to 20 percent of patients. Typically, the damage to the kidneys continues to progress, but so slowly that the patient is without symptoms; the only evidence of kidney damage may be the presence of protein and red and white blood cells in the urine.

A normal life may be possible for 20 or 30 years, until the kidneys can no longer function. At that time, patients must receive dialysis or a kidney transplant is necessary to prolong life.

Incontinence

Urinary incontinence is the loss of voluntary bladder control. It occurs frequently in children and in older people.

Causes

Most often, incontinence is caused by some underlying condition, such as obstruction, infection, or inflammation of any portion of the urinary tract. Successful treatment of the underlying cause clears up the problem.

Stress incontinence is the leakage of urine on coughing, sneezing, straining, or laughing. This type of incontinence is common in women whose pelvic muscles have been weakened by childbirth.

Treatment

Although the first step in treating incontinence is to detect and correct any underlying problem, it is important to remember that many children do not establish complete bladder control before they are four or five years old. Children of any age may have occasional accidents, especially if they are ill or exhausted.

Persons who have problems with incontinence can help themselves by going to the bathroom often and regularly, by arranging their sleeping and living quarters near bathrooms, and by wearing clothes that can be removed quickly and easily. It may also help to keep a bedpan or urinal next to the bed and to drink only a small amount of water, if any, before going to bed.

Drugs are available to aid in controlling urination in certain conditions. Stress incontinence can usually be surgically corrected.

Kidney failure

Kidney failure occurs when certain abnormalities within the kidneys prevent them from functioning normally, leading to chemical imbalances and the buildup of toxic (poisonous) substances and fluid within the body. This can eventually lead to organ damage and possibly death.

There are two forms of kidney failure. In the acute form, there is a sudden malfunction of the kidneys, leading to a rapid buildup of toxins and fluid within the body, often within several hours. In the chronic form of kidney failure, there is a slow, progressive deterioration of kidney function, leading to a buildup of toxins and fluid, often occurring over several months or years.

Causes
Numerous conditions can cause kidney failure. High blood pressure, kidney stones or other urinary tract blockage, adverse reactions to chemicals or drugs, serious injury, infectious disease, shock after surgery, heart attack, blood transfusion with incompatible blood, severe dehydration, complications during pregnancy, immunologic disease, and congenital (existing from birth) kidney defects may all lead to kidney failure.

Symptoms
The most characteristic symptoms of kidney failure are a reduction in the volume of urine and edema (excessive accumulation of fluid in the tissues). As a result, the feet and hands and the area around the eyes may swell and become puffy. The urine may be bloody or cloudy in appearance.

More generalized signs of kidney failure include drowsiness and fatigue, loss of appetite, diarrhea, nausea, dry skin, and difficulty in breathing. Delirium, coma, and death will eventually occur in untreated cases.

Diagnosis

Analysis of blood and urine samples is commonly used to diagnose kidney failure. Urine tests may show that white blood cells, sugars, or protein have slipped through the normally efficient filtering system of the kidneys. Similarly, when the kidneys are not filtering waste materials from the blood, blood analysis will detect waste products remaining in the blood. X-ray studies, ultrasound scans of the kidneys, or cystoscopy may identify structural abnormalities or blockage of the kidneys.

Treatment

In the case of acute kidney failure, treatment begins with diagnosing and correcting the cause of the kidney damage and restoring normal kidney function as rapidly as possible. For example, shock may be treated with intravenous fluids, drugs, and, in some cases, blood transfusions.

Rest is essential as the kidneys recover. Limiting fluid intake, except in cases of unusual fluid loss from diarrhea or vomiting, may prevent congestive heart failure due to kidney overload. Physicians often recommend a low-protein diet due to the inability of the kidneys to process the waste products of protein metabolism.

Should these measures prove ineffective, the patient may be helped by dialysis. Dialysis is a process that cleans and filters toxic substances from the blood with an artificial kidney machine. Most dialysis patients receive treatment by traveling to the hospital three times a week. However, newer portable techniques allow more freedom for dialysis patients.

In the case of chronic kidney failure, destruction of the kidney has progressed so much that treatment cannot bring kidney function back to normal. Treatment of these patients involves dialysis and a diet low in salt and protein. Dialysis will offer a chance to prolong life, but it is not a cure; only surgically replacing the damaged kidneys can cure the condition. In recent years, methods of matching kidney donors with recipients have improved, thereby limiting transplant rejection and serious complications. Today, kidney transplants have a high rate of success.

Kidney stones

Kidney stones are deposits of mineral or organic substances

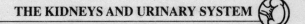

that form in the kidneys. When abnormally high levels of certain minerals, such as calcium, are in the urine, they may condense into hard masses, forming stones in the kidneys or urinary tract. The stones may be as small as a tiny pebble or as large as a walnut.

Causes

Increased levels of calcium in urine may come from drinking excessive quantities of milk. Eating foods rich in vitamin D, which helps the body absorb calcium, can also contribute to an overaccumulation of calcium. In addition, fractured bones can release extra calcium, which may condense into stones in the kidneys.

Certain disorders encourage buildup of mineral deposits in the kidneys. Gout is a joint disease that results from high blood levels of uric acid (a waste product from the breakdown of protein), which can crystallize into stones in the urine.

Urinary infections that impede bladder function can also cause retention of urine, which then harbors higher concentrations of elements that can solidify into stones. In addition, overactive parathyroid glands (endocrine glands that regulate calcium absorption) permit increased mineral absorption.

Middle-aged men and persons with gout or chronic urinary tract infections are more susceptible to the development of kidney stones. However, in many cases, it is not possible to pinpoint the cause of the kidney stones.

Symptoms

Kidney stones may be present for years and never produce any symptoms. Problems arise when a stone becomes so large that it obstructs or irritates a part of the kidney or causes problems as it passes out of the kidney. Symptoms include severe pain and tenderness over the affected kidney, frequent and painful urination, blood in the urine, nausea, fever, chills, and extreme exhaustion.

A more serious condition can develop if a stone becomes lodged in a ureter. It produces excruciating pain across the back, abdomen, and reproductive organs. If blockage occurs in the urethra, urine output decreases. The trapped urine may back up, distending and injuring the urinary tract. This situation requires immediate medical treatment.

Kidney stones that are too small to be noticed may still

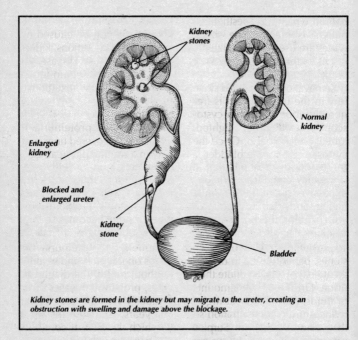

Kidney stones are formed in the kidney but may migrate to the ureter, creating an obstruction with swelling and damage above the blockage.

cause damage to the urinary tract.

Diagnosis

To determine the type of kidney stone formation, a physician analyzes samples of the patient's blood and urine. Analysis of stone fragments or the actual stone is critical in determining the exact chemical imbalance. An ultrasound or X-ray study may reveal the location and nature of the stones.

Treatment

Treatment is aimed at keeping the patient well hydrated and as comfortable as possible until the stone is passed.

For kidney stones too large to pass, surgical removal may be necessary. A new, nonsurgical method of treating kidney stones called extracorporeal shock-wave lithotripsy is becoming more widely available. With this technique, tiny shock waves are pulsed into a water bath in which the anesthetized patient is placed. The shock waves are used to pulverize the stones so that they can pass out of the urinary tract.

Removal of an impacted stone low in the urinary tract is frequently done through a cystoscope (a flexible, lighted, tubelike instrument). Once the cystoscope is in the bladder, a tiny guide wire attached to a basket is inserted into the ureter and withdrawn, with the stone inside.

Prevention
To prevent recurrence of kidney stones, patients need to drink a great deal of fluid to dilute their urine. Drinking large amounts of fluids, particularly at night, reduces urine concentration so that stones cannot form. Surplus water can also flush the system of any small stones. For individuals with excess calcium, uric acid, or other minerals in their urine, medication and dietary therapy can be helpful in preventing kidney stone recurrences.

Proteinuria

Excessive proteinuria (protein in the urine) is a symptom of kidney problems.

Causes
Proteinuria can be caused by, among other conditions, kidney malfunction, heart disease, the consumption of certain foods, pregnancy, and overexertion.

Symptoms
Most cases of proteinuria in adults are discovered unexpectedly in a routine physical. Usually, the person will have experienced no symptoms and will be essentially healthy, with no evidence of kidney disease.

Treatment
Treatment of proteinuria depends on its cause and severity. In about half of the diagnosed cases, proteinuria ceases spontaneously within a year to several years. There are instances in which the patient continues to lose greater and greater amounts of protein in the urine. Eventually, the condition may cause high blood pressure and kidney failure.

Pyelonephritis

Pyelonephritis is an inflammatory condition of both the kidney tissue and the renal pelvis (the funnel-shaped expansion of the upper end of the ureter where it joins the kidney).

There are two types of pyelonephritis, descending and ascending. In the descending type, the bacteria reach the kidney through the bloodstream, infecting first the kidney tissues themselves and then moving downward to infect the renal pelvis of the kidney. In the more common ascending type, the bladder is infected first, and the infection then spreads upward to the kidney.

Causes
Most cases of pyelonephritis are caused by bacterial infection. Conditions that increase the likelihood of such an infection include scars from previous infections, urinary tract infections, abnormal growth of the prostate gland, kidney stones, tumors, stagnation of urine due to backflow from the bladder, diabetes mellitus (excess sugar in the bloodstream), and pregnancy.

Symptoms
Symptoms of acute pyelonephritis include fever, back pain, difficulty in urinating, a burning sensation on urination, mental confusion, nausea, vomiting, and in extreme cases, loss of consciousness. Although some cases of chronic pyelonephritis can be traced to an initial attack, many patients will have no evidence of past or current infections.

Treatment
Acute pyelonephritis is treated with antibiotics given orally or intravenously. Recurrent episodes should be treated with an appropriate antibiotic. Chronic pyelonephritis requires careful management and frequent re-evaluation. Patients are generally treated with an antibiotic even during periods when they feel no symptoms and usually receive long-term therapy.

THE ENDOCRINE SYSTEM

The endocrine system comprises a number of glands that produce hormones with a varied array of vital functions. Hormones are chemical substances that are secreted by organs or by cells of organs in one part of the body and are carried by the bloodstream to other organs or tissues, where they control or regulate the development or function of those structures.

Endocrine glands are also called *ductless glands,* because they secrete hormones directly into the bloodstream. In contrast, exocrine glands release their secretions through ducts (for example, the sweat glands produce fluid that flows to the skin's surface through tiny tube-like sweat ducts).

Hormones can be considered chemical messengers. They are targeted at specific cells in the body, and their arrival in those cells causes specific activities to occur. One of the major tasks of hormones is to coordinate the activities of organ systems. For example, when a person has to run, the hormone epinephrine acts on the heart to increase its rate and force of contraction; it acts on the blood vessels to increase blood flow to the muscles and decrease blood flow to the gastrointestinal tract. Hormones also help control the type and rate of body growth and metabolism, and they help the body maintain a consistent internal environment.

The endocrine system has a large influence on the way we feel and act. In turn, our energy and other needs in any given situation set the activity of the endocrine system. This feedback relationship is crucial in maintaining our general well-being.

Adrenal glands

The adrenal glands are critical to normal body functions, such as maintenance of fluid balance, reaction to stress, and reproduction. There are two adrenal glands, each of which lies above a kidney. The adrenal glands have two distinct parts: the cortex (outer layer), which

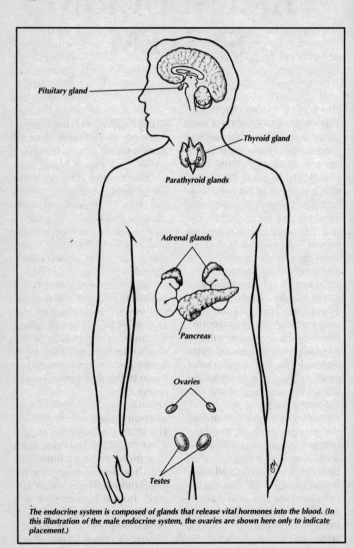

The endocrine system is composed of glands that release vital hormones into the blood. (In this illustration of the male endocrine system, the ovaries are shown here only to indicate placement.)

secretes steroid hormones, and the medulla (inner part), which secretes epinephrine and norepinephrine.

There are more than 30 steroid hormones produced by the adrenal glands. These hormones serve to regulate a wide array of processes throughout the body. Epinephrine and norepinephrine are responsible for the changes in heart rate, blood pressure, and level of usable glucose (a form of sugar) that are necessary to cope with stress.

Pancreas

The pancreas is located in the rear center of the abdominal cavity, behind the stomach. Specialized cells in the pancreas produce two hormones, insulin and glucagon, needed to maintain stable blood sugar levels in the body. Insulin helps body cells use glucose for energy, thereby reducing the amount of sugar in the bloodstream. To balance this action, the hormone glucagon stimulates the liver to release its stored sugar into the blood, thereby raising the blood sugar levels.

The pancreas also functions in digestion. Nonendocrine cells in the pancreas produce special chemicals called enzymes, which are secreted directly into the small intestine through ducts. These enzymes help break down proteins, carbohydrates (sugars and starches), and fats in the small intestine.

This dual activity of the pancreas means that it functions as both an endocrine and an exocrine organ.

Pituitary gland

The pituitary gland is a small organ located just beneath the base of the brain, between the two frontal lobes and directly above a cavity called the sphenoid sinus. It is sometimes called the master gland because all other endocrine glands come under its control. Its job is to receive messages about the need for a particular hormone and to secrete either the hormone or substances that cause the manufacture and release of the hormone.

The anterior (front) lobe of the pituitary gland secretes somatotropin (growth hormone), which affects the body's general growth; thyrotropic hormone (thyroid-stimulating hormone), which acts on the thyroid gland to stimulate production of thyroid hormones; adrenocorticotropic hormone (ACTH), which stimulates the adrenal cortex; follicle-stimulating hormone and luteinizing hormone, which are necessary for maturation and release of egg and sperm cells; and prolactin, a hormone that acts on the mammary glands to promote the secretion of milk.

The posterior lobe of the pituitary gland secretes oxytocin, which stimulates smooth muscle tissue to contract (and is of critical importance during childbirth) and vasopressin, a hormone that regulates by acting on the kidneys.

Sex glands

The primary responsibility for hormone production for the reproductive system lies with the testes (male sex glands) and ovaries (female sex glands).

The testes are two oval organs in the scrotum (the pouch of skin behind the penis). The testes produce sperm and sex hormones that govern the male secondary sex characteristics, including the growth of facial hair.

The two ovaries are located in the pelvis. The ovaries secrete the hormones estrogen and progesterone, which govern ovulation (monthly release of an egg from an ovary) and the female secondary sex characteristics, such as breast development.

Thyroid and parathyroid glands

The thyroid gland is located at the front of the neck above the top of the breastbone. It consists of two main lobes on either side of the trachea (windpipe) that are connected by a narrow band of tissue called the isthmus. The hormones secreted by the thyroid influence the rate of metabolism (the chemical processes in the body having to do with energy production).

The four parathyroid glands are located on the back and side of each lobe of the thyroid gland. Their secretion, parathyroid hormone, controls calcium levels in the blood.

Addison disease

Addison disease is a condition that occurs when the adrenal cortex fails to produce enough of its hormones.

Causes

Formerly, the cause of this disease was often tuberculosis or a fungal infection. However, in recent years, the disease is more likely to be idiopathic (of unknown cause). One theory is that most cases are due to autoimmune destruction of the adrenal cortex (that is, the body produces antibodies against its own tissues). Other known causes of Addison disease include partial destruction of the adrenal cortex by cancer, surgery, degeneration of the tissue, or deposition of a substance called amyloid.

A similar condition, known as secondary adrenal insufficiency, is caused by failure of the pituitary gland to produce enough adrenocorticotropic hormone (ACTH), which stimulates the adrenal cortex to produce its hormones.

Symptoms
Early symptoms of Addison disease are weakness, fatigue, and a tendency to become faint when rising suddenly from a bed or chair. Increased pigmentation of the skin, producing a "tan" all over the body, on exposed and unexposed areas alike, with even darker pigmentation on creases and bony pressure points, occurs in most cases. In certain places, the tan may be broken by completely white patches, known as vitiligo. Black freckles appear on the forehead, face, shoulders, and neck. There may be skin discoloration around the nipples, and the mucous membranes of the mouth may have dark-blue patches.

Symptoms that may appear later include weight loss, dehydration (excessive loss of body fluids), low blood pressure, and sometimes nausea, vomiting, diarrhea, dizziness, an inability to get or stay warm, and a loss of appetite.

The most alarming symptoms are those of a condition called adrenal crisis, which requires immediate attention and hospitalization. Signs of this are extreme weakness; severe pains in the lower back, abdomen, or legs; shock (collapse of the circulatory system); and renal shutdown (kidney failure). Such a crisis may be brought on by severe stress, such as infection, injury, or surgery. It can also be caused by a loss of salt through perspiration during hot weather.

Diagnosis
One laboratory sign of Addison disease is a high level of ACTH but a low level of cortisol (one of the adrenal gland hormones) in the blood. This indicates that the pituitary gland is working overtime, stimulating the adrenal cortex with ACTH to produce cortisol, but that the cortex is failing to produce it.

Treatment
The basic treatment for Addison disease is to provide steroid

hormones, principally cortisone, to replace those not being produced by the adrenal cortex. An additional steroid drug may be prescribed to promote retention of salt, and thereby water, in tissues and blood, so that the low blood pressure of severe Addison disease can be avoided.

The outlook for patients receiving hormone treatment is excellent. Continued medical supervision is necessary to prevent emergencies caused by a sudden withdrawal of treatment or by an increased need for hormones because of infection, injury, surgery, pregnancy, or other stress on the body. It is important to avoid infection, but should infection occur it is necessary to treat it as soon as possible. At all times, patients should carry a card or wear a bracelet describing the condition and the need for cortisone. It is also critical to take the medication exactly as prescribed and to be monitored by a physician who can increase or decrease the dosage as the need arises.

Corticosteroids

Corticosteroids are hormones produced in the cortex of the adrenal glands in response to stimulation by adrenocorticotropic hormone (ACTH), which is secreted by the pituitary gland. There are more than 30 corticosteroids, which regulate essential processes throughout the body. They are divided into three groups: mineralocorticoids, glucocorticoids, and androgens (male sex hormones).

Natural forms
Mineralocorticoids are involved in maintaining salt and water balance in the body. Without these hormones, the tissues and blood would become depleted of salt and water; the resultant decrease in blood volume would cause a drop in blood pressure that could lead to shock (collapse of the circulatory system).

Glucocorticoids help regulate the body's use and reserves of sugars and proteins, among other complex metabolic processes. They also participate in the inflammatory response and the body's reaction to stress. The most important of these hormones is cortisol, which plays a major role in protein breakdown and formation, blood sugar control, and reduction of inflammation. Cortisol is also necessary to mount an effective response against severe stress resulting from disease or injury.

Androgens (which are also produced in the testes) stimulate the development of the male secondary sex characteristics, such as beard growth and increased muscle mass.

Drug forms

Pharmacologic preparations of both ACTH and corticosteroids are used to treat disease in the same way that the natural hormones would; they also act as substitute or supplemental hormones for patients who have lost the ability to manufacture their own. The primary difference is that ACTH acts less directly and more generally than corticosteroid drugs. ACTH stimulates the adrenal glands to enlarge and secrete more of all the steroids that they produce, rather than any one specific hormone. Corticosteroid drugs can be administered to the part of the body that needs them most. For example, a dab of hydrocortisone cream will eliminate a rash, and a hydrocortisone injection will diminish the swelling of a painful knee joint, generally with little effect on the rest of the body. Sometimes, however, corticosteroids are considered for generalized use throughout the body. Corticosteroids have an advantage over ACTH in that they can be taken by mouth and may be given in doses that far exceed what the adrenal glands can produce. ACTH must be injected because it would otherwise be destroyed by digestive enzymes, which do not affect the corticosteroids.

Cushing syndrome

Cushing syndrome is a group of abnormalities resulting from an excess of the hormones produced by the cortex of the adrenal glands. The hormones produced in excess are chiefly cortisol, which has many complex functions; various hormones that regulate the body's use of sugars and proteins; male sex hormones; and a hormone that controls the distribution of fluids and salts in the body.

Causes

In most cases, Cushing syndrome is caused by excess production of adrenocorticotropic hormone (ACTH), which is normally manufactured by the pituitary gland to stimulate production of hormones by the adrenal glands. This excess of

ACTH can be caused by an ACTH-producing tumor in another organ, such as the lung or pancreas; by overmedication with ACTH or corticosteroid drugs; by tiny, nonmalignant ACTH-producing tumors on the pituitary gland; or by a tumor (usually nonmalignant) on the adrenal gland. The effect of too much ACTH, for whatever reason, is overgrowth of tissue in the adrenal cortex, resulting in overproduction of all its hormones. Since these hormones regulate essential processes throughout the body, excess production causes widespread disorders.

Symptoms

One of the most obvious signs of Cushing syndrome is the moon-shaped face, caused by excess fluid in the tissues. Because of deposition of excess fat, the trunk of the body is obese (although the arms and legs are thin), and there are fat pads over the shoulders and neck, producing a "buffalo hump." Purple "stretch marks" on the skin (usually of the abdomen), poor wound healing, easy bruising, muscle weakness, fractures in weakened bones, and emotional instability may also be part of the syndrome. Hairiness, acne, and decreased or absent menstruation may occur in women, due to the increase in male hormones. Diabetes and high blood pressure are also very common.

Diagnosis

Diagnosis of Cushing syndrome requires measurement of adrenal cortex hormones in the blood and urine. In healthy people, cortisol levels in the blood are high on awakening but decrease during the day; in the person with Cushing syndrome, cortisol levels are high all of the time. Various tests can determine whether the cause of the syndrome is a tumor of the pituitary gland (in which case the disorder is known as Cushing disease) or a tumor on the adrenal gland or elsewhere. Tumors on the adrenal glands may be identified by X rays, ultrasound, and computed tomography (CT). CT scans and other special X rays of the head can often locate tumors of the pituitary gland.

Treatment

Cushing syndrome is treated by restoring a normal balance of hormones. This may involve surgery, radiation treatments, or drugs. Tumors on the adrenal glands are removed by surgery.

If there is a tumor on just one adrenal gland, the other gland usually shrinks and ceases normal productivity. Hormone supplements are usually given before surgery and must be taken for weeks or months after surgery until the second gland recovers normal function. In a rapidly worsening case of Cushing syndrome in which the cortex is greatly enlarged on both sides, methods of treatment include chemotherapy (drug treatments), radiation treatments of the pituitary gland (to weaken it and lower its output of ACTH), or removal of any adenomas (nonmalignant growths) on the pituitary gland. The removal of the adrenal glands is usually a last-resort measure. In this case, the patient must take daily supplements of adrenal cortex hormones for the rest of his or her life.

If Cushing syndrome is being caused by production of ACTH by a cancerous tumor in a part of the body other than the adrenal glands, the cancer is removed, if possible. However, in many cases it is inoperable, so drugs to suppress production of the adrenal glands are given.

Cushing syndrome is a very serious, possibly fatal, disease unless it is detected and treated early. The outlook is best for those whose condition is caused by noncancerous growths and who receive early treatment.

Those who must take replacement hormones after treatment should carry a medical identification card and immediately tell their doctor about any infections, injuries, or stressful situations that might require an increase in hormone dosage. They should also report signs of underdosage, such as weakness, dizziness, or fatigue, as well as signs of overdosage, such as swollen tissues and rapid weight gain. Anyone whose adrenal glands have been removed must always take replacement hormones; stopping these medications for any length of time is fatal.

Diabetes mellitus

Diabetes mellitus, which is often referred to as sugar diabetes, is a condition in which the body is unable to properly process carbohydrates (sugars and starches), which are the body's major source of energy.

Cause

Normally, digestion causes carbohydrates to release a form of sugar called glucose into the

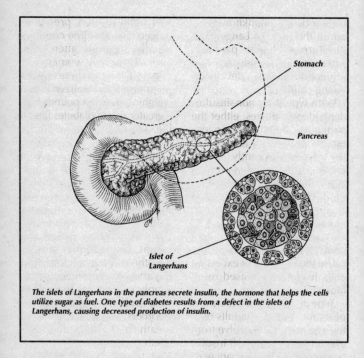

The islets of Langerhans in the pancreas secrete insulin, the hormone that helps the cells utilize sugar as fuel. One type of diabetes results from a defect in the islets of Langerhans, causing decreased production of insulin.

blood. As the blood glucose level rises, the pancreas is stimulated to secrete the hormone insulin. Insulin acts to reduce the sugar content in the blood by transporting glucose from the blood to body cells, where it is used for fuel, or to the liver, where it is stored until needed.

When the pancreas produces insufficient insulin or the body cannot use the insulin it manufactures, diabetes results. The glucose concentration in the blood increases because glucose circulates throughout the body without being absorbed. Eventually, the kidneys filter glucose from the blood, and urine carries the excess sugar from the body.

Types

There are two major forms of diabetes. Type I (or insulin-dependent) diabetes results

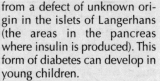
from a defect of unknown origin in the islets of Langerhans (the areas in the pancreas where insulin is produced). This form of diabetes can develop in young children.

With type II (or non–insulin-dependent) diabetes, either the pancreas functions inadequately or the body is unable to use insulin efficiently. Sometimes, a shortage of insulin-receptor cells (sites throughout the body where the interaction of glucose and insulin occurs) allows the insulin to remain in the bloodstream. Obesity often contributes to the problem because the presence of excess fat cells leads to increased resistance to insulin.

Type II diabetes, which appears most often in adults over the age of 40, may evolve from a gradual slowing of insulin production within the pancreas. In addition, other disorders of the endocrine system may cause hormonal imbalances that disturb glucose regulation.

Research shows that people who have a family history of type II diabetes may have a greater tendency to acquire the condition. Women are more likely to be affected, but for all adults, the risk of developing type II diabetes doubles with every decade after the age of 40.

In some women, pregnancy triggers diabetes. The condition usually subsides after childbirth. However, women who show signs of diabetes during pregnancy and deliver babies weighing over ten pounds have a greater risk of diabetes later in life.

Complications

Although patients with diabetes can usually control the condition, untreated diabetes can lead to serious complications. Extremely high blood sugar levels place great strain on other organs. Diabetes may accelerate atherosclerosis (clogging of the arteries). Insufficient blood supply contributes to heart attack, stroke, kidney disease, eye disorders, impotence, gangrene (death of tissue), and even death.

Symptoms

Symptoms of type I diabetes are excessive thirst and urination, fatigue, altered vision, fainting, irritability, and slow healing of cuts and bruises. Weight loss may occur despite constant hunger and voracious eating.

The same symptoms may signal type II diabetes, or no symptoms may appear at all. Physicians frequently detect this form when they perform routine examinations or tests for other problems.

Diagnosis

Doctors can diagnose diabetes by analyzing blood samples for elevated sugar concentrations. They may also test blood and urine for excess ketones, the chemical by-products of the breakdown of fat for energy. Since people with diabetes do not use glucose normally, their bodies burn fat for fuel, and as a result, ketones are eliminated in the urine.

Treatment

Both forms of diabetes mellitus require a treatment plan that maintains normal, steady blood glucose levels. Once blood sugar levels have been brought under control with insulin injections, diet, or medication, a person with diabetes can usually lead a relatively normal life.

Type I diabetes requires injections of insulin to maintain blood sugar levels evenly throughout the day. If the blood glucose concentration rises, imbalance may be signalled by weakness, fatigue, and thirst. These symptoms mean that more insulin is needed. However, if blood glucose concentration falls too low, an insulin reaction sets in, causing dizzi-

ness, hunger, fatigue, headache, sweating, trembling, and (in severe cases) unconsciousness. A quick remedy for this problem is to give the person simple sugar, such as is found in orange juice and some kinds of candy. This should be done only if the person is conscious and alert, however; nothing should be given by mouth to an unconscious or semiconscious person, because of the risk of choking.

Ideally, a doctor can prevent these fluctuations of sugar levels by coordinating the type and timing of insulin injections with meal content and energy output. A special diet is important to balance daily insulin injections. Young children with diabetes, in particular, need sufficient calories to grow and develop normally. Insulin requirements for persons with type I diabetes differ greatly. Some patients may maintain balanced blood sugar levels with one insulin injection taken before breakfast. Other patients may require several insulin injections per day. Insulin requirements may change as the patient grows older, undergoes surgery, becomes pregnant, or develops an unrelated illness.

Many people with type II diabetes can regulate their condition with proper diet; some require insulin injections. Sometimes, oral antidiabetic drugs, which work by stimulating the pancreas to produce more insulin or by stimulating the insulin receptors, may be prescribed.

Special attention to diet is critical for diabetes control. Overweight individuals need to lose weight. Thereafter, emphasis is on eating balanced meals that will sustain the recommended weight. Fats need to be limited to reduce susceptibility to atherosclerosis, and the diet should be low in simple sugars. The diet should include plenty of fibrous roughage, such as is contained in fruits, vegetables, and whole grains; fiber in the diet has been shown to reduce or slow sugar absorption in the digestive tract. A doctor can provide a medically approved diet plan, with enough flexibility to allow the diabetic patient to share in regular family meals while meeting his or her special dietary needs.

With either type of diabetes, follow-up is important to plan diet, determine changes in insulin dosage (in type I), and monitor blood for sugar levels. Testing urine for sugar has been shown to be inaccurate, and the availability of home blood glucose monitoring has all but replaced urine sugar testing for most diabetic patients. For individuals with type I diabetes, however, urine ketone testing is still important.

It has been shown in recent years that meticulous control of blood glucose levels can delay or prevent many of the complications of diabetes mellitus. Therefore, strict adherence to the regimen prescribed by the physician is of major importance.

Goiter

A goiter is an enlargement of the thyroid gland, which appears as a large swelling at the front of the neck.

Causes

Goiter may be caused by a lack of dietary iodine, which is necessary for the production of thyroid hormone. If there is a deficiency in iodine, the thyroid gland enlarges in an attempt to satisfy the body's demand for more hormone. When this situation occurs, the cells in the gland enlarge but do not increase in number.

At one time, goiter was common in areas where there is a lack of iodine in the soil and water. Since the ocean is the basic source of iodine, inland areas were the most deficient and had the highest number of goiter cases (in the United States, the Great Lakes region was such an area; in Europe, inhabitants of mountainous inland regions in the Alps often suffered from iodine deficiencies). In recent times, however, the use of iodized table salt has largely solved this problem.

Some forms of goiter are associated with an overactive thyroid gland; that is, one that produces more hormone than the body needs. Other forms of

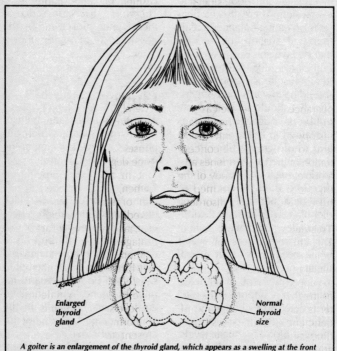

Enlarged thyroid gland

Normal thyroid size

A goiter is an enlargement of the thyroid gland, which appears as a swelling at the front of the neck.

goiter are associated with an underactive thyroid gland.

Symptoms

Often, the only symptom is swelling in the neck. If the thyroid is overactive, nervousness, weight loss, bulging eyes, rapid heartbeat, and high blood pressure may be noted. If the thyroid is underactive, sluggishness, weight gain, dry skin and dry hair, and fatigue may be present.

Diagnosis

The diagnosis is made primarily on the basis of the classic appearance and, in some cases of iodine deficiency, the dietary history of the patient. Blood tests to determine the concentration of thyroid hormones and a nuclear medicine study of the thyroid may be performed to rule out other thyroid disorders.

Treatment

The chief objective of goiter treatment is reduction of the swelling. The first step is usually to suppress the overfunctioning of the thyroid gland. If the goiter is caused by simple iodine deficiency, small doses of iodine can be given. Sometimes, administering synthetic thyroid hormone, in an attempt to halt the increased efforts by the gland to produce the natural hormone, will reduce the enlargement. If treatment is started early enough, surgery to remove portions of the enlarged gland can be avoided. Surgery may be necessary if the size of the goiter interferes with normal breathing by pressing on the windpipe or if its appearance is cosmetically undesirable.

Hirsutism

Hirsutism is excessive hair growth or hair growth in areas that are not usually hairy. In general, this condition is due to a hormonal imbalance.

Causes

Some degree of hirsutism is present in about 30 percent of women, and it may be a symptom of some other disorder. Hereditary tendencies, however, account for a large percentage of cases of hirsutism in women. It is thought, though, that hirsute women may have hair follicles that are hypersensitive to normal female androgen levels. (Androgen is a male sex hormone, but it is normally present to a lesser extent in women.)

In some cases, hirsutism is only one sign of virilization

(masculinization), which is characterized by acne, balding, and increased muscle mass. This condition may be due to overactive adrenal glands (which secrete some sex hormones), ovarian tumors, adrenal tumors, or use of steroid medications. However, the majority of hirsute women are not masculinized.

A common cause of hirsutism is polycystic ovaries; in this condition, the presence of numerous cysts on the ovaries leads to infrequent or absent menstruation and ovulation, obesity, and enlarged ovaries. Hirsutism is also seen in Cushing syndrome, a condition that in women is characterized by excessive fat tissue in the face, neck, and trunk; absence of menstruation; convex (outward) curvature of the spine; high blood pressure; and muscular weakness. Mild hirsutism also appears in young girls with underactive thyroid glands. Absence of or damage to the pituitary gland, anorexia nervosa (self-inflicted starvation), and use of some drugs can also cause hirsutism.

Symptoms
The only symptom of hirsutism is excessive growth of hair in men or women or growth of hair in normally hairless areas in women (for example, on the face, neck, breasts, chest, and abdomen). The hair may be soft and fine or coarse, depending on many factors.

Diagnosis
Diagnosis is usually confirmed through visual examination and medical history. Tests measuring various hormone levels in the blood may also be given.

Treatment
The treatment of hirsutism is based on removing the cause. For example, adrenal hyperplasia (an abnormal increase in the number of cells in the adrenal gland) can be suppressed by corticosteroid drugs. Patients with polycystic ovaries can be treated with low-dose estrogen birth control pills or with other drugs.

Removing the cause does not always diminish the hair growth, however, and hair removal may be desired for cosmetic reasons. The only safe, permanent local treatment is electrolysis (destruction of individual hair follicles with an electric current). Other measures, such as plucking, shaving, waxing, or using a depilatory wax or chemical, will mask the problem temporarily.

Prevention

Other than prompt diagnosis and treatment of the primary cause or underlying disorder (provided there is one), there are no known preventive measures against hirsutism.

Hyperthyroidism

Hyperthyroidism generally encompasses several different disorders with the common feature of excessive production of thyroid hormone. The two most common forms of hyperthyroidism are Graves disease and toxic multinodular goiter.

Causes

The production of thyroid hormone is normally regulated by the pituitary gland, which secretes thyroid-stimulating hormone (TSH) when a need for thyroid hormone is present and decreases secretion of TSH when it senses an adequate supply of the hormone. Generally speaking, some malfunction occurs in hyperthyroidism, and the thyroid is no longer sensitive to this regulatory mechanism. Graves disease is probably caused by the presence of an abnormal chemical stimulator of thyroid hormone production. In toxic multinodular goiter, nodules of thyroid tissue form, and secrete abnormally large amounts of thyroid hormone, independent of the amount of hormone in the body.

Symptoms

Because thyroid hormone is involved in so many vital processes, including maintenance of body temperature, conversion of food to energy, and regulation of growth and fertility, the effects of an excess of that hormone are many and varied. The symptoms common to all forms of hyperthyroidism include rapid heartbeat, weight loss despite increased appetite and food intake, generalized hyperactivity, tremors (shakiness), increased sweating, severe nervousness and emotional instability, alteration of menstruation and fertility, and muscle weakness.

In addition to these symptoms, patients with Graves disease often have bulging eyes. Their skin is characteristically warm, moist, and velvety, and there may be areas of raised, thickened, sometimes itchy skin on the legs and feet with the texture of orange peel. The thyroid gland is frequently enlarged, smooth, and soft. This disease occurs most often in

405

those in their 30s and 40s. It is more common in women than in men.

In toxic multinodular goiter, the thyroid gland is lumpy but not uniformly enlarged. This condition occurs most often in the middle-aged and elderly.

Diagnosis

The diagnosis of hyperthyroidism is made on the basis of the patient's medical history and findings from a physical examination and various laboratory studies. Significant elevation of the level of thyroid hormone in the blood can be detected with special blood tests. The diagnosis can be further established through the use of nuclear medicine scans obtained after the injection of radioactive iodine, which becomes concentrated in the thyroid gland. The nuclear medicine study yields not only a picture of the gland but also an estimate of the degree of hyperactivity.

Treatment

Specific treatment of hyperthyroidism depends on which condition is present. However, treatment of the hyperthyroid state in general has several common elements. The drug propranolol, a beta-blocker, is commonly used to help prevent the effects of the hormonal overstimulation that greatly contributes to the tremors, increased heart rate, and sweating. This drug, although it diminishes symptoms, does not decrease the amount of thyroid hormone being produced. Therefore, an antithyroid drug, such as propylthiouracil, is necessary. Antithyroid drugs work by actually interfering with the production of thyroid hormone. However, this is usually only a temporary solution; when the drug is stopped, the excess production sometimes resumes. The definitive therapy for hyperthyroidism is the destruction or removal of most or all of the thyroid gland. This is achieved by using radioactive iodine or surgery.

Graves disease is usually first treated by blocking hormonal overstimulation with propranolol. Simultaneously, an antithyroid drug is started. This drug may be maintained for a long period of time. If relapse occurs (which it frequently does) or if the level of thyroid hormone is not normalized, the question then is how to reduce the amount of thyroid tissue. Whether surgery or radioactive iodine is used depends on many complex factors. Both treatments frequently result in too little thyroid hormone in the blood, but this problem is easily remedied by supplementation with synthetic thyroid hormone.

Hypoglycemia

Hypoglycemia is the state of having an abnormally low blood glucose level. (Glucose is a sugar released into the blood as a result of digestion of carbohydrates.)

The two main forms of this condition are reactive hypoglycemia and fasting hypoglycemia. To understand how both forms occur, it is helpful to understand how glucose levels are normally regulated.

During digestion, elevated blood glucose levels trigger the secretion of the hormone insulin from the pancreas. Insulin acts to reduce the sugar level in the blood by helping body cells absorb the glucose for fuel.

Reactive hypoglycemia
Reactive hypoglycemia is caused by oversecretion of insulin and consequent rapid lowering of blood glucose levels in response to ingestion of glucose. Reactive hypoglycemia is also known as postprandial (after

meals) hypoglycemia, because it occurs specifically in response to ingestion of food.

The specific causes of reactive hypoglycemia are unknown in most cases. However, certain persons—for example, those in the early stage of adult-onset diabetes mellitus and patients who have had part or most of the stomach removed surgically—are particularly susceptible to reactive hypoglycemia.

Fasting hypoglycemia
Fasting hypoglycemia is caused by insufficient production of glucose or overutilization of the glucose present in the blood. Often, these two factors combine to severely depress the blood glucose level. An insulin-producing tumor on the pancreas can also cause fasting hypoglycemia. Because alcohol disturbs the normal mechanisms of sugar storage and release within the liver, heavy drinkers are at greater risk of developing the disorder. Fasting hypoglycemia can also occur in anyone who has not eaten for an unusually long interval, but this is a temporary situation.

Symptoms
The symptoms of both types of hypoglycemia include fatigue,

407

nervousness, perspiration, dizziness, headache, hunger pangs, visual impairment, and accelerated heartbeat. The condition may also cause anxiety, difficulty in concentrating, confusion, and blackouts. If sugar deprivation continues unchecked, severe hypoglycemia may produce convulsions (short-term loss of consciousness, accompanied by jerking muscle movements) or deep coma (prolonged loss of consciousness).

True hypoglycemia is an uncommon condition. Since many of the symptoms of anxiety and hypoglycemia are alike, the two conditions are often confused.

Diagnosis

To diagnose hypoglycemia, a doctor analyzes a blood sample to detect abnormally low sugar levels. Blood drawn during an attack of the condition allows the most accurate assessment, since symptoms can then be correlated with actual blood glucose levels.

Treatment

Treatment for hypoglycemia is often aimed at the underlying cause of the disease. For example, surgical removal of a pancreatic tumor or adjustment of a diabetic patient's insulin dosage

may be necessary. In most cases of reactive hypoglycemia, however, there is no known cure for the tendency of the pancreas to overproduce insulin when it is not needed. The most effective treatment is to avoid all foods that generate attacks.

A good diet for a patient who is susceptible to episodes of hypoglycemia is one that is low enough in sugar and starches to moderate the reaction of the pancreas to sugar intake and rich enough in protein to help maintain gradual elevations of blood sugar. Eating several smaller meals a day, rather than three large meals, may also help to keep blood sugar levels stable.

Hypothyroidism

Hypothyroidism is a disorder in which an underactive thyroid gland produces too little thyroid hormone.

Causes

Hypothyroidism can result from chronic (long-term) thyroid inflammation or a deficiency of thyroid-stimulating hormone, which is secreted by the pituitary gland. Autoimmune disorders (in which the immune system attacks the body's own tissues) are also a common cause of hypothyroidism. In addition, heredity may play a role in the development of the condition. Women seem more prone to thyroid disorders, and in some women, pregnancy triggers the hormonal imbalance. Hypothyroidism can also develop after suppression or partial removal of the thyroid gland as treatment for hyperthyroidism (a condition that results when an overactive thyroid gland produces too much thyroid hormone).

Symptoms

Because thyroid hormone influences every tissue in the body, the effects of having too little of the hormone are many and varied. People with hypothyroidism may be overweight, easily exhausted, and subject to recurrent infection. They may be constipated, intolerant of cold, have dry skin and hair, exhibit puffiness of the hands and face, and suffer depression. Women may also experience menstrual disorders.

Diagnosis

The diagnosis of hypothyroidism is based on laboratory tests of the blood. Determination of levels of thyroid hormone is fundamental. Cholesterol levels may also be measured. A special nuclear medicine study (the injection of radioactive iodine) may be performed.

Chronic hypothyroidism may cause symptoms of reduced general body functioning. Anemia (deficiency of red blood cells) may result from diminished function of the bone marrow, where red blood cells are formed. Heart rate may decrease, and reflexes may become sluggish. The physician's evaluation of growth patterns often provides the first clue to the diagnosis of hypothyroidism in young children.

Treatment

Since hypothyroidism develops from a shortage of thyroid hormone, the most effective treatment is generally thyroid hormone supplementation. Supplements are either natural hormones extracted from the thyroid glands of animals or synthetic hormones. Both types control the problem, but the newer, synthetic forms are much more efficient, and their effects are more easily regulated. Although treatment provides the necessary hormone control, hypothyroidism often continues throughout life, and the patient may require lifelong follow-up to monitor treatment.

Contrary to popular belief, the correction of hypothyroidism will not cause an obese person to lose a significant amount of weight.

Ketosis

Ketosis is an abnormal condition that occurs when the body burns fat instead of glucose (the form of sugar that is the body's chief source of energy) and, as a result, produces more of the chemical substances called *ketones* than is normal.

Causes

Ketones are the by-product of the chemical process that occurs when fat is broken down to produce energy. Under normal circumstances, ketones are broken down into carbon dioxide and water by the liver and other organs. In ketosis, the body is producing more ketones than it can process. The buildup of ketones disrupts the chemical balance of the body; if left unchecked, this condition can prove fatal.

Ketosis occurs most often in persons with insulin-dependent diabetes mellitus, a disorder in which the pancreas produces little or no insulin (a hormone secreted into the bloodstream to regulate glucose levels). This deficiency prevents the body from absorbing enough glucose and forces it to obtain its energy by burning fat. If ketosis is allowed to progress in a diabetic patient, a condition called diabetic ketoacidosis may occur. This is a life-threatening disorder that involves severe dehydration and coma.

Ketosis is also a consequence of starvation (and the self-induced starvation of excessive dieting), in which the body must rely on stores of fat for energy. Ketosis or ketoacidosis can also occur with excessive intake of alcohol.

Symptoms

The most common symptoms are a slightly sweet breath odor (similar to the smell of acetone or nail-polish remover), extreme dryness of the mucous membranes, weight loss, increased thirst and urination, weakness, abdominal pains, generalized aches, nausea and vomiting, and breathlessness.

Diagnosis

Ketosis is diagnosed by testing the glucose and ketone levels in blood or urine. A urine test, although somewhat less accurate, may also be used to detect the condition.

Treatment

In insulin-dependent diabetics, administration of insulin corrects diabetic ketoacidosis. Diabetics are especially susceptible to ketosis before their condition is diagnosed, while they are fighting an infection, or when they neglect their diet or medication. Treatment of ketosis caused by starvation consists of feeding the patient substances that contain sugar or administering glucose solution intravenously. Alcoholic ketoacidosis is treated in a similar manner, usually with the addition of vitamin supplements.

Pituitary disorders

Because of the vital role of the pituitary gland in regulating many body functions, disorders of this gland (often caused by tumors) can result in disastrous abnormalities in growth and body maintenance.

Persons who have excessive secretion of growth hormone by the anterior lobe during the years in which the skeleton is growing become giants; those who have deficient secretion at that time become dwarfs. If oversecretion occurs after a person has become an adult, a condition called acromegaly results, in which the victim's hands, feet, jaws, and facial bones grow disproportionately large.

A condition known as diabetes insipidus (which is not related to the more common diabetes mellitus) is due to a malfunction of the posterior lobe. In this disorder, a deficiency of the pituitary hormone vasopressin results in abnormally high urinary output of water. Control can be regained with the use of synthetic vasopressin to inhibit excessive water release.

THE MALE REPRODUCTIVE SYSTEM

The male reproductive system consists of those structures in the male body designed to create life. The reproductive system includes the two testes, a network of ducts, the seminal vesicles, the prostate gland, and the penis.

The testes are two oval glands located in the scrotum (the pouch of skin that hangs behind the penis). They produce the male sex hormone testosterone and sperm (male reproductive cells). Sex hormones control the secondary male sex charac-

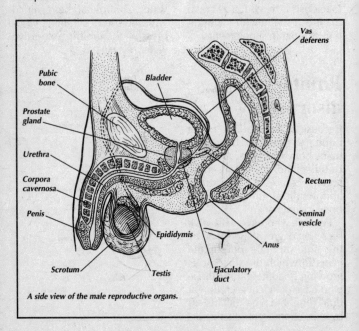

A side view of the male reproductive organs.

teristics (such as growth of the penis and of body hair, voice change, and increased muscle mass), which begin to appear at puberty.

The testes discharge sperm into the epididymis, the first structure in the duct system. Other passageways include the two vasa deferentia (the plural of vas deferens), the ejaculatory duct, and the urethra (the tube that connects the bladder to the outside of the body).

The epididymis runs along the top and side of each testis. Inside the epididymis are several ducts that conduct sperm from the testis into the vas deferens. The vas deferens loops up into the body before descending into a duct in the seminal vesicle. This duct joins the ejaculatory duct, which extends

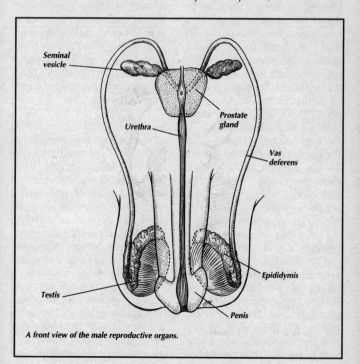

A front view of the male reproductive organs.

413

through the prostate gland, and enters the upper segment of the urethra. At different times, the urethra functions as a passageway for urine and for sperm.

As sperm travel through the duct system, they combine with fluids from the seminal vesicles, the prostate gland, and the urethra to form semen. The two seminal vesicles, which lie near the underside of the urinary bladder, discharge a thick, sticky fluid. The prostate gland is a small, doughnut-shaped organ that completely surrounds the urethra. The prostate gland secretes an alkaline substance that makes up the major portion of seminal fluid. The sperm are protected from acid (present both in the male urethra and in the vagina) by the alkalinity of the prostatic secretions. Sperm are also capable of the greatest mobility when in a slightly alkaline medium. Proper prostate secretion is thus essential to effective sperm action.

The penis is the external organ that propels sperm into the female during sexual intercourse. During sexual excitement, the corpora cavernosa (large internal spaces within the penis) become filled with blood, making the penis rigid enough to enter the vagina (the entryway to the female reproductive tract). The semen, which is formed in the urethra, then travels out of the penis during ejaculation.

Gynecomastia

Gynecomastia is excessive development of the breasts in a male. Breast enlargement is a normal, short-term occurrence in some newborn boys, whose breasts enlarge in response to female hormones they receive from their mother during pregnancy. The condition may also appear at puberty, when a boy's body is undergoing normal hormonal changes.

Causes
In most cases, gynecomastia is the result of too much estrogen (a female sex hormone) in the boy's body. Breast enlargement at birth and at puberty usually occurs because the estrogen level has not yet adjusted to normal (both sexes have estrogen in their bodies). Abnormal gynecomastia occurs when some condition, such as a tumor of one of the testes or an estrogen-secreting tumor of one of the adrenal glands, results in abnormally high levels of estrogen. Some medications can also cause gynecomastia.

Symptoms

In addition to the obvious enlargement of the breasts, symptoms may include tenderness in the breasts and, in extreme cases, secretion of milk.

Treatment

Gynecomastia should always be brought to the attention of a doctor. It is especially important that tumors of the adrenal or pituitary glands or testes be ruled out or treated. Such tumors are usually removed surgically. In severe or prolonged cases, the excess breast tissue can be removed by plastic surgery, with little visible scarring. In most cases, patients can be reassured that the condition is temporary. Especially in need of such reassurance are teenage boys, who are often embarrassed and fearful that they are abnormal.

Hydrocele

A hydrocele is an abnormal collection of fluid around a testis, which is noticeable as a soft mass in the scrotum. The term *hydrocele* literally means a sac of water.

There is normally a double-layered covering around each testis. Within these two layers,

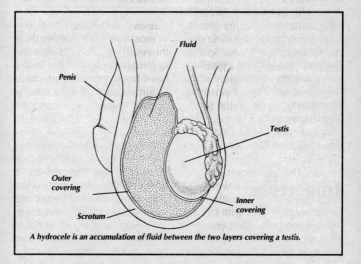

A hydrocele is an accumulation of fluid between the two layers covering a testis.

415

there is usually just enough fluid for lubrication. Occasionally, however, the amount of fluid is increased, causing swelling around the testis.

Causes
If the hydrocele is caused by an injury or inflammation in the scrotum, it is a secondary hydrocele. If there is no apparent cause, it is a primary hydrocele.

Symptoms
The most obvious symptom is the swelling. Although hydroceles are usually painless, pain may also be present.

Treatment
A small, painless hydrocele often requires no treatment. Care must be taken not to dismiss a hydrocele for something more serious. Only a physician can make the diagnosis. Therefore, any scrotal mass merits immediate medical attention. The treatment for a hydrocele is surgical removal of the fluid. The condition can recur.

Impotence

Impotence is the inability to achieve and maintain an erection, which is necessary for the penis to penetrate the vagina during sexual intercourse. The corpora cavernosa of the penis normally fill with blood during sexual excitement, which causes the penis to become rigid and erect. Impotence is a partial or total impairment of this function.

Types
There are two types of impotence: primary impotence, in which a man is never able to have an erection adequate for sexual intercourse; and secondary impotence, in which a man quite often fails to complete intercourse to the satisfaction of both partners. Secondary impotence is the more common type.

Many men experience temporary impotence at some point in their lives, but chronic (recurring) impotence can lower a man's self-esteem and put a strain on his marriage or social relationships.

Causes
Impotence can be caused by either physical or psychological problems. Impotence may be brought on by stress related to a job, fear of causing pregnancy, unresolved conflicts about sexuality, or fear of sex after a heart attack or major surgery. Drug and alcohol abuse are also

among the leading causes of impotence.

Physical factors known to trigger impotence include the following: an imbalance in the hormonal system that causes a decrease in production of testosterone (the male hormone necessary for an erection); the use of certain drugs for the treatment of high blood pressure, particularly diuretics and beta-blockers; diseases of the nervous system, such as multiple sclerosis; structural abnormalities of the penis; injury to the penis; and malfunctioning of the circulatory system, which can interfere with the blood flow to the penis. Vascular problems (including those from diabetes) may also be associated with symptoms.

Symptoms

The major symptom of impotence is inability to attain or maintain erection of the penis for sexual intercourse. This may be accompanied by a lack of interest in sex, but it does not necessarily mean infertility (the inability to father a child).

Diagnosis

Several tests can help to diagnose the cause of impotence. A blood test will show whether adequate levels of testosterone are present. With a blood pressure cuff specially designed to wrap around the penis and an ultrasound study (a technique that uses sound waves to create images of internal structures), blood vessel problems in the penis can often be detected. Another test registers the size of erections that naturally occur during sleep; if erections do not occur during sleep, a physical cause, rather than an emotional one, is likely.

Treatment

To determine if certain medications might be the cause of impotence, prescription drugs may be replaced or eliminated one at a time. If impotence has a physical basis, a number of treatments are available. Injections of testosterone and other hormones may relieve some problems. Surgery may be necessary to repair the arteries and veins that carry blood to and from the penis.

The use of penile implants is a successful new treatment for impotence, with several varieties now in use. One is a silicone rod that is implanted in the corpora cavernosa, resulting in a permanent partial erection. Another is a flexible silver wire surrounded by silicone, which allows manipulation of the penis to an erect position for intercourse. A third model consists of balloonlike cylinders implanted in the corpora cavernosa and connected to a container of fluid; with the use of a hand pump, the cylinders may be filled with the fluid, in much the same way that blood normally fills the penis during an erection.

Counseling by a psychologist or trained sex therapist may be recommended for men whose impotence seems to stem from emotional problems. Counseling may also help those with physical disorders learn to deal with their impotence.

Prevention

Avoiding the abuse of alcohol and drugs, as well as eliminating or coping with stress, should help to prevent at least some episodes of secondary impotence.

Prostatitis

Located just below the bladder, the prostate is a small, doughnut-shaped male sex gland that surrounds the neck of the bladder and the urethra. The main function of the prostate is to produce fluid for semen, which transports sperm.

Prostatitis is an infection or inflammation of the prostate. It predominately affects older men, usually in the form of chronic (recurring) flare-ups. Though not generally a serious disorder, prostatitis can be irritating and uncomfortable because it may disrupt normal urination. Advanced cases of prostatitis may cause a sudden total blockage of urine flow, requiring emergency treatment before the backup of urine can cause damage to the bladder and kidney.

Causes

Sexually transmitted diseases and urinary tract infections are the most common underlying causes of prostatitis.

Symptoms

Symptoms, when present, can include any of the following: fever, chills, urinary frequency, frequent urination at night, difficulty urinating, burning or painful urination, low-back pain, joint or muscle pain, tender or swollen prostate, blood in the urine, or painful ejaculation.

Diagnosis

Prostatitis is diagnosed by an examination of the prostate to check its size, shape, and firm-

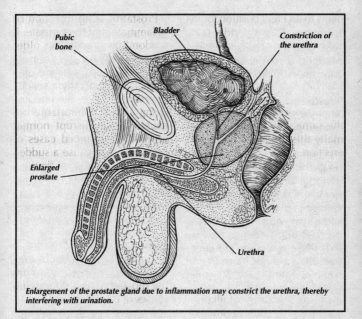

Bladder

Pubic bone

Constriction of the urethra

Enlarged prostate

Urethra

Enlargement of the prostate gland due to inflammation may constrict the urethra, thereby interfering with urination.

ness. A simple procedure, called a digital rectal examination, allows the physician to estimate whether the prostate is enlarged or has lumps or other areas of abnormal texture. An infected prostate will be tender to the touch; when it is massaged by the doctor, pus cells will be forced out and will then appear in the urine. A culture of the urine specimen will be examined for bacteria, although very often no bacteria are identified in a case of chronic prostatitis. However, a urinalysis

may show some evidence of infection, and if a trace of blood is present, the urine may be additionally tested for the presence of malignant cells.

Enlargement of the prostate can be diagnosed by means of a procedure called an intravenous pyelogram (IVP), in which dye is injected into a vein in the arm and allowed to travel through the bloodstream to the kidneys and urinary bladder and out through the penis. The dye may show enlargement or obstruction in the ureters.

The patient will then be asked to urinate; if the IVP shows a large quantity of urine left in the bladder, a partial obstruction can generally be diagnosed.

Treatment
Most prostate infections can be treated quite successfully with antibiotics. Chronic nonbacterial prostatitis, however, is not treated with antibiotics. An individual may find that taking hot baths, drinking water, and a change in diet helps to alleviate some symptoms. While there is no scientific evidence proving that these remedies are effective, they are not harmful and some people experience relief from symptoms while using them.

Urethritis

Urethritis is an infection or inflammation of the urethra (the tube that runs through the penis and connects the bladder to the outside of the body). Urethritis is the most common condition affecting the male reproductive system.

Causes
Two sexually transmitted diseases, gonorrhea and chlamydia, are the most common causes of urethritis in both men and women. Irritation may also be caused after sexual intercourse by chemicals contained in vaginal spermicides and douches.

Symptoms
The most common symptoms of urethritis are burning during urination and a creamy white or yellow discharge from the penis. Unlike a bladder infection, urethritis does not cause an increase in the frequency of urination.

Diagnosis
Urethritis is diagnosed by an examination of the penis to check for discharge. The doctor will then take specimens of the discharge for examination under a microscope and for bacterial culture.

Treatment
Infections of the urethra are treated with antibiotics. A person who has urethritis should abstain from sexual activity until a full course of antibiotics has been taken and until all tests indicate that the infection is no longer present.

Every sexual partner of the infected person needs to be examined and, if necessary, treated.

Prevention
Urethritis can be prevented by avoiding sexual contact with someone who is infected with either gonorrhea or chlamydia. Using condoms also helps reduce the risk of contracting these infections. If urethritis is caused by chemical irritation from vaginal spermicides or douches, these substances should be avoided or a condom should be used.

THE FEMALE REPRODUCTIVE SYSTEM

The female reproductive system consists of those structures within the female body that are designed to create and nourish new life. The system includes the ovaries, fallopian tubes, uterus, cervix, and vagina.

Although the breasts, or mammary glands, are actually a type of sweat gland, their function (supporting new life) is closely related to that of the reproductive system. For that reason, disorders affecting the

breasts will also be considered in this chapter.

The reproductive process begins in the ovaries. The ovaries are small, egg-shaped glands located in the lower abdomen. These glands control the cyclic functions of the reproductive system—ovulation and menstruation. Ovulation is the monthly production and release of a mature egg (occasionally two or more eggs). This process and other reproductive

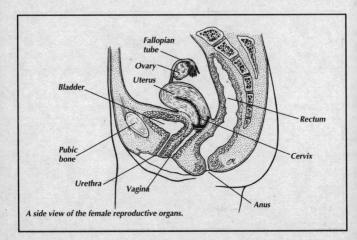

A side view of the female reproductive organs.

functions are regulated by two hormones, estrogen and progesterone, which are secreted by the ovaries. Estrogen regulates the secondary sex traits of body hair growth, breast development, ovulation, and menstruation. Progesterone is responsible for preparing the uterus for pregnancy, as well as contributing to enlargement of the breasts during pregnancy and milk production after childbirth. The two hormones coordinate to control the menstrual cycle.

Once an egg has been released, it travels through the fallopian tubes, which extend from each ovary into the uterus. Their reproductive function is to contain the egg until fertilization (union of an egg and a sperm, or male sex cell) takes place and to provide a passageway leading the sperm to the egg and the fertilized egg to the uterus.

The uterus is a pear-shaped, hollow organ that is normally about the size of a lemon. Its muscular walls are lined with rich, soft tissue called the endometrium. Each month, the lining adds layers in anticipation of receiving a fertilized egg. Should fertilization occur, the lining nourishes the fertilized egg in the uterus until birth. However, if the egg remains unfertilized, the uterus sheds the endometrium and the

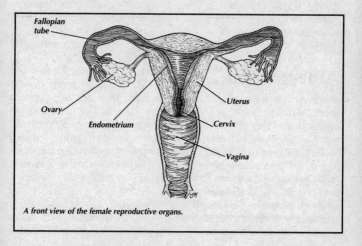

Fallopian tube

Ovary

Endometrium

Uterus

Cervix

Vagina

A front view of the female reproductive organs.

egg, which leave the body as menstrual discharge.

The cervix is a narrow structure with an inch-long canal connecting the lower end of the uterus to the upper portion of the vagina. This canal is the conduit for sperm on their way to fertilize an egg and for menstrual discharge and babies as they pass out of the uterus.

The vagina, or birth canal, is a passageway leading from the cervix to the outside of the body. In the average adult woman, it measures four to five inches in length. Although the vaginal walls are normally close together, they separate to accommodate the infant during childbirth and the erect penis during sexual intercourse. The vagina produces secretions that lubricate and cleanse it.

Amenorrhea

Amenorrhea is the absence of menstruation. There are two categories of this disorder. Primary amenorrhea is the failure to begin menstruating by the age of 16. Secondary amenorrhea, the more common of the two conditions, is the absence of three or more periods in a row in a woman who has been menstruating for some time. Primary amenorrhea is specifically defined at the age of 16 and can go on indefinitely. Secondary amenorrhea is usually a temporary condition; the periods generally resume when the underlying cause for the interruption has been corrected.

Causes
Primary amenorrhea can be caused by an endocrine gland disorder (such as hyperthyroidism or hypothyroidism); genetic abnormalities; damaged or missing ovaries, uterus, or vagina; or an excessively thick hymen (the membrane that usually covers the vaginal opening in women who have not yet had sexual intercourse), which blocks the outflow of the menstrual discharge.

Secondary amenorrhea is caused most commonly by pregnancy. It can also be triggered by strenuous sports training, poor nutrition, drastic weight gain, jet lag, certain medications (including corticosteroids, tranquilizers, and birth control pills), major surgery or serious disease, emotional shock, or the loss of a large percentage of body fat.

Symptoms
Primary amenorrhea is commonly accompanied by abnor-

mal or inhibited physical development; the young girl may fail to develop breasts or body hair, indicating that a genetic disorder may be preventing her from attaining sexual maturity. These girls are also usually short in height.

Secondary amenorrhea has no symptoms other than the absence of menstrual periods.

Diagnosis

Diagnostic evaluation of both types of amenorrhea will probably include a test to rule out pregnancy, tests to detect genetic or hormonal disorders, and X rays or ultrasound studies.

Treatment

Primary amenorrhea may be treated with an extensive hormone therapy program to stimulate physical development. If the cause is a thick hymen, a minor surgical procedure may be performed. Some cases of primary amenorrhea, however, are untreatable (for example, those caused by structural abnormalities of the reproductive organs).

Secondary amenorrhea may be treated with a hormone that will trigger ovulation and reestablish the menstrual cycle. However, quite often this condition will reverse itself without treatment, especially if the cause is merely an interruption in the patient's normal routine, an emotional upset, or pregnancy.

Prevention

Maintaining good nutritional habits and a normal weight and avoiding overly strenuous sports can probably be beneficial in preventing secondary amenorrhea. No specific precautions can be taken, however, to prevent primary amenorrhea.

Cystocele

A cystocele is a protrusion into the vagina of a portion of the urinary bladder.

Cause

A cystocele is usually the result of damage to the wall of fibrous tissue that normally separates the vagina and the bladder. Such an injury often occurs during childbirth and may happen with the birth of a baby of any size. However, women who have never given birth may also develop a cystocele. A cystocele may not appear until menopause, when the damaged area is weakened further by lack of estrogen, permitting the rear and base portions of the

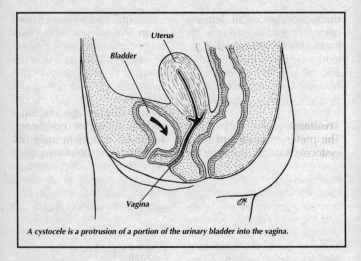

A cystocele is a protrusion of a portion of the urinary bladder into the vagina.

bladder to protrude into the vagina. A portion of the rectum (the final part of the large intestine), the small intestine, or the urethra (the tube through which urine leaves the body) may also bulge into the vagina. Prolapse of the uterus (in which the uterus drops through the vagina and in very severe cases protrudes through the vaginal opening) may occur.

The protrusion of the bladder into the vagina creates a pool of stale urine in the bladder, which cannot be easily emptied, and as a result becomes a breeding ground for bacteria. Cystitis (inflammation of the bladder), signaled by painful

and difficult urination, often results.

Symptoms
A woman with a cystocele may feel a fullness in the vagina and may find it difficult to empty her bladder completely. However, many women afflicted with a cystocele may have no recognizable symptoms at all.

Diagnosis
Diagnosis is made by examining the inside of the vagina. If a bulge can be seen in front of the cervix, a cystocele is suspected. Also, if a catheter inserted into the bladder after urination can draw out more

than two ounces of leftover urine, the diagnosis is even more likely. If a special X-ray study in which dye is injected into the bladder reveals a bulged-out section of the bladder, the diagnosis is confirmed.

Treatment

The preferred treatment for a cystocele is surgery to repair the damaged wall and put the protruding section of bladder back in its original place. A pessary (a device inserted into the vagina to support it and reduce the cystocele) may be used in women who cannot or do not wish to undergo surgery. A cystocele does not always require treatment. However, if frequent bouts of cystitis occur, some form of treatment will be necessary to relieve discomfort.

DES

Diethylstilbestrol (DES) is an artificial estrogen (female sex hormone) used to treat a variety of disorders. For nearly three decades, this drug was frequently prescribed to prevent miscarriage. In 1971, however, the Food and Drug Administration banned its use for this purpose because it had been found to be ineffective.

Use of DES has been linked to an increased incidence of adenocarcinoma of the vagina (a rare cancer of the glandular cells of the reproductive organs) in the daughters of the several million women who took it to prevent miscarriage and other complications of pregnancy. Testicular cancer in male offspring has also been associated with maternal DES use. People exposed to DES before birth also have a higher than average incidence of benign (noncancerous) growths, structural changes involving the reproductive organs, and infertility problems. These abnormalities usually appear in the late teens to early 30s. Although the incidence of serious complications is small, physicians strongly advise that people who were exposed to DES before birth be routinely examined to detect any abnormalities.

Because of the potential problems, DES should not be taken by a woman who is pregnant or suspects that she is pregnant. DES may be used safely by nonpregnant women to treat a variety of disorders, including certain vaginal conditions and estrogen deficiency that may occur at menopause or after the surgical removal of the ovaries. Since DES is a hormone that may produce a variety of effects in the body, its use must always be supervised by a physician.

Dilation and curettage

Dilation and curettage, also called a *D&C,* is a surgical procedure in which the cervix of the uterus is dilated (expanded) and the endometrial lining of the uterus is scraped with a curette (a loop-, ring-, or scoop-shaped instrument with a long handle).

Purpose

This procedure is often used in the diagnosis of diseases of the uterus (such as cancer) and to halt excessive bleeding. It is also used to perform an abortion and may be employed after a miscarriage (involuntary expulsion of a fetus before it is able to live on its own) to remove any remains of tissue and thereby lower the risk of hemorrhage and infection.

Dilation alone may be performed to enlarge the passageway out of the uterus. This might be done if a severely narrowed cervix is causing painful menstruation because of re-

stricted flow of menstrual fluid. For treatment of this problem, multiple dilations may be necessary since the cervix will often become narrow again after several months.

The procedure

A D&C is a relatively minor procedure, seldom requiring hospital admission. Because the rectum should be empty before the procedure, an enema may be given; the urinary bladder should also be emptied.

The procedure is performed in an operating room under sterile conditions. Anesthesia may be general (the patient is put to sleep) or local. The patient rests on her back with her feet in stirrups. The surgeon inserts metal dilators of progressively larger sizes into the cervix until it is open enough to permit the insertion of the surgical instruments.

A curette is used to remove endometrial tissue. Special forceps may also be used to remove tissue. When the operation is finished, an absorbent pad is placed over the entrance to the vagina. The pad is checked every 15 minutes for two hours, and excessive bleeding is reported to the physician.

Mild painkillers should be enough to control discomfort

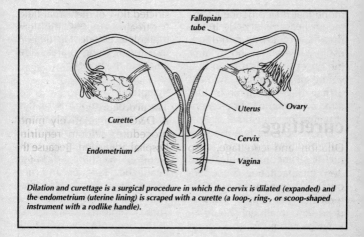

Dilation and curettage is a surgical procedure in which the cervix is dilated (expanded) and the endometrium (uterine lining) is scraped with a curette (a loop-, ring-, or scoop-shaped instrument with a rodlike handle).

from the operation. If there is pain in the abdomen that cannot be relieved in this way or that is continuous or sharp, it should be reported immediately. Some difficulty in urinating is to be expected immediately after the procedure.

In most cases, the patient stays in bed for one to two hours after surgery. Most women return home several hours after the procedure or the next day. A return to many daily activities is possible immediately, and in a week all normal physical activities may be resumed. Sexual intercourse and use of tampons are not recommended, however, until after the follow-up visit to the doctor (usually about two weeks after the procedure).

Risks
The principal risks of a D&C are hemorrhage, infection, and perforation (puncture) of the uterus. The latter is more likely during pregnancy, when the uterine walls are especially soft and thin.

Dysmenorrhea

Dysmenorrhea is the term for painful menstruation. It occurs most commonly in teenagers and in women who have never been pregnant.

There are two types of dysmenorrhea. Primary dysmenorrhea is a recurring condition, usually beginning shortly after the onset of menstruation in a young girl. Secondary dysmenorrhea develops later in life, after a woman has been menstruating for some time.

Dysmenorrhea is not a serious condition, but it can be annoying, uncomfortable, and even incapacitating. Since secondary dysmenorrhea usually indicates that another disorder is present, treatment should always be sought for this condition.

Causes

The cause of primary dysmenorrhea is thought to be the release of prostaglandins from the lining of the uterus shortly before the beginning of a menstrual period. (Prostaglandins are substances that, among other functions, stimulate uterine contractions.) The resulting contractions constrict blood vessels in the uterus, causing pain in the same way that a decrease in blood supply to the heart causes chest pain. The reason for this excessive production of prostaglandins is not known. Secondary dysmenorrhea is usually a result of another reproductive problem, such as fibroid tumors, a narrow cervix, or endometriosis (the displacement of tissue from the uterine lining to areas elsewhere in the body).

Symptoms

The major symptoms of dysmenorrhea are cramps and pain in the lower abdomen, possibly extending around to the back. Nausea, vomiting, diarrhea, headache, fatigue, and nervousness are mainly associated with primary dysmenorrhea. These symptoms usually appear at the beginning of, or slightly before, the menstrual period, and may last several hours or several days.

Diagnosis

Diagnostic evaluation will include a complete physical examination as well as medical and menstrual histories. If the symptoms have been present from the onset of menstruation at puberty, primary dysmenorrhea is usually the diagnosis. If the symptoms appeared suddenly in a woman who has been menstruating for some years, secondary dysmenorrhea can be assumed. In that case, further diagnostic evaluation of the reproductive organs will then be necessary to identify the underlying disorder. Ultrasound examinations (in which the echoes of sound waves are used to create images of internal structures) or X-ray studies often prove useful.

Treatment

Primary dysmenorrhea has been treated successfully with nonsteroidal anti-inflammatory drugs (such as ibuprofen, naproxen, meclofenamate, diflunisal, and mefenamic acid), which, when taken just before a period is to begin, act to suppress the production of prostaglandins and thereby reduce the intensity of the contractions that cause pain.

Secondary dysmenorrhea is treated by correcting the problem that is causing it. For instance, if endometriosis is the underlying problem, it may be treated with hormone therapy or surgery, thereby relieving the dysmenorrhea as well.

Home remedies often help to ease menstrual pain and relieve pressure. These include placing a hot-water bottle or heating pad on the abdomen, taking hot baths, and lying on the back with the knees bent. A woman who experienced dysmenorrhea before pregnancy may find that the problem is lessened after childbirth, possibly because of enlargement of the cervix or destruction of some nerve fibers in the uterus.

Dyspareunia

Dyspareunia is difficulty or pain for a woman during intercourse.

Causes

Dyspareunia may be caused by a resistant hymen (the membrane that usually covers the opening to the vagina in virgins) or by inflammation of or injury to the vagina, the urethra (the tube that carries urine from the bladder to the outside), the vulva (the structures around the opening to the vagina), or the anus. It can be the result of formation of scar tissue around an episiotomy (a surgical cut to enlarge the opening of the vagina immediately before childbirth) or surgery to repair the vagina. Other physical causes include tight muscles in the area around the vagina, an "hourglass" contraction of the vagina, a divided vagina, inflammation of the cervix, prolapsed (fallen) uterus, infected fallopian tubes, and endometriosis.

Inadequate lubrication of the vagina is a common cause of dyspareunia. This deficiency may be due to inadequate arousal of the woman before insertion of the penis or to menopause, which is accompanied by a decrease in vaginal secretions and thinning of the vaginal lining. Unconscious tightening of the vaginal muscles, called vaginismus, is another possible cause—perhaps the result of fear, unreadiness or unwillingness to perform the sex act, or other psychological reasons. Improperly fitted or improperly lubricated birth control devices (condoms or diaphragms) and an allergy to spermicides are other causes.

Symptoms
Pain during or after sexual intercourse is the primary symptom of dyspareunia.

Diagnosis
Diagnosis is made on the basis of both a physical and an emotional evaluation. In some cases, physical abnormalities can be detected during the physical examination. In other cases, careful inquiry into the patient's emotional state and sexual history may reveal factors that account for the discomfort.

Treatment
Treatment for dyspareunia is correction of any underlying disease, injury, or structural defect, if such a problem exists. For some couples, counseling by a psychiatrist or sex therapist may be helpful.

Water-soluble lubricating jelly (not petroleum jelly), obtainable in any drugstore, provides a good vaginal lubricant. Estrogen creams can be used along with water-soluble jelly to restore lubrication to a dry vagina after menopause. Soothing creams and temporary avoidance of intercourse can relieve the soreness of dyspareunia.

Endometriosis

Endometriosis is a condition in which tissue from the endometrial lining of the uterus becomes detached and grows in the abdominal cavity outside the uterus. It occurs only in women of childbearing age, especially in women between the ages of 30 and 40 years.

Cause
During each menstrual cycle, the endometrium normally thickens and swells in preparation for possible pregnancy. If no pregnancy occurs, portions of endometrial tissue break down and pass out of the uterus

as part of the menstrual flow. When endometriosis develops, displaced endometrial tissue continues to swell and bleed each month in an abnormal location, but the blood has no outlet. The body responds to the presence of this accumulated blood by surrounding it with scar tissue, which builds up month after month, until blood-filled pockets, or cysts, are formed on the affected organs.

The exact cause of endometriosis is not known, but several conditions are thought to lead to its development: Menstrual blood may flow backward through the fallopian tubes and into the abdominal cavity; the cervix or vagina may be blocked, so that the menstrual blood cannot flow out normally; or surgery or another condition may lead to the displacement of some tissue from the uterus.

Symptoms
The symptoms of endometriosis are pain immediately before, during, or immediately after the menstrual period; pain during intercourse; discomfort in the

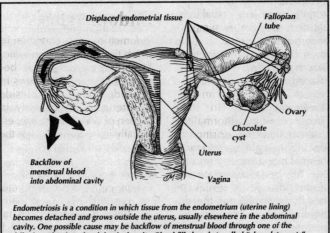

Endometriosis is a condition in which tissue from the endometrium (uterine lining) becomes detached and grows outside the uterus, usually elsewhere in the abdominal cavity. One possible cause may be backflow of menstrual blood through one of the fallopian tubes into the abdominal cavity. Blood filled pockets called "chocolate cysts" sometimes form when scar tissue surrounds accumulations of blood and displaced endometrial tissue.

lower urinary tract or intestine; irregular or excessively heavy menstrual flow; bleeding from the rectum; blood in the urine; and infertility. Some women may experience all of these symptoms, while others may experience only one or two.

Diagnosis

Diagnostic evaluation begins with a complete medical and menstrual history. Pelvic examinations may be performed—once during menstruation and once between periods—to investigate the changes in the reproductive organs during the cycle. The doctor may also perform a laparoscopy, in which a lighted, tubelike instrument is inserted into the lower abdomen through a tiny incision, which will allow a view of displaced tissues.

Treatment

Treatment of this disorder consists of halting the condition, reducing the pain, and restoring normal menstruation and fertility. The best way to halt endometriosis is to modify the body's natural hormonal secretions with drugs in order to stop menstruation and ovulation for some time, thus allowing the endometrial tissue to shrink. Naturally, the patient will be

unable to become pregnant during this type of drug therapy, but since endometriosis often causes infertility, many patients are already unable to conceive.

Three types of drugs are usually used in this treatment. Birth control pills, as well as several other medications that modify female hormonal secretions, are sometimes prescribed in doses high enough to stop menstruation and ovulation. However, an excessive dosage often brings with it undesirable side effects, such as nausea, fluid retention, and blood clotting.

A synthetic hormone called danazol creates a condition similar to menopause, causing menstruation and ovulation to stop and the endometrial tissue to shrink almost immediately. Danazol does not have some of the side effects associated with other hormonal drugs. However, it is relatively expensive and is not effective in all cases.

The newest form of treatment is a nasal spray that causes the brain to stop producing hormones that cause ovulation and menstruation. As with the use of danazol, the nasal spray causes endometrial tissue to shrink almost immediately. If drug therapy is unsuccessful, surgery may be necessary, involving either the removal of scar tissue and endometrial tissue or, in advanced cases, the removal of the uterus and ovaries, rendering the patient sterile. Endometriosis may be destroyed by using very precise medical lasers. This form of therapy has been used to dissolve areas of endometriosis while leaving surrounding normal tissue unharmed.

Fibrocystic breast disease

Fibrocystic disease is a condition in which benign (noncancerous) lumps form in the breast, either temporarily or for the duration of the childbearing years.

This condition is not dangerous in itself, but it has been found that women with certain forms of breast lumps may be two to four times more likely to develop breast cancer than are other women. To complicate matters, the presence of these benign lumps makes it difficult to detect any new, possibly dangerous growths.

Cause

The exact cause of fibrocystic disease is not known. However, the tendency to develop it may be inherited. Also, it is seen more often in women who have never breast-fed a child; the reason for this is not known.

Symptoms

The most noticeable symptom of this disorder is the presence of the lumps, which may take the form of either solid masses or fluid-filled sacs called *cysts*. Large cystic lumps near the surface can be moved about freely, unlike cancerous lumps, which are usually firmly attached to surrounding tissue. Changes in hormonal secretions during the menstrual period tend to increase the size of the lumps slightly, which causes additional pain, but the size of the cysts decreases after the period. Other symptoms include a slight discharge from the nipple and persistently heavy and tender breasts, not only before and during menstruation (as is commonly seen in healthy breasts) but all the time.

Diagnosis

Diagnostic evaluation will begin with a physical examination. Mammography (a special X-ray study of the breasts) and ultrasound are often done to determine whether the lumps are fluid-filled cysts or solid masses. If they are found to be

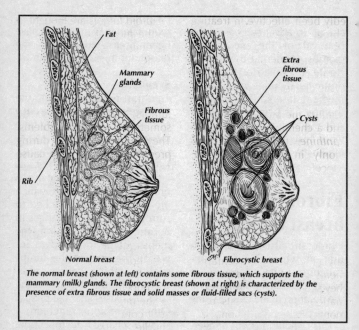

The normal breast (shown at left) contains some fibrous tissue, which supports the mammary (milk) glands. The fibrocystic breast (shown at right) is characterized by the presence of extra fibrous tissue and solid masses or fluid-filled sacs (cysts).

solid, a biopsy (the removal of a small piece of tissue for analysis) may be performed to detect the presence of cancerous cells.

Treatment

Fibrocystic disease often requires no treatment. In some cases, the lumps disappear in a few months. Cysts that are unusually large or particularly bothersome may be drained of their fluid by the insertion of a hollow needle in a procedure called *aspiration*. If there are many small lumps or if there is continuous development of new ones, other forms of treatment may be necessary to prevent the formation of cysts. Birth control pills may be prescribed, since they act to equalize the concentration of hormones in the body throughout the monthly cycle; however, birth control pills have also been found to cause cysts in some women. Large doses of vitamin E (taken under a doctor's supervision) have reportedly been effective in treating fibrocystic disease.

Prevention

Relieving or preventing fibrocystic disease may be promoted by discontinuing or drastically limiting the intake of nicotine and a chemical called *methylxanthine,* found most commonly in coffee, tea, cola, chocolate, and some cold medications. Because certain forms of breast lumps carry a greater risk of breast cancer, women with lumps should have a physical examination at least twice a year. They should also report any new growths or enlargements of existing lumps, and they should perform self-examination of their breasts each month after menstruation.

Fibroid tumors

Fibroid tumors are solid, noncancerous growths composed of smooth muscle fibers and connective tissue that grow in the walls of the uterus or out from the uterus. Only rarely do they appear on the cervix. Occasionally, they fill the entire uterus, push through the cervix, and appear in the vagina. These tumors usually grow slowly and vary in size and shape.

Fibroid tumors are thought to be the most common type of abdominal tumor, found in about 25 percent of all women over the age of 30 (more frequently in black women). Cancer rarely develops in fibroid tumors; however, they do sometimes cause problems. They tend to enlarge during pregnancy, which can cause complications as the fetus grows.

Causes

The cause of fibroid tumors is not known, but their growth seems to be related to the female hormone estrogen, since these tumors rarely appear before puberty and tend to recede by the menopause years. They most commonly appear in the middle to late reproductive years, when the estrogen level is at its peak.

Fibroid tumors may occur along with other disorders, such as endometriosis (the displacement of tissue from the uterine lining to areas elsewhere in the body) or pelvic inflammatory disease.

Symptoms

Common symptoms of fibroid tumors are dysmenorrhea (pain during menstruation) and gushing or flooding of the menstrual

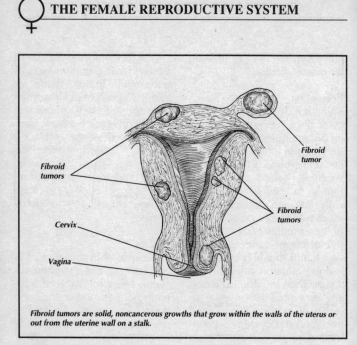

Fibroid tumors are solid, noncancerous growths that grow within the walls of the uterus or out from the uterine wall on a stalk.

flow. Occasionally, there is abdominal pain; however, pain is not usually a symptom unless a complication develops. If fibroid tumors become very large, they may press on surrounding organs, such as the intestines and bladder, which may result in constipation or frequent urination. If they extend into the uterus, heavy and prolonged menstrual periods may result. If the tumor is advanced, the abdomen may be noticeably enlarged. Sometimes, however, these tumors cause no symptoms.

Diagnosis

Diagnostic evaluation begins with a physical examination and may include curettage (scraping the uterus walls) or endometrial biopsy (removal of some tissue from the lining of the uterus) to test for cancer. X rays and ultrasound may also be used to establish the location, size, and nature of the tumor.

Treatment

Fibroid tumors may require no treatment at all, other than regular checkups with the doctor.

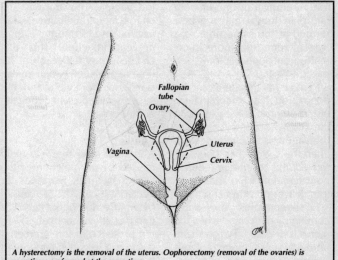

A hysterectomy is the removal of the uterus. Oophorectomy (removal of the ovaries) is sometimes performed at the same time.

Fibroid tumors that are causing complications may require one of two types of surgery. Removal of the tumor (called a *myomectomy*) is usually recommended for women in their early reproductive years whose symptoms are somewhat mild and who desire a future pregnancy.

Removal of the uterus (called a *hysterectomy*) is usually recommended for older women who have completed their families and for women who do not want to become pregnant in the future.

Hysterectomy

Hysterectomy is the surgical removal of the uterus, which causes the termination of menstruation and the inability to bear children.

A hysterectomy may be either total or partial. Total hysterectomy entails removal of the entire uterus, including the cervix. Partial hysterectomy, which is rarely done today, involves removal of only the body of the uterus but not the cervix. Oophorectomy (removal of one or both ovaries) and salpingectomy (removal of one or both fallopian tubes) may be performed at the same time as a hysterectomy (for more information on oophorectomy, see pages 449-450.)

Removal of the uterus can be done through an abdominal incision or through the vagina. In the latter procedure, the top of the vagina is stitched together after the uterus has been removed; this technique requires no external incision and, therefore, leaves no external scar.

Hysterectomies are most commonly performed when the uterus is diseased. Symptomatic fibroid tumors, uterine prolapse (falling of the uterus out of its normal position), and cancer of the uterus are common reasons for a hysterectomy.

Contrary to common belief, a hysterectomy, in and of itself, does not interfere with, or diminish the pleasure of, sexual intercourse. Nor does a hysterectomy cause a woman to gain weight.

Leukorrhea

Leukorrhea is an abnormal discharge from the vagina. All women have some normal discharge in the form of mucous secretions from the cervix and the vagina. This normal discharge helps to lubricate the vagina and, to some extent, prevent infection. This discharge is most noticeable at the time of ovulation (when an egg is released from the ovary), but it is generally present during the entire menstrual cycle.

Causes
Abnormal discharge is usually caused by an infection of the vagina by fungi, parasites, or bacteria. It can also be caused by an infection of the cervix, a tumor or other abnormal growth, the presence of foreign matter (such as a forgotten tampon) in the vagina, or an inflammation of the vagina caused by chemicals in douches or contraceptive creams or jellies.

Symptoms
An abnormal vaginal discharge usually is heavy, is accompanied by itching of the genital organs and anal area, and has a disagreeable odor.

Diagnosis
To diagnose the cause of the discharge, the doctor will perform a pelvic examination and will often take a sample of the discharge for microscopic examination. Sometimes a culture of the discharge may also be

performed so that the organism causing the problem can be grown in the laboratory and identified.

Treatment

Once the cause of the abnormal discharge has been identified, specific steps are taken to treat it. If the discharge is caused by a bacterial infection, oral antibiotics or antibiotic vaginal creams may be prescribed. Specific oral drugs or vaginal preparations will be prescribed if the discharge is caused by a type of yeast or trichomonad (a single-celled parasite). In some cases, a biopsy of the cervix or vagina may be required if the doctor suspects that a tumor may be causing the discharge.

Douching with vinegar and water or other solutions available without a prescription generally will not cure the discharge, even though symptoms may improve for a few days. A woman with an abnormal vaginal discharge should consult her doctor rather than attempt to treat herself.

Mastectomy

Mastectomy is the surgical removal of a breast or part of a breast, usually as a treatment for cancer.

Types

There are several types of mastectomy, each characterized by which muscles, glands, and other tissues are surgically removed.

- Lumpectomy—surgical removal of the tumor along with some of the surrounding breast tissue
- Partial mastectomy—surgical removal of the tumor along with as much as one half of the breast
- Simple mastectomy—surgical removal of the entire breast
- Modified radical mastectomy—surgical removal of the entire breast plus the armpit lymph nodes
- Radical mastectomy—surgical removal of the entire breast, the armpit lymph nodes, and the muscles below the breast
- Extended radical mastectomy—surgical removal of the entire breast plus additional tissue in the chest, as well as the armpit lymph nodes and chest muscles
- Super-radical mastectomy—surgical removal of the same tissues and muscles as in the extended radical mastectomy, as well as some tissues and lymph nodes in the neck

441

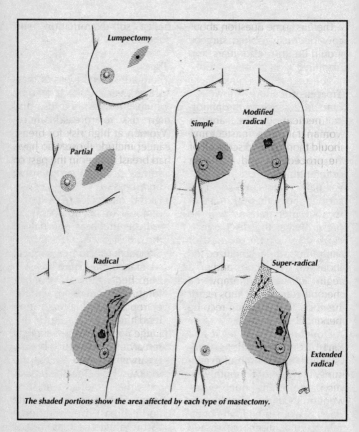

The shaded portions show the area affected by each type of mastectomy.

Choice of type

The type of mastectomy to be performed is determined by a multitude of factors, including the location, size, and type of tumor. The age and general health of the patient are also extremely important.

A biopsy (removal of a small tissue sample for microscopic examination) will be performed before the mastectomy. In addition, other tests may be done to determine if the cancer has spread to other areas of the body.

There is some question about how extensive the surgery should be. In recent years, the modified radical mastectomy has become the most frequently chosen procedure. However, there are differences of opinion in medical circles, and a woman facing a mastectomy should thoroughly discuss all of the procedures and available options with her doctor.

Treatment

The operation is performed while the patient is under general anesthesia. Afterward the patient remains hospitalized for about two to five days and may begin radiation therapy or chemotherapy. Checkups every three to six months are recommended.

Early detection

Establishing the habit of examining her breasts monthly is very important for every woman. With this simple routine, a woman can often detect a cancerous lump before cancer cells can spread beyond the breast. The effectiveness of breast self-examination is shown by the high percentage of breast tumors that are discovered by patients themselves during a monthly breast self-examination. (For instructions on breast self-examination, see page 559–561.)

Many experts recommend annual mammography (X-ray examination of the breasts) for women over the age of 50 and for younger women who are at high risk for breast cancer. (Women at high risk for breast cancer include those who have had breast cancer in the past or who have a mother or sister who has had the disease.)

Menopause

Menopause is the normal, natural stage in a woman's life when her menstruation and ovulation cycles stop, ending her reproductive years. Also called the *climacteric,* or the change of life, menopause occurs around age 50 but can start anywhere between age 35 and 60.

Cause

Scientists do not fully understand what causes menopause. They believe it is triggered when the ovaries stop responding to the sex hormones that are secreted by the pituitary gland. The subsequent decline in the production of the female hormone estrogen sets off the bodily changes.

Symptoms

During the years immediately preceding the onset of menopause, menstrual periods may become irregular and menstrual flow scanty.

Other physical symptoms of menopause include hot flashes (a warm and flushed feeling over the face, neck, and chest that lasts a few minutes and recurs throughout the day), excessive perspiration, dryness in the vagina (which can lead to painful or difficult sexual intercourse), pounding heartbeat, joint pains, headaches, itching skin, increased facial hair, and decreased armpit and pubic hair.

Nonphysical symptoms of menopause include depression, anxiety, irritability, apprehension, decreased ability to concentrate, lack of confidence, and insomnia.

The duration of symptoms ranges from a few weeks to more than five years. Not every woman experiences the same changes, other than an end to menstruation; about 25 percent notice no other changes, 50 percent discern some physical or psychological symptoms, and the other 25 percent are troubled by very uncomfortable or distressing menopausal symptoms.

Diagnosis

It is important not to attribute all physical changes to menopause to the point of overlooking the symptoms of some disease. This is a good time to schedule an examination and discuss the bodily changes with a doctor. A woman should see a doctor immediately if she starts to bleed in between menstrual periods, bleeds excessively, or has another period six months or more after they have apparently stopped.

Treatment

The primary treatment for the physical symptoms of menopause is replacement of the female sex hormones (commonly estrogen or a combination of estrogen and progesterone in the form of an oral tablet). Estrogen in the form of a vaginal cream may be prescribed specifically to treat vaginal dryness. The lowest effective dose is administered because of possible side effects. Any treatment merely lessens the discomfort of menopause; it cannot stop or slow down the process. Because of the many beneficial effects of hormone replacement therapy, most physicians now believe that it should continue for the remainder of the patient's life.

Estrogen is not usually given to women with severe circulatory or liver disorders and is carefully controlled when prescribed to those with diabetes, epilepsy, or heart or kidney disease. Progesterone is not prescribed for women with liver disease and is carefully controlled in those with asthma, epilepsy, or heart or kidney disease. The benefits and hazards should be discussed with a doctor; other medication is available to treat certain menopausal symptoms in women who cannot take hormones.

Treatment for the psychological or emotional symptoms may include tranquilizers, antidepressants, sleeping pills, or psychotherapy. During this time, it may also be difficult for a woman to face the aging process and its physical ramifications—the end of the childbearing years and a sense of uselessness because of a possible decrease in family responsibilities. Some form of counseling may be helpful in such a situation.

Fertility and the need to practice birth control at this stage depend upon a woman's age at the time of her last period. In general, a woman under the age of 50 may still be able to conceive for up to 24 months after the date of her last period; over 50, conception may be possible for up to one year.

After menopause, a woman is more liable to suffer osteoporosis (a disease that makes bones porous and brittle). This can often be prevented or controlled with estrogen therapy and calcium supplementation under medical supervision. The risk of heart attack also increases after menopause; estrogen therapy helps to decrease that risk.

Menorrhagia

Menorrhagia refers to an abnormally long or heavy menstrual flow, often accompanied by the passing of blood clots.

The condition, which is especially common in women in their late 30s and 40s, seldom indicates the existence of a serious disorder. However, it may result in iron deficiency anemia.

Causes

Menorrhagia is a common problem, often caused by a disturbance in the hormones controlling the menstrual cycle. It can also be caused by fibroid tumors in the uterus, inflammation of the pelvic region, and underactivity of the thyroid gland.

Diagnosis

If abnormal menstrual flow continues or recurs or if there is any chance of pregnancy, a physician should be consulted. The physician may perform a number of tests (including a Pap test) to determine whether there is a serious underlying cause. Biopsy (removal of a small tissue sample for laboratory examination) of the cervix or the uterine lining may be performed to check for cancer or other abnormalities. The physician may also do a blood test to check for iron-deficiency anemia.

Treatment

It is suggested that women who experience this disorder try to reduce the level of their activities during menstruation and be sure to get enough iron so that they will not become anemic.

Hormones (estrogen and progesterone) may also be used to control heavy bleeding if the underlying problem is a hormonal disturbance. Hysterectomy may be necessary in severe cases that do not respond to estrogen therapy and in cases of extensive fibroid tumors.

Menstruation

Menstruation is the monthly breakdown and discharge of portions of the endometrial tissue that lines the uterus.

The normal process

Endometrial tissue thickens during each menstrual cycle to prepare the uterus for possible pregnancy. Approximately midway through the cycle, ovulation occurs. Ovulation is the process by which an ovary produces and releases an egg. The fingerlike projections at the end of the nearby fallopian tube sweep the egg into the tube, where it begins inching toward the uterus. If the egg is fertilized by a sperm, the fertilized egg moves to the uterus and becomes implanted in the rich uterine lining, where it grows for the next nine months. If the egg does not become fertilized, the thickened endometrial tissue breaks down and passes, along with the unfertilized egg, out of the cervix, through the vagina, and out of the body as the menstrual discharge. This monthly cycle is controlled by estrogen and progesterone, secreted by the ovaries.

Young women usually start menstruating and ovulating at puberty, which usually oc-

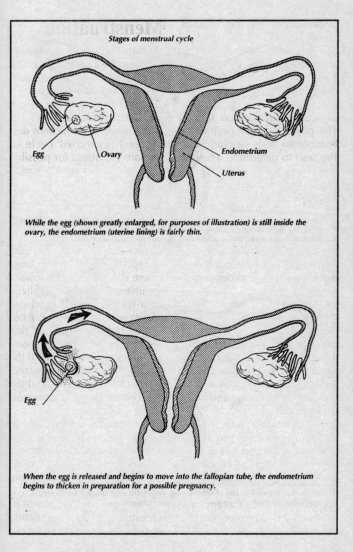

Stages of menstrual cycle

Egg | *Ovary*

Endometrium

Uterus

While the egg (shown greatly enlarged, for purposes of illustration) is still inside the ovary, the endometrium (uterine lining) is fairly thin.

Egg

When the egg is released and begins to move into the fallopian tube, the endometrium begins to thicken in preparation for a possible pregnancy.

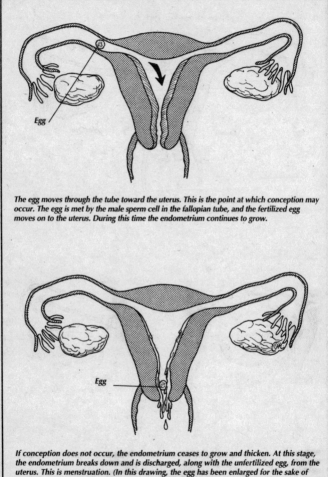

The egg moves through the tube toward the uterus. This is the point at which conception may occur. The egg is met by the male sperm cell in the fallopian tube, and the fertilized egg moves on to the uterus. During this time the endometrium continues to grow.

Egg

Egg

If conception does not occur, the endometrium ceases to grow and thicken. At this stage, the endometrium breaks down and is discharged, along with the unfertilized egg, from the uterus. This is menstruation. (In this drawing, the egg has been enlarged for the sake of illustration; normally the egg is only visible under a microscope.)

curs between the ages of 9 and 14. Thereafter, they normally menstruate and ovulate about once every month (except while pregnant) until they reach menopause.

Menstrual disorders

Menstruation may be accompanied by complications of varying degrees of seriousness. Most women will experience at least one such problem at some point in their reproductive lives. The most common problems are dysmenorrhea (painful menstruation), amenorrhea (the absence of one or more menstrual periods), and premenstrual syndrome (a complex of physical and emotional symptoms that appear in the days before the period begins).

For many years, the symptoms of these disorders have been attributed to emotional factors. Research has shown, however, that most symptoms are caused by very real physical changes, and many new methods of treatment have been developed.

Although the disorders themselves are generally not dangerous, they can be physically and emotionally incapacitating. Furthermore, they may be symptoms of disease in the reproductive organs. Therefore, to be on the safe side, medical treatment for distressing symptoms accompanying menstruation should always be sought.

Oophorectomy

Oophorectomy is the surgical removal of an ovary. An oophorectomy is a major operation, usually performed through either a vertical or a horizontal incision in the abdominal area, but occasionally performed through the vagina.

Removal of one ovary is called a *unilateral oophorectomy*. A salpingectomy (removal of all or part of the nearby fallopian tube) is usually performed at the same time. Removal of both ovaries is called a *bilateral oophorectomy*. A bilateral oophorectomy ends a woman's ability to conceive children and brings on menopause (if it has not already occurred). A hysterectomy (removal of the uterus) is generally performed in conjunction with a bilateral oophorectomy, because the uterus has no purpose without both ovaries and, if left, can later harbor tumors.

Purpose

Oophorectomy is used to correct a number of conditions in

which the ovaries are the site of the trouble, including benign (noncancerous) and malignant (cancerous) ovarian cysts and tumors. In women with recurrent cancer or endometriosis, oophorectomy is performed to stop the production of hormones that aggravate the condition. Breast cancer, as well, may be dependent on hormones to grow; about one-third of women with breast cancer show a decrease in breast cancer growth after removal of their ovaries.

Pros and cons

Some physicians recommend a bilateral oophorectomy when a hysterectomy must be performed. There are pros and cons when it comes to removing healthy ovaries. Arguments for their removal are that it reduces the risk of ovarian cancer; that a small number of women will develop painful cystic ovaries, which would necessitate a second operation; and that for a woman in her 40s, the ovaries will naturally stop functioning within a few years anyway. Arguments against routine oophorectomy are that it causes the premature onset of menopause, which brings with it a greater risk of osteoporosis (loss of bone mass) and heart attack;

that the abrupt end of hormone production is less natural than the gradual tapering off of natural menopause, provoking severe menopausal symptoms, such as hot flashes and vaginal shrinkage.

If a woman is in her childbearing years, her doctor will make every effort to save healthy ovarian tissue. Because the ovaries are fed by an excellent blood supply, they heal quickly and even a small bit of preserved ovarian tissue will function, secrete hormones, and release eggs. The woman remains fertile and avoids early menopause.

In women past menopause, for whom fertility is no longer an issue and in whom the ovaries no longer produce estrogen, both the ovaries and the uterus are commonly removed even if only one of the ovaries is abnormal.

Ovarian cysts

An ovarian cyst is an abnormal swelling or saclike growth on an ovary.

Ovarian cysts may be filled with liquid or may contain a semifluid substance. Most cysts are small, but they can vary in size from less than an inch in diameter to as large as 15 to 20 inches in diameter. Depending on their size, type, and location, they can cause severe pain and complications or no symptoms at all. They are common among women between the ages of 20 and 50 and can grow alone or in groups, on one ovary or both. Approximately 85 percent are benign (noncancerous).

Causes

The origin of most ovarian cysts is unknown. In some instances, they develop from an abnormal egg. Others originate as eggs in polycystic ovaries (ovaries in which the eggs are not released after they mature). Still others are related to abnormalities in the ovary. Women with endometriosis (the displacement of tissue from the uterine lining to elsewhere in the body) tend to develop growths on the ovaries.

Dermoid cysts, which are most often found in women under the age of 30, arise from the ovarian cells that produce the eggs and may contain fragments of hair, teeth, bone, and sweat and oil glands.

Complications

Cysts can rupture during sexual intercourse, a fall, childbirth, or surgery, or for no apparent reason. The resulting effect depends on how irritating the cystic fluid is to the surrounding tissues. The situation can be dangerous if the fluid is infected, cancerous, or extremely irritating. Also, in response to the injury caused by cystic fluid, surrounding tissues may produce adhesions (fibrous, scarlike material).

Symptoms

Symptoms of ovarian cysts vary with the type of growth. Some cause no symptoms and are discovered during a routine pelvic examination.

Ovarian cysts can cause painless swelling in the lower abdomen; pain during sexual intercourse; frequent urination (if they press against the bladder); irregular vaginal bleeding; or pain, nausea, and fever (if the cysts rupture or grow on stalks that become twisted). Excessive and abnormal body hair growth and the development of acne may result from hormonal imbalances caused by polycystic ovaries.

Diagnosis

Ovarian cysts are diagnosed by pelvic examination, ultrasound (a technique that uses sound waves to create an image of

451

internal structures), or laparos-copy (a surgical procedure in which a tubelike instrument is inserted through the abdominal wall to view the pelvic organs). The condition can be difficult to diagnose accurately because the symptoms can resemble those of acute appendicitis or other abdominal problems. In addition, it can be hard to determine if a cyst is malignant and if it is actually on the ovary rather than on some other organ.

Treatment

Cysts that are small, are not creating any problems, or are likely to disappear on their own require no treatment. If treatment is necessary, however, cysts can be removed surgically. Removal of ovarian cysts involves either taking out the entire ovary (oophorectomy) or taking out only the cyst (cystectomy).

If the ovarian cyst is found to be cancerous, it is necessary to remove both ovaries, both fallopian tubes, and the uterus, since the cancer may have spread from the ovarian cyst to these other structures. This procedure is also performed if an ovarian cyst is found after menopause, because these cysts are often cancerous.

Ovulation

Ovulation is the process by which an ovary produces and releases an egg.

The egg develops within the ovary in a small, fluid-filled sac called a *follicle*. When the egg is mature, this sac ruptures, releasing the egg from the ovary. The fingerlike projections on the nearby fallopian tube sweep the egg into the tube, where it begins to inch toward the uterus. If the egg is fertilized by a sperm, the fertilized egg moves along the tube to the uterus and becomes implanted in the rich uterine lining, where it grows for the next nine months.

If the egg does not become fertilized, the uterine lining breaks down and passes, along with the unfertilized egg, out of the cervix, through the vagina, and out of the body as the menstrual discharge.

Ovulation is regulated by a complex system of hormonal and chemical secretions from the ovaries, the hypothalamus (part of the brain), and the pituitary gland (the master gland, which controls most hormonal secretions). Ovulation and menstruation begin during puberty, which usually occurs between the ages of 9 and 14, and

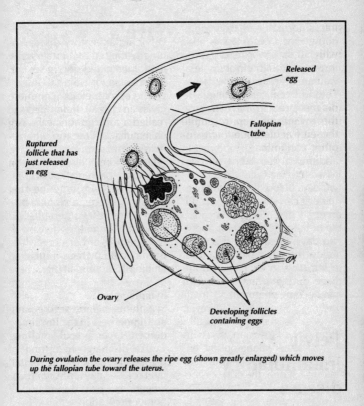

During ovulation the ovary releases the ripe egg (shown greatly enlarged) which moves up the fallopian tube toward the uterus.

continues every month (except during pregnancy) until menopause (around age 50).

One way to recognize when ovulation is happening is to take the body temperature with a basal thermometer (a special thermometer that will show even slight changes in body temperature) before rising in the morning. In most women, the body temperature rises slightly soon after ovulation occurs each month and does not return to normal until the menstrual flow begins. Another way is to count 14 days forward from the first day of the last menstrual period in an average 28-day cycle (count 15 days for a cycle

453

that is normally 29 days long, 16 days for a cycle that is normally 30 days long, and so on). However, this method is less accurate than the thermometer method because the length of the menstrual cycle can vary from month to month. Some women feel abdominal cramps during ovulation.

A sperm that has been released into the vagina as long as two days before the release of a ripe egg can still fertilize it; and an egg, once released, is capable of being fertilized for about two days. Because of this variability, there is a period of four to ten days in each menstrual cycle during which a woman can become pregnant.

Pelvic inflammatory disease

Pelvic inflammatory disease (PID), or *salpingitis*, is an inflammation of one or both of the fallopian tubes. Although the term is widely used to refer to infections of other organs in the pelvic cavity, pelvic inflammatory disease properly refers only to an inflammation of the fallopian tubes.

Causes

Pelvic inflammatory disease is usually caused by certain bacteria transmitted during sexual intercourse or vaginal infections. Two of the most common causes of pelvic inflammatory disease are gonorrhea and chlamydia, both sexually transmitted diseases.

Under normal circumstances, the cervix prevents bacteria in the vagina from entering the uterus. However, a woman becomes more vulnerable to pelvic inflammatory disease if the opening of her cervix has been dilated by recent surgery, childbirth, or miscarriage.

Symptoms

Symptoms include severe pain and tenderness in the lower abdomen, fever, a foul-smelling vaginal discharge, menstrual irregularities, pain during sexual intercourse, nausea, vomiting, fatigue, and pain during urination or defecation.

Diagnosis

It is important to seek medical attention as soon as symptoms occur, so that the infection can be treated. The physician will perform an examination and take a sample of fluid from the cervix to identify the infecting organism.

Complications

If PID is not diagnosed and treated early, the infection can cause abscesses (pus-filled cavities) to form in the fallopian tubes or around the ovaries. The inflammation can also damage and irreversibly scar pelvic tissues. If the fallopian tubes are blocked, conception can become impossible. The infection can also result in septicemia (in which bacteria enter the bloodstream and are spread to other parts of the body) and in peritonitis (inflammation of the membrane lining the pelvic and abdominal cavities).

Treatment

The doctor will prescribe antibiotics to fight the infection and aspirin or other painkillers for pain relief. The woman may be advised to rest in bed, abstain from sexual intercourse, and apply heat to the lower abdominal area. In some cases, the woman may have to enter the hospital to receive antibi-

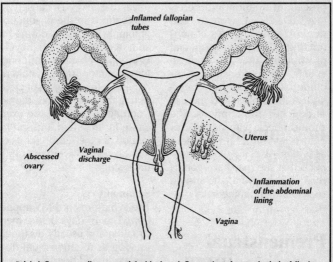

Pelvic inflammatory disease, or salpingitis, *is an inflammation of one or both the fallopian tubes, which can lead to an ovarian abscess, an inflammation of the abdominal lining, and blockage of the fallopian tubes. Vaginal discharge is a common sign of the condition.*

otics intravenously. Laparoscopy or surgery to drain blocked tubes or abscessed tissue may be performed. If the damage is too extensive, the fallopian tubes, the uterus, and the ovaries may have to be removed surgically.

Prevention
When the cervix is dilated for any reason, a woman is more susceptible to PID for several weeks. Since the cervix is dilated in childbirth, abortion, miscarriage, and the surgical procedure dilation and curettage (D&C), a woman can minimize her chances of contracting PID by taking special precautions after any of those events. Such precautions include avoiding sexual intercourse, tub baths, and the use of douches and tampons. She should check with her doctor before resuming any of these activities. Also, if a woman suspects that she may have gonorrhea or chlamydia, she should seek treatment immediately.

Premenstrual syndrome (PMS)

Premenstrual syndrome (PMS) is a term used to encompass the varying complex of physical and emotional symptoms experienced by some women during the week before their menstrual period begins. In the past, this and other menstrual problems were thought to be caused by emotional instability or hysteria, but current research, while not yet offering conclusive findings, indicates that there are physical reasons for such disorders.

Cause
Many medical researchers believe that PMS is caused by fluctuations in the production of female hormones during the course of the menstrual cycle. Hormonal changes influence the amounts of salt and fluid retained in the body, especially during the week before the period begins. Neither the exact cause for this fluid and salt retention nor the reason for its effect on certain women is fully understood.

Symptoms
The symptoms of PMS appear from 5 to 14 days before menstruation and usually disappear as soon as the menstrual flow begins. In addition to nervousness and irritability, a bloated or puffy feeling that results from edema (fluid retention) often

characterizes this disorder. Other possible symptoms include depression, headache, fatigue, tenderness in the breasts, and acne.

Diagnosis
The diagnosis of premenstrual syndrome is based on a physical examination and the woman's menstrual history. The occurrence of any of the symptoms with some regularity before each menstrual period and their disappearance soon after menstrual flow begins are the key diagnostic clues.

Treatment
At present, there is no single or sure remedy for the discomforts of premenstrual syndrome. Depending on the symptoms present, various medications can be helpful. The edema is often treated by reducing salt intake or by taking diuretics, medications that help to eliminate excess fluid from the tissues by increasing the production of urine. The avoidance of methylxanthines (chemicals contained in coffee, tea, cola, chocolate, and certain medications) will often help reduce headache and irritability. Tranquilizers and psychological counseling may be recommended for patients in whom PMS causes emotional distress. Research has shown the antidepressant fluoxetine (Prozac) to lessen symptoms of PMS in some women. A balanced diet, moderate exercise, and adequate rest may also be beneficial in treating PMS.

Prevention
A reduction of salt intake may help to prevent the initial fluid retention that often accompanies PMS.

Self-treatment with diuretics without the advice of a physician is not recommended.

Prolapse of the uterus

Prolapse is a collapse, descent, or other change in the position of an organ in relation to surrounding structures. Prolapse of the uterus may be one of three types of prolapse:
- First-degree prolapse, in which the uterus sags downward so that the cervix is flush with the entrance to the vagina
- Second-degree prolapse, in which the cervix is outside the vagina
- Third-degree prolapse, in which the entire uterus is outside the vagina

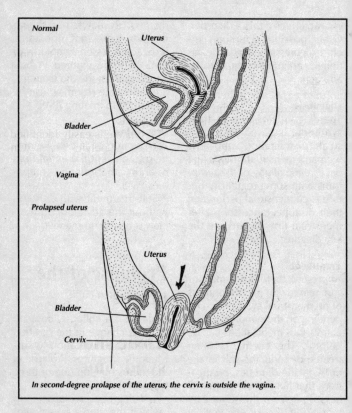

Normal

Uterus

Bladder

Vagina

Prolapsed uterus

Uterus

Bladder

Cervix

In second-degree prolapse of the uterus, the cervix is outside the vagina.

Cause
Prolapse of the uterus occurs when the muscles and ligaments that normally hold the uterus in place become stretched or slack. Prolapse of the uterus is most often due to a long or difficult childbirth or multiple childbirths.

Symptoms
There may be a feeling of heaviness in the vagina, backache, or inability to control urination.

Diagnosis
Prolapse of the uterus is apparent to a physician during a pelvic examination.

Treatment

It is especially important to treat prolapse of the uterus because it can make childbirth difficult and may damage other organs. In mild cases, the patient may find that exercises for the muscles of the pelvic floor are helpful. If the prolapse is the result of injury or stress, surgical repair may be indicated, in which the uterus is returned to its proper place.

If the prolapse is due to disease or swelling, the underlying disorder must first be controlled before the uterus can be returned to its original position. In some cases, a pessary (a plastic ring or donut) is inserted into the vagina to hold the uterus in its proper position.

Rectocele

Rectocele is a condition in which a part of the rectum protrudes into the vagina.

Cause

The usual cause of this condition is a weakening of the back wall of the vagina due to the stretching caused by childbirth.

Symptoms

A minimal protrusion may produce no symptoms or only a mild pressure sensation during bowel movements. In more severe cases, however, chronic constipation and painful bowel movements may frequently occur.

Diagnosis

A rectocele is easily identified during a pelvic exam. On straining or coughing, the rectum may be found to bulge into the vagina.

Treatment

Rectocele is not a dangerous condition and generally requires no treatment. If severe constipation or painful bowel movements develop, surgical repair is often curative.

Toxic shock syndrome

Toxic shock syndrome (TSS) is a rare, sometimes fatal condition that develops very suddenly and progresses rapidly when a bacterial infection spreads through the bloodstream. The disorder was first defined in 1978, when its link to the use of tampons was suspected. Most of the reported cases have occurred in women under the age of 30 who use extra-absorbent tampons. A significant number of these cases have been fatal.

Cause

Most researchers believe that TSS occurs when the bacteria *Staphylococcus aureus* enters the bloodstream and produces a toxin (poison) that causes leaks in blood vessel walls, allowing blood to seep into the tissues. This results in a sudden, very dangerous drop in blood pressure, shock, and sometimes death.

In serious cases, low blood pressure and weakening of the cell membranes can leave the victim susceptible to further complications, such as heart and liver damage. Often, the body cannot produce enough antibodies (protective substances) to fight off the invasion of organisms through the weakened cell membranes, so TSS can easily recur.

Although the use of tampons is considered a definite risk factor, tampons do not actually cause the disease but rather promote the growth of bacteria that leads to the disorder. The tampons swell to fill the vagina and thereby inhibit the elimination of blood, creating a breeding ground for infection. Also, if tampons are left in the vagina for long periods of time, the chances for infection are increased. Tampon applicators, moreover, may scratch the walls of the vagina, allowing bacteria to enter.

Since about 25 percent of cases now occur in men and nonmenstruating women, it is clear that the bacteria can enter the body in ways other than through the vagina. In these cases, TSS often occurs when the body has been weakened by major surgery, severe burns, or boils or abscesses. Also, women who have recently given birth are at a higher risk of contracting TSS because the vagina is more susceptible to the invasion of bacteria at this time.

Symptoms

TSS produces high fever, vomiting, diarrhea, a sunburnlike rash, peeling of skin on the soles of the feet and the palms of the hands, blurred vision, and disorientation.

Diagnosis

The occurrence of the high fever, the characteristic rash, low blood pressure, and involvement of several organ systems strongly points to the diagnosis of TSS. Cultures of the blood and mucous membranes will be performed to search for evidence of infection by *Staphylococcus aureus.*

Treatment
Emergency medical treatment should be sought immediately. This condition requires hospitalization, during which the patient is given therapy similar to that administered to poisoning victims. Fluids or blood transfusions are given to raise blood pressure, an ice blanket is used to reduce fever, and antibiotics are administered to fight the infection.

Precautions
The best precaution is probably to discontinue or limit the use of tampons. Tampons can still be worn safely, but they should be changed every three to four hours and alternated with sanitary napkins as often as possible, especially before going to sleep.

Vaginitis

Vaginitis is an inflammation of the vagina, usually marked by burning and itching of the external genital organs.

Causes
Vaginitis is most commonly caused by an imbalance of the microorganisms normally present in the vagina, resulting when some factor causes one of the strains to reproduce more quickly than the others. The microorganisms most often involved are the fungus *Candida albicans,* the bacterium *Hemophilus vaginalis,* and the protozoan (one-celled organism) *Trichomonas vaginalis.* Possible causes of overgrowth of microorganisms include the use of birth control pills, which produce changes in the vaginal lining; the use of certain antibiotics, which may kill some types of bacteria but allow others to flourish; the presence of a warm, moist environment (such as may be created by wearing tight pants or panty hose, nylon underwear, or a wet bathing suit), which acts as a breeding ground for infection; and, particularly for infection by *Hemophilus vaginalis* or *Trichomonas vaginalis,* the introduction of an infectious microorganism through sexual contact with an infected individual. Vaginitis tends to occur more often in the summer, because excessive heat and moisture are known to promote the disease.

One variety of the disease, called *noninfectious vaginitis,* is not caused by overproduction of microorganisms, but rather by direct irritation of the vagina by some outside agent, such as the chemical irritation that arises from the excessive use of douches, feminine hygiene sprays, bubble baths, and talcum powder.

Pregnant women and those who have diabetes or gonorrhea (a sexually transmitted disease) are at a higher risk of developing vaginitis than other women.

Symptoms

Infection by *Candida albicans* causes severe itching of the external genital organs and pain during intercourse. Because of the thick, white vaginal discharge, which resembles cottage cheese in texture and has a "yeasty" odor, this condition is commonly known as a *yeast infection*. This is the type of vaginitis most frequently contracted by pregnant women and women with diabetes.

Infection by *Hemophilus vaginalis* causes a grayish, foul-smelling discharge.

The presence of *Trichomonas vaginalis* is indicated by itching and burning, a greenish-white discharge, and foul odor. These symptoms are likely to appear during or immediately after menstruation.

Noninfectious vaginitis is characterized only by irritation and dryness, usually with no discharge.

Diagnosis

Vaginitis is diagnosed by determining which microorganism is causing the infection. Microscopic examination of a sample, or smear, of vaginal secretions is used to make the diagnosis.

Treatment

Treatment varies according to the type of microorganism. Fungal infections are generally treated with an antifungal cream, which is applied directly to the vagina, or as a vaginal suppository (forms of which are now available without a doctor's prescription).

Bacterial infections are treated with antibiotics, administered either orally or as vaginal suppositories. Because bacterial infections can be transferred between sexual partners, both individuals are usually treated with oral antibiotics.

An oral antibiotic called metronidazole is given to women with protozoan infections and to their partners. Because some studies have linked this drug to cancer and genetic damage in laboratory animals, metronidazole should not be taken during the first half of pregnancy.

Noninfectious vaginitis is usually treated simply by avoiding the irritants that can cause it, such as perfumed soaps, chemical sprays, and scented bathroom tissue, and by not wearing tight-fitting clothing.

Prevention

Some types of vaginitis can probably be prevented by using only nonscented, white toilet paper; wearing cotton underwear and loose-fitting pants; avoiding the overuse of douches, feminine hygiene sprays, and scented toiletries; and having any sexual partner use condoms.

PROBLEMS OF COUPLES

A couple can encounter health problems in three areas: contraception (birth control), infertility, and sexually transmitted diseases (also called *venereal disease*). Decisions or problems in all three areas affect both partners.

Although sex is a topic that arouses considerable curiosity and interest, it is also surrounded by many myths and misconceptions that can lead to needless anxiety. Fortunately, societal attitudes have been changing, and there is now more free and open discussion about subjects that used to be considered taboo.

The best approach to solving any problem includes two ingredients: an understanding by both partners of how the male and female reproductive systems work and a willingness to communicate openly and honestly with each other.

Responsibility for these areas of health should not be shouldered by either the man or the woman alone. Both partners need to work together to weigh consequences, consider alternatives, and provide mutual support.

Birth control
Couples who want to delay or prevent pregnancy can choose from several different kinds of contraceptives: physical devices (intrauterine devices), barrier methods (condoms, cervical caps, diaphragms), chemical methods (spermicides, sponges, pills, implants), a combination of barrier and chemical methods (diaphragm with a spermicide), permanent birth control (vasectomy for men and blocking of fallopian tubes for women), and abstinence from intercourse during the woman's fertile period.

Some birth control methods require a doctor's prescription; others can be purchased over the counter. Methods vary in effectiveness, convenience, and safety. It's a good idea for a couple to discuss with a doctor the advantages and disadvantages of the various methods of birth control, especially the side effects, ease of use, and reliability. Choose the birth control method that best suits your needs as a couple; what works well for one couple may not appeal to another.

Infertility

About one of every five couples who want to conceive a child is unsuccessful at doing so. If pregnancy does not occur after a year of regular sexual intercourse without contraceptives, the couple may want to consider a consultation with an obstetrician/gynecologist or a urologist who specializes in infertility.

During the last ten years or so, medical science has made tremendous inroads into diagnosing and treating causes of infertility and has given new hope to childless couples. Improved testing procedures, new drugs that stimulate ovulation, new methods of fertilizing a woman's egg both inside and outside of the body, and surgical techniques that can correct female or male structural problems or reverse sterilization procedures have enabled many couples to become parents.

Sexually transmitted diseases

One of the risks of intimate sexual contact, especially for men and women who have more than one partner, is infection with a sexually transmitted disease (STD), or venereal disease (VD). Despite improved diagnosis and treatment for these diseases, their incidence has increased, probably because of the sexual freedom of the last 20 years, which has resulted in large part from more reliable birth control.

Sexually transmitted diseases are caused by organisms that thrive in the warm, moist environment of the reproductive system and are transmitted by sexual contact.

Gonorrhea is the most prevalent of the sexually transmitted diseases, but herpes, syphilis, and chlamydia are common enough to be of concern to sexually active people. With the exception of herpes, these diseases can be cured. (A consequence of delaying treatment is permanent sterility, however.)

Acquired immunodeficiency syndrome (AIDS) is a serious sexually transmitted disease in which the body's natural defense system is disabled, allowing organisms that are normally fought off to become deadly (see page 29).

STDs are particularly serious for pregnant women. The diseases can be transmitted to a

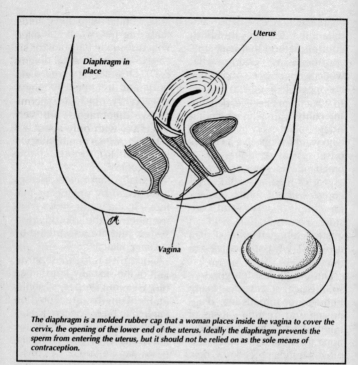

The diaphragm is a molded rubber cap that a woman places inside the vagina to cover the cervix, the opening of the lower end of the uterus. Ideally the diaphragm prevents the sperm from entering the uterus, but it should not be relied on as the sole means of contraception.

baby while it is passing through the birth canal and can critically affect the child.

If you do become infected with any of these diseases, you must abstain from further sexual contact until the problem has been controlled. Any sexual partners need to be informed of the possibility of infection and must seek treatment, whether or not symptoms develop.

Birth control

Birth control, also called *contraception*, is the voluntary prevention of pregnancy. A variety of methods are available. Couples who use no contraceptive method have an 80 to 90 percent chance of achieving pregnancy over a 12-month period, provided that they have no underlying infertility problem.

Condom

A condom is a thin rubber or synthetic sheath that a man fits over his erect penis just before sexual intercourse. A condom used alone is about 70 percent to 90 percent effective, depending on the care with which it is used.

Several problems can occur with the use of the condom, however. Tiny holes or tears may develop in the sheath, causing leakage of sperm. Also, when the penis is withdrawn from the vagina after intercourse, the condom sometimes breaks or partially unrolls inside the vagina, releasing sperm.

However, a latex condom used regularly with a spermicide is approximately 95 percent effective in preventing pregnancy. Condoms have the great advantage of being readily available in any drugstore without a prescription. Latex condoms also have the advantage of helping to prevent the spread of many types of sexually transmitted diseases, including acquired immunodeficiency syndrome (AIDS).

Diaphragm

The diaphragm is a molded rubber cap that the woman places inside the vagina to cover the cervix. The diaphragm blocks sperm from entering the uterus. It must be inserted before intercourse and left in place for six hours afterward. Diaphragms are available in different sizes and must be fitted by a physician. When used with spermicides, diaphragms are very effective, with only about a 3 percent chance of pregnancy.

Cervical cap

The cervical cap is a molded rubber cap that fits over the outside of the cervix. While the diaphragm covers both the cervix and the back of the vagina, the smaller cervical cap fits only over the cervix. Like a diaphragm, the cervical cap blocks sperm from entering the uterus. It must be inserted for each act of intercourse and left in place for six to eight hours afterward. Cervical caps come in different sizes and must be fitted by a physician. Their effectiveness is similar to that of the diaphragm. The cervical cap contains spermicide.

Spermicide

Spermicide is a chemical foam, cream, suppository, or jelly applied to the woman's vagina to kill sperm. A spermicide should be used in conjunction with a condom or diaphragm; used alone, a spermicide is only 75 to 85 percent effective. Some disadvantages of a spermicide are that it must be applied before each individual act of sexual intercourse, it has chemical odors, and it may cause irritation of the vagina. A chief advantage is that spermicides are readily available at drugstores without a prescription.

Contraceptive sponge
The contraceptive sponge is a disposable, spongelike device saturated with spermicide. The sponge is inserted into the vagina up against the cervix, where the device works by continuously releasing spermicide for up to 24 hours. Additional applications of spermicide are not necessary, even for multiple acts of intercourse. There are other advantages as well: The sponge is available without a prescription; unlike a diaphragm, the sponge does not have to be fitted; and the sponge can be inserted ahead of time, which allows greater spontaneity in sex. The sponge has been found to be about 85 percent effective.

Some side effects are associated with the use of the sponge. Cases of local irritation or allergic reaction have been reported; however, these have been mild and infrequent. There

is also concern that the sponge could become a breeding ground for infection, especially if used improperly. You should consult your doctor about the contraceptive sponge and its proper use before trying this method of birth control.

IUD
The intrauterine device (IUD) is a small plastic device inserted into the woman's uterus by a physician. The IUD has a string attached to it that hangs into the cervix, so that the woman can check to be sure that the IUD is still in place. Most researchers believe that the IUD prevents pregnancy by causing changes in the uterine lining that disrupt the normal environment of an egg. For the woman who can use an IUD, the advantages are great, because she does not have to worry about contraception each day. The effectiveness rate is high, with less than a 1 percent chance of pregnancy.

However, there are several disadvantages to the use of an IUD. Severe menstrual cramps and increased menstrual bleeding may follow the insertion of an IUD. Sometimes these side effects lessen after a month or two. In other cases, severe cramps and prolonged bleeding continue, and the physician

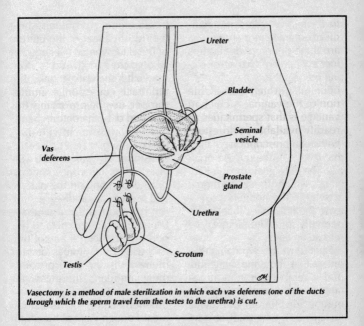

Vasectomy is a method of male sterilization in which each vas deferens (one of the ducts through which the sperm travel from the testes to the urethra) is cut.

may advise removal of the IUD. The IUD is also thought to increase the probability of pelvic infections within the first few months following insertion.

Sterilization

A woman may be sterilized by an operation that blocks the fallopian tubes (the structures through which eggs travel from the ovaries to the uterus). A man may be sterilized by a procedure called a *vasectomy*, in which each vas deferens (one of the two ducts through which the sperm travel from the testes to the urethra) is cut. These procedures may be reversed but only by complicated surgery, which is not always successful. Therefore, physicians recommend sterilization only when a couple has decided, without reservation, that they desire no further pregnancies.

Oral contraceptives

Oral contraceptives, or birth control pills, are one of the

469

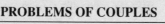

most effective reversible methods of contraception. A woman taking the pill properly has less than a 1 percent chance of getting pregnant.

The pill—which is available by prescription only—uses synthetic female hormones (estrogen and progestin) to override the natural hormonal regulation that results in the release of an egg. The pill signals the pituitary gland, which directs hormonal activity in the body, not to release the hormones that would normally stimulate the ovary to release an egg.

Each day the woman takes one pill, at about the same time of day, removing it from a container that has the required number of pills for one cycle (usually 21). One to three days after she takes the last pill for that cycle, her menstrual period begins. Menstrual periods may be lighter in flow, and cramps may be reduced or absent.

If she forgets to take one pill or more, menstrual bleeding may begin. In that case, she should continue taking the pills daily, but she should also use another contraceptive method, such as a condom, until after her next regular period.

Birth control pills are not recommended for women with a history of high blood pressure, blood-clotting problems, hepatitis, or cancer of the uterus or breast. A woman over age 35 who smokes is advised to stop smoking if she wants to take the pill. Birth control pills should not be taken by a woman who suspects she may be pregnant. In addition, women with diabetes, epilepsy, heart disease, or thyroid disease may be advised not to take birth control pills, depending on the nature and severity of the disease.

It is important for a woman taking birth control pills to report to her doctor if any of the following symptoms occur: blurred vision; severe chest pain; sudden shortness of breath; abdominal pain; unusual bleeding or bruising; breakthrough vaginal bleeding (spotting); changes in menstrual flow; pain in the calves; depression; difficult or painful urination; enlarged or tender breasts; hearing changes; increase or decrease in hair growth; migraine headaches; numbness or tingling; rash; skin color changes; swelling of the feet, ankles, or lower legs; vaginal itching; weight changes; or yellowing of the eyes or skin.

Hormonal implants
The newest form of contraception is the hormonal implant.

With this method, six small plastic rods containing the synthetic female hormone progestin are inserted with a needle under the skin of the upper arm or forearm. The hormone is gradually and slowly released from the plastic rods, thus preventing ovulation. This method is effective for about five years from the time the implants are inserted. The major advantage of this method is that the woman does not need to remember to take birth control pills or use a spermicidal agent or diaphragm before each sexual act. Disadvantages include the high cost of the implants, possible infection at the site of insertion, irregular menstruation, and the necessity for surgical incisions on the arm when the implants need to be removed. Hormonal implants are about as effective as oral contraceptives.

Natural family planning
Natural family planning is based on calculating when ovulation (release of an egg from one of the woman's ovaries each month) occurs. The couple then abstains from intercourse during the fertile period.

A man's sperm can live in a woman's body for about two days. The egg can live for about 24 hours after ovulation. A few days are added to this fertile period for safety's sake, because it is so difficult to determine just when ovulation occurs. All told, a couple needs to abstain from intercourse seven to ten days a month in order to have the greatest chance of preventing pregnancy.

There are three methods a woman can use to determine when she ovulates. The temperature method is one of the most reliable. Each morning on awakening and before getting out of bed, she takes her temperature with a special basal temperature thermometer (which measures temperatures only between 96°F and 100°F) and records it on graph paper. Near the middle of the menstrual cycle, the temperature may drop slightly (indicating that ovulation is about to occur) and then rise rapidly and continue to climb for the next three days. The temperature will not return to preovulation levels until the beginning of the menstrual period. The "safe" days to have sexual intercourse are from four days after the sudden rise in temperature until three or four days after the end of the period. It is important to become familiar with the menstrual cycle by recording the

471

temperature levels for several months before relying on this method of birth control.

The mucus method may also help determine the time of ovulation. Each morning the mucus from the vagina and cervix is examined. Cervical mucus undergoes changes as hormone levels vary during the course of the cycle. To detect these changes, the vaginal area is blotted each morning with a facial tissue, and then the mucus is tested between the thumb and forefinger. After the menstrual period, there will be several days with no mucous discharge. This is followed by several days of a thick, sticky yellow or white discharge. There will then be one or two days when the mucus becomes transparent and very slippery, with the consistency of raw egg whites. The mucus will form a string between the thumb and forefinger. This is when ovulation occurs. After ovulation, the mucus again becomes thick and sticky, or there may be no mucus at all. The fertile period begins with the thick, sticky yellow or white discharge and continues until about three days after the phase when the mucus has the consistency of egg whites. Intercourse should be avoided during this time. In other words, the safe period is from three days after the slippery mucus stage to about three days after the end of the menstrual period. The use of certain medications (such as antihistamines), which alter mucus production throughout the body, will make determination of ovulation by the mucus method difficult, however.

The calendar method is also an option for women. A record of menstrual cycles is kept for one year or more. The doctor will then use the record to figure out the most likely day of ovulation, based on the fact that the average woman menstruates 14 days after she ovulates. However, any individual woman may vary from that average, so the calendar method is not a precise system.

Natural family planning does not require the use of mechanical aids or drugs. The effectiveness rate for this kind of birth control is currently up to about 80 percent, depending on the care with which the techniques are followed. However, even in women with regular cycles, fluctuating factors such as illness, fatigue, stress, and use of certain drugs can delay ovulation or cause the techniques used to determine ovulation to be inaccurate, thereby throwing off the most careful calculations.

Chlamydia

Chlamydia trachomatis is a species of sexually transmitted bacteria that affects the reproductive organs in both men and women. Like other STDs, chlamydia is a highly contagious illness spread primarily through direct sexual contact.

Complications
Left untreated, chlamydia can lead to prostatitis (inflammation of the prostate gland, where seminal fluid is produced) and epididymitis (inflammation of the ducts leading from the testes) in men and to pelvic inflammatory disease (an inflammation in the pelvic cavity affecting the fallopian tubes) and infertility in women. Chlamydia can also be transmitted from a mother to her baby during childbirth, resulting in ear infections and pneumonia in the newborn; it has also been linked to an increased risk of stillbirths and sudden infant death syndrome (SIDS).

Cause
Chlamydia is caused by the organism *Chlamydia trachomatis*, which is transmitted by direct sexual contact with an infected person. It displays symptoms similar to those of gonorrhea.

Symptoms
Sometimes no symptoms are evident. In other cases, there is a discharge from the penis or vagina, pain and burning during urination, and other symptoms similar to those of gonorrhea. In fact, chlamydia can often occur with gonorrhea, so if symptoms persist after treatment for gonorrhea, they may be due to chlamydia.

Diagnosis
A physician can test for the presence of chlamydial infection by taking a sample of secretions from the penis or cervix. Results of this test can be obtained in as little as 30 minutes. Since gonorrhea can produce the same symptoms as chlamydia, the doctor will usually find it necessary to test for both infections.

Treatment
Penicillin has no effect on chlamydia, so this disease is treated with another antibiotic, such as doxycycline, tetracycline, or erythromycin. This is why treatment of gonorrhea with penicillin will not affect a coexisting case of chlamydia.

A person who has chlamydia or any other STD should abstain from sexual activity until all tests have indicated that the disease is no longer present. Every sexual partner of the infected person needs to be examined and, if necessary, treated for chlamydia.

Prevention
Chlamydia can be prevented by avoiding sexual contact with someone who has the disease. Because the chances of contracting chlamydia or any other sexually transmitted disease increase with the number of sexual partners a person has, limiting the number of partners is the first step toward prevention of sexually transmitted diseases. Using condoms also helps to reduce the risk of contracting chlamydia.

Genital warts

Genital warts (known medically as *condylomata acuminata*) are caused by human papillomavirus (HPV). These viral growths appear on the external genital organs. The condition is considered to be an STD.

If left untreated, genital warts can grow quite large, causing discomfort during sexual intercourse, urination, and bowel movements. Genital warts are seen more frequently in uncircumcised men than in those who have been circumcised. Scientists now believe that some viruses that cause genital warts may, over a period of several years, lead to the development of certain genital tumors such as cancer of the cervix and cancer of the penis. Close follow-up and regular Pap smears are therefore necessary.

Pregnancy may make genital warts grow faster, but they usually shrink after the baby is born. They may even become large enough during pregnancy to block the birth canal, making a cesarean delivery (through an incision in the walls of the uterus and abdomen) necessary. The wart virus can be transmitted from a mother to her child during birth, sometimes causing the development of warts within the throat of the baby.

Cause
Genital warts are caused by direct sexual contact with an infected person. About 60 percent of all those exposed to genital warts will develop the condition. However, the warts will not appear until six weeks to eight months after the initial exposure.

Symptoms

The only symptom of genital warts is the warts themselves, which appear most frequently on the penis, vagina, vulva (the structure surrounding the opening of the vagina), and anus. They may also be found in the mouth or on the cervix. Genital warts are soft, moist, and pink, occurring alone or in clusters; cluster formations tend to resemble cauliflower in their uneven, puffy appearance. Genital warts are seldom painful, but they can be irritated by sexual intercourse; in fact, the warts often grow on the parts of the sex organs that receive the most friction during sexual intercourse.

Diagnosis

Because their appearance is so distinctive, a physician can usually diagnose genital warts by a simple physical examination. If there is any doubt, a sample of tissue from the wart can be tested to rule out other disorders, such as cancerous growths or the warts that often accompany syphilis (another STD). Sometimes the physician may use a magnifying instrument called a colposcope to detect small genital warts that may not be visible to the naked eye.

Treatment

Small genital warts are sometimes treated with a drug called podophyllin, which is applied directly to the warts and then washed off several hours later. More than one application may be necessary. Because podophyllin is toxic in large quantities, very large or persistent warts are often removed by cryotherapy (a process in which liquid nitrogen is used to freeze the growths, which then fall off); by heat treatments, which dry out and destroy the warts; or by laser therapy, which vaporizes the growths.

A person who has genital warts or any other STD should abstain from sexual activity until all tests have indicated that the disease is no longer present. As is the case with all other STDs, every sexual partner of the infected person needs to be examined and, if necessary, treated.

Prevention

Genital warts can be prevented by avoiding sexual contact with someone who has the condition. Because the chances of contracting this and other STDs increase with the number of sexual partners a person has, limiting the number of partners is the first step in prevention.

Using condoms also helps to reduce the risk of contracting genital warts.

Gonorrhea

Gonorrhea is one of the most frequently reported STDs. It is a highly contagious bacterial infection spread primarily through direct sexual contact.

Gonorrhea predominantly affects the penis in men, the cervix in women, and the throat and anus in both sexes. Left untreated, it can lead to a generalized blood infection, sterility, arthritis, and heart trouble. Additionally, in men it can spread throughout the prostate gland and the ducts of the reproductive system, causing painful inflammation.

Gonorrhea can also lead to eye infections if the genital secretions come in contact with the eyes—for instance, if a person rubs his or her eyes after handling infected genital organs. Because the infant passes through the potentially infected birth canal during the birth process, every state requires that a few drops of penicillin or erythromycin be placed in the eyes of all newborns to prevent infection and possible blindness.

Symptoms

In women, this disease may have no symptoms, but in many cases, it is marked by a discharge from the vagina and urethra and by frequent, painful urination. Gonorrhea may lead to pelvic inflammatory disease (PID), which results when the infection extends to the fallopian tubes; the scar tissue that forms may block the tubes, preventing conception and sometimes causing sterility. The symptoms of PID include fever, chills, vaginal discharge, and vomiting.

The primary symptom of gonorrhea in men is a yellowish discharge from the penis within two to ten days of exposure to the disease, accompanied by painful and burning urination.

Gonorrhea of the anus is marked by a bloody or mucus-filled discharge from the anus and pain during bowel movements. Gonorrhea of the throat may have no symptoms or may reveal itself only as a scratchy, sore throat or a severe, flame-red sore throat.

Diagnosis

Diagnosis is made by taking a sample of the discharge, examining it under a microscope to identify the infection, and confirming the diagnosis by per-

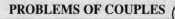

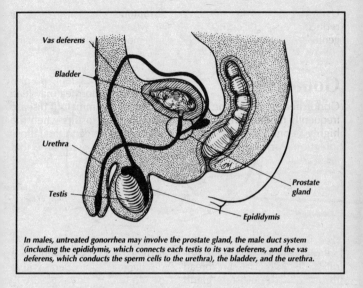

In males, untreated gonorrhea may involve the prostate gland, the male duct system (including the epididymis, which connects each testis to its vas deferens, and the vas deferens, which conducts the sperm cells to the urethra), the bladder, and the urethra.

forming a culture (a technique in which the sample of the discharge is placed in a special substance that encourages the growth of bacteria).

Treatment

Gonorrhea is usually treated with penicillin or tetracycline. These antibiotics can be either injected or taken orally.

Men being treated for gonorrhea should avoid alcoholic beverages, because recent studies have shown that drinking may increase the chances of developing an inflammation of the urethra (the canal leading from

the urinary bladder through the penis).

While under treatment, the patient should abstain from sexual activity until further tests have confirmed that gonorrhea is no longer present. This testing is usually done two weeks after the beginning of treatment. If signs of the disease are still present, drug therapy can be reinstated with a different antibiotic.

A culture to detect a chlamydial infection is usually performed along with the culture to detect gonorrhea (since symptoms of the two infections are the same). If chlamydia is

477

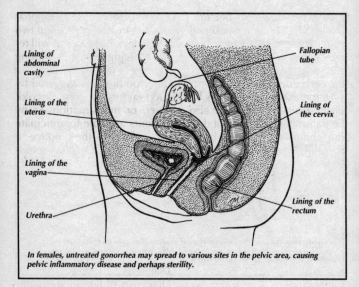

Lining of abdominal cavity

Lining of the uterus

Lining of the vagina

Urethra

Fallopian tube

Lining of the cervix

Lining of the rectum

In females, untreated gonorrhea may spread to various sites in the pelvic area, causing pelvic inflammatory disease and perhaps sterility.

found, it can be treated with an antibiotic.

Every sexual partner of the infected person should be examined and, if necessary, treated.

Prevention

Gonorrhea can be prevented by avoiding sexual contact with someone who has the disease. Because the chance of contracting this and other STDs increases with the number of sexual partners a person has, limiting the number of partners is the first step in prevention. Using condoms also helps to reduce the risk.

Herpes

Herpes is a highly contagious illness spread primarily through direct sexual contact.

Herpes can be treated but not cured. Its symptoms appear briefly and then disappear; the disease lies dormant in nerve cells, but it may be reactivated by stress or illness. It is believed to be contagious only during active periods, when blisters are present. Persons taking drugs that suppress the body's immune system (for instance, cancer or organ transplant patients) are at a higher risk of contracting herpes, because their bodies are in a weakened state. There is also some evidence that links genital herpes with a higher rate of cancer of the cervix in women.

Herpes is spread primarily by direct sexual contact. It can also be transmitted to an infant during childbirth, causing brain damage or death. Therefore, if a woman shows signs of the active disease while in labor, the baby will be delivered by cesarean section (through an incision in the walls of the uterus and abdomen), rather than through the vagina, where the herpes blisters may be present.

Cause
Herpes is caused by herpes simplex virus type 2, which is similar to the virus (herpes simplex virus type 1) that causes cold sores and fever blisters on the lips.

Symptoms
The predominant symptom of herpes is the outbreak of painful, itching blisters filled with fluid on and around the external sexual organs. Women may have a vaginal discharge. Symptoms vaguely similar to those of the flu may accompany these outbreaks, including fever and fatigue.

The blisters will disappear without treatment in about two to ten days, but the virus will remain, lying dormant among clusters of nerve cells until another outbreak is triggered by such factors as stress, a cold, fever, or menstruation. Many patients are able to anticipate an outbreak—they notice a warning sign, a tingling sensation called a prodrome, of the approaching illness. Herpes is thought to be contagious only during actual outbreaks, so sexual activity should be avoided while blisters or other symptoms are present.

Diagnosis
Diagnosis of herpes is accomplished by microscopic examination and culture of the fluid contained in the blisters.

Treatment
Unlike other STDs, herpes cannot be cured, because any medication that will attack the virus while it lies dormant in the nerve cells will also damage the nerve cells. However, there is treatment for acute outbreaks now available that involves the use of either the antiviral drug acyclovir or laser therapy, both of which will heal blisters, reduce pain, and, most important, kill large numbers of the

herpes virus organisms. Acyclovir has also been found to reduce the reproduction of the virus in initial outbreaks, thus possibly lessening the number of subsequent outbreaks. It should be noted, however, that to be effective, therapy must be started immediately after the first sores appear. Every sexual partner of the infected person needs to be examined for the herpes virus and, if necessary, treated.

Prevention

Herpes can be prevented by avoiding sexual contact with an infected person whose disease is in its active period. Because the chances of contracting this or any other STD increase with the number of sexual partners a person has, limiting the number of partners is the first step toward prevention. Using condoms also helps to reduce the risk.

Infertility

Infertility is defined as a couple's failure to conceive a child after one year of regular sexual intercourse without birth control. In about 40 percent of all cases of infertility, the problem lies with the man; in 60 percent, it lies with the woman or with both partners.

Infertility is not sterility. The term infertility implies that the condition can be treated and reversed—that it may be a temporary problem. The term sterility is applied to a permanent, irreversible inability to have children.

Recent research has shown that a woman's fertility drops off significantly between the ages of 31 and 35 and continues to decline thereafter until menopause, when it ceases altogether. A man's fertility also declines after the age of 40, although men can remain fertile until old age.

Causes of male infertility

One of the major causes of male infertility is a low sperm count. It is measured by the number of active sperm present in a milliliter (there are approximately five milliliters in one teaspoon) of semen (the fluid ejected from the penis during intercourse). An average sperm count is 90 million or more sperm per milliliter. A count of at least 40 to 60 million is thought to be necessary for fertilization; when the count is less than 20 million, it is unlikely that the man can father a child (although, since only one sperm is needed to fertilize an egg, it is still possible).

A low sperm count can be caused by low levels of testosterone (the male sex hormone); by exposure to chemicals, pesticides, or radiation; by engaging in sexual intercourse too frequently, which depletes the sperm supply too quickly; and by heat (which slows sperm production) generated by wearing tight underwear or pants, sitting for long periods in hot cars or trucks, or working near ovens and kilns.

Infertility can also result if sperm cannot propel themselves through the female reproductive tract to reach the egg, or if sperm are irregularly shaped (only sperm with oval-shaped heads can fertilize an egg).

In addition to problems with the sperm themselves, male infertility can be caused by any obstruction in the tubes that convey the sperm from the testes (the male sex organs where sperm are produced) to the penis. Infertility may also be caused by varicose veins in the scrotum (the pouch containing the testes), perhaps because the increased blood flow in these swollen veins brings extra heat to the area, or by a local infection or injury; the infertility problem will probably reverse itself when the condition is corrected. In addition, surgical removal of part of the prostate gland (one of the organs in which most of the fluid in semen is produced), as well as the use of certain drugs for high blood pressure, can lead to retrograde ejaculation (a disorder in which the semen is passed backward into the bladder, to exit with the urine, rather than out through the penis).

Causes of female infertility

A woman may be infertile because of a variety of conditions. It may be that she is not ovulating (releasing an egg each month); this is true in about 25 percent of all cases of female infertility. The fallopian tubes (through which the eggs travel on their way from the ovaries to the uterus) may be obstructed, often as a result of pelvic inflammatory disease (PID), which irritates the tubes and causes scar tissue to form. PID can develop as a reaction to an IUD (intrauterine device used for birth control), an STD, or an infection of the lower reproductive tract. Endometriosis (the displacement of tissue from the uterine lining to elsewhere in the body) may also cause the formation of scar tissue that

481

blocks the fallopian tubes. An imbalance of the female hormones estrogen and progesterone or of other hormones secreted from the pituitary or thyroid glands can interfere with the reproductive cycle. A cervix that creates an environment that in some way prevents sperm from surviving may also be the cause of the infertility.

Diagnosis

Diagnosis of an infertility problem will usually begin with physical examinations and complete medical and sexual histories of both partners.

A fresh sample of the man's semen will be examined under a microscope to determine the quantity and quality of the sperm. The results of the exam will provide a sperm count and will also indicate whether the sperm are adequately mobile and whether the heads of the sperm are oval, both characteristics that are necessary for conception.

To determine whether ovulation is taking place in the woman, the basal body temperature (the body temperature on awakening, before eating or drinking) will be taken every morning for several months. If the temperature rises by 0.6°F to 1.0°F for a few days in the middle of the menstrual cycle, ovulation is probably taking place. An endometrial biopsy, in which a sample of the lining of the uterus is obtained for examination, can also indicate whether ovulation is occurring and whether hormonal secretion is normal.

Obstruction of the fallopian tubes can be diagnosed by injecting a dye into the reproductive tract and then taking an X-ray examination. Another test consists of injecting carbon dioxide gas into the fallopian tubes and waiting for the patient to feel pain in the upper part of the body, indicating that the gas is passing through the fallopian tubes and that there are no obstructions.

A cervix that creates an environment that prevents sperm from surviving can be identified by a microscopic examination of the mucus in the cervix. (The exam is performed shortly after sexual intercourse to determine the rate of sperm survival.) Endometriosis is diagnosed by inserting into the abdomen a laparoscope (a small, lighted instrument), through which the doctor can actually see the uterus, fallopian tubes, ovaries, and any displaced endometrial tissue that may be causing the infertility.

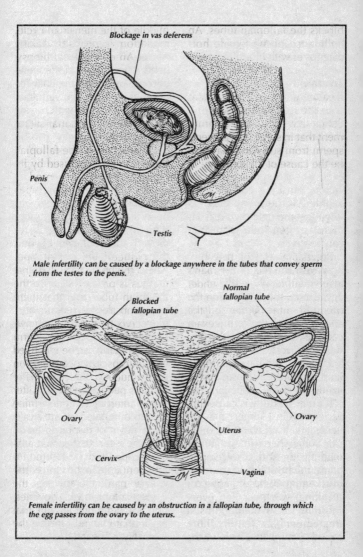

Male infertility can be caused by a blockage anywhere in the tubes that convey sperm from the testes to the penis.

Blockage in vas deferens

Penis

Testis

Normal fallopian tube

Blocked fallopian tube

Ovary

Ovary

Uterus

Cervix

Vagina

Female infertility can be caused by an obstruction in a fallopian tube, through which the egg passes from the ovary to the uterus.

483

Hormonal imbalances in both men and women can be diagnosed with blood tests.

Treatment
Treatment for a low sperm count caused by a testosterone deficiency is usually hormone therapy to increase testosterone levels. If the low sperm count is due to chemicals, radiation, or excess heat, exposure to these factors must be corrected or avoided. If the sperm count is low for some unknown reason, there is often little more that can be done.

Pregnancy is still possible, however. The techniques used involve artificially fertilizing an egg from the woman with sperm from the partner or from another man. The fertilization can take place inside the woman's body or outside the body, in which case the fertilized egg is then transferred to inside the body.

If male infertility is caused by varicose veins, surgery may be necessary. If an obstruction exists somewhere in the tubes leading to and through the penis, microsurgery to open the blockage may be used to correct the problem.

Failure to ovulate is often treated with a fertility drug called clomiphene, which stimulates production of the hormone that regulates ovulation. About 60 percent of the patients who receive clomiphene become pregnant; the chances of multiple births are very low. A stronger drug, which is a combination of certain pituitary gland hormones, may also be prescribed, but it carries with it a greater likelihood of multiple births.

Obstructed fallopian tubes may require microsurgery to open the blockage or a procedure in which an egg is removed and replaced beyond the point of the obstruction, where it may be fertilized normally. A cervix that prevents the survival of sperm can be treated with the female hormone estrogen, which stimulates the increased production of mucus that is necessary to transport the sperm. Sometimes sperm can be placed directly into the uterus, bypassing the cervix completely. Endometriosis can be treated by the surgical removal of displaced tissue and the scar tissue that has formed around it. Hormonal imbalances can be corrected with hormone therapy.

Test-tube, or in vitro, fertilization is a technique in which an egg is removed from the woman's ovary and then placed in a test tube or special sterile dish containing the man's sperm. Once the egg has been fertilized, it is placed into the woman's uterus, where it will continue to grow. This technique is used primarily in women whose blocked fallopian tubes cannot be opened by surgery.

Another new technique used to treat infertility is called gamete intrafallopian transfer (GIFT). In this procedure, clomiphene or another fertility drug is given to the woman to stimulate ovulation. When an egg is produced by the ovary, it is removed via laparoscopy and immediately mixed with sperm from the man. This sperm-egg mixture is then transferred by laparoscopy into a fallopian tube, where fertilization may then take place normally. Fertilization occurs in the woman's body and not in a test tube. GIFT is a complicated and expensive procedure that should be used only by couples who have not been able to conceive using standard treatments for infertility.

Although recent advances in treating infertility have led to greater and greater success, about 15 percent of all female infertility problems and about 10 percent of all male problems remain undiagnosed and therefore untreatable.

Artificial insemination

Artificial insemination is the introduction of semen (the fluid containing sperm) into a woman's vagina or uterus by means other than sexual intercourse (usually with a special syringe) at or before the time of ovulation in the hope of achieving fertilization. The semen may be from the woman's partner or from a donor.

Artificial insemination using semen from the partner is sometimes done when he has a low sperm count—that is, when there are not enough sperm per unit of fluid to be likely to fertilize an egg. To obtain enough sperm, several collections may be made over a period of days or weeks; the sperm obtained is frozen, pooled, and used in one insertion. Artificial insemination may also be used when one or the other partner cannot perform the act of sexual intercourse, perhaps because of a physical condition or an emotional problem.

Artificial insemination using semen from a donor can be an alternative to adoption when the man cannot father a child, whether because of low sperm count, absence of sperm, poor quality of sperm, lack of motion by sperm, or inability to perform sexual intercourse. It may also be considered when the man carries a genetic defect that he does not want to transmit to the child.

Syphilis

Syphilis is one of the most widely known sexually transmitted diseases. It is a serious, highly contagious disease that is primarily spread by direct sexual contact. Although in the United States the number of reported cases of the disease fell in the 1940s and '50s, that trend has reversed itself, and the number of cases has steadily grown since then. In addition, many undiagnosed and untreated cases of syphilis are presently believed to exist.

If the disease is untreated and given the time to do damage, it can affect almost every organ system. The brain, bones, spinal cord, heart, and reproductive organs are all subject to severe injury from syphilis. The disease can be fatal if it is allowed to progress. It can also cause blindness, heart disease, and brain damage. One form of neurologic damage that can be caused by syphilis produces psychotic symptoms. The dire consequences of untreated syphilis can also affect an infected fetus while still in the womb. The disease in this case is called *congenital syphilis*. Syphilis in a woman who is pregnant must be treated before the 18th week of the pregnancy. This early treatment will prevent the disease from being passed to the fetus.

Cause

The cause of syphilis is a spiral-shaped bacteria called a *spirochete*. The organism travels directly through intact mucous membranes, such as those found in the genital and urinary tract, and enters the bloodstream or lymphatic system. It can also be passed from a pregnant woman to her fetus, causing congenital syphilis. A recently infected pregnant woman has a 75 to 95 percent chance of passing the disease to the fetus. Once in the system of either an adult or a fetus, it can incubate for several weeks before producing any discernable symptoms.

Stages and symptoms

Syphilis is a progressive disorder that passes through three stages: primary, secondary, and tertiary.

Primary syphilis is characterized by the appearance of a painless, open sore (called a chancre) 10 to 90 days after exposure to the disease. As a rule, there is usually only one sore, appearing most commonly on the genital organs, but also at times on the rectum, cervix, lips, tongue, fingers, or anywhere that direct contact was made. The chancre first appears as a red bump, sometimes surrounded by a red ring that oozes clear fluid; it soon turns into a painless ulcer and disappears within several weeks without treatment. Although the chancre is gone, the disease is still active in the body.

Secondary syphilis usually appears within six weeks to six months of initial contact. Symptoms resembling those of the flu (fever, sore throat, headache, fatigue, aching joints, and enlarged lymph nodes) are common. Secondary syphilis is also characterized by extremely contagious red or reddish-brown erosions that can be seen on the lining of the mouth, the penis, the external female sex organs, the anus, and warm, moist areas, such as the underarms; by growths resembling warts in the genital area (not to be confused with the more common nonsyphilitic genital warts); and by a rash on the palms of the hands or the soles of the feet in the form of round, reddish spots that occur in patches and do not itch. These sores, growths, and rashes heal within three to six weeks without treatment, and the disease enters the third stage.

At the beginning of the third stage, all symptoms disappear, and the disease becomes latent (present but not showing symptoms) for a time. The patient appears to be healthy, and the disease is probably no longer contagious (except in the case of pregnant women, who can still pass it on to their offspring). This latent stage can last indefinitely, but in about one-third of patients the disease will most likely progress, and the entire body may come under siege. The brain, bones, spinal cord, and heart may be affected, resulting in blindness, brain damage, heart disease, or even death.

Diagnosis

Syphilis is diagnosed on the basis of the patient's medical and sexual history and findings from a physical examination, blood tests, and microscopic examination of a sample taken from the sores or rash areas. Several blood tests may be nec-

PREGNANCY AND CHILDBIRTH

This chapter considers the normal course of the childbearing process—from conception to childbirth—as well as common disorders that may arise during pregnancy.

CONCEPTION

Conception is the union of a sperm cell from the father with an egg from the mother to begin a new life.

Ovulation

During the course of her life, the average woman produces 350 to 400 eggs, or ova. The two organs in which the eggs are produced, known as ovaries, are located near the top and on either side of the uterus. Ducts known as fallopian tubes conduct the eggs toward the uterus. At the midpoint of the average 28-day menstrual cycle, an egg matures in one of the ovaries, is expelled from the ovary during the process called ovulation, and starts to travel through the nearby fallopian tube toward the uterus. The egg is propelled by the waving action of tiny hairlike structures, known as cilia, that line the tube. If the egg meets a sperm cell en route, conception may occur.

Fertilization

Sperm cells—which look like tadpoles through a microscope—originate in the man's testes. At the climax of sexual intercourse, an average of 300 million to 500 million sperm cells, contained in a teaspoonful of thick white fluid, spurt from the tip of the man's penis deep into the woman's vagina. Immediately, the sperm start swimming forward, propelled by their long, waving tails and aided by contractions of the muscles of the woman's vagina and uterus. The goal of the sperm is to swim through the cervix, into the uterus, and up one of the fallopian tubes to fertilize an egg.

Millions of sperm are killed by the acidic secretions of the vagina and the cervix or become trapped by mucus in the vagina. (During the middle of the woman's menstrual cycle, when the egg is moving along a fallopian tube, the secretions are thinner, less acidic, and less of a barrier; also, there are alkaline chemicals in the fluid accompanying the sperm, which act to neutralize the woman's acidic secretions.) The vast majority of sperm fail to pass through the uterus and up one of the fallopian tubes. During most of the woman's menstrual cycle, both tubes are empty and the sperm find nothing to fertilize. Only for a few days is an egg present in one of the tubes, and then it may be reached by only a few of the millions of sperm cells that began the journey. The sperm completely surround the egg, their tails waving furiously in an attempt to force their pointed heads into the female cell. Finally, one succeeds. The tail detaches, and the head moves toward the center of the egg. In seconds, a chemical change comes about in the egg that prevents the entry of any other sperm. Conception has occurred.

The fertilized egg

Unlike all other cells in the body, the sperm and the egg each contain only 23 chromosomes (chromosomes are the chemical "blueprints" that together determine all of the inherited characteristics of an individual; all of the other cells contain twice that number). In the first 12 hours after conception, the 23 chromosomes from the mother and the 23 chromosomes from the father join to form a new nucleus of 46 chromosomes. This is the basic unit from which the new individual will develop.

During the next four or five days, as the fertilized egg, or zygote, drifts down the fallopian tube and into the uterus, the original cell divides and subdivides into anywhere from 16 to 48 cells. In another two or three days, the growing cluster of cells becomes implanted in the nourishing, blood-rich lining of the mother's uterus, which soon forms the beginning of a placenta around the baby-to-be, called an *embryo* at this stage. (The placenta is the structure through which oxygen and nutrients pass from the mother to the fetus and through which carbon dioxide and other waste products pass from the fetus to the mother.) Within about 17 days of conception, the placenta begins blood circulation to the embryo. In the embryo, various cells are specializing to form different parts of the body.

By the end of the seventh week of pregnancy, all of the basic structures of the body have been formed. The developing embryo now is called a *fetus.*

PREGNANCY

Pregnancy is the condition that exists in a woman between the time one of her eggs is fertilized by a sperm and the time her child is born.

Physical changes

During normal pregnancy, many changes take place in a woman's body. The abdomen expands, and the breasts enlarge, grow sensitive, and prepare to produce milk for the baby. Blood volume increases by up to 30 percent. Breathing proceeds more from the chest and less from the abdomen. The bladder is pushed higher into the abdomen because of the increased abdominal space taken up by the growing fetus. The amount of blood flowing through the kidneys increases by 25 percent to 40 percent, because wastes must be eliminated from both the mother and

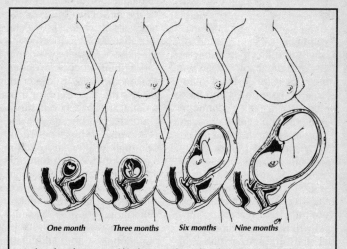

One month   Three months   Six months   Nine months

As the unborn fetus grows within the uterus, the mother's body changes both internally and externally.

fetus. There is a slight increase in the acidity of the saliva (this may be one of the causes of the nausea and vomiting that are so common). The nipples and external genitalia may darken, and brown spots or splotches may appear on the skin. A hormone called *relaxin* causes the ligaments (connective tissues that link bones together at joints) to loosen during the tenth or twelfth week of pregnancy; this will be particularly important in the pelvic area because it will allow greater flexibility at the time of delivery. Many of the glands increase in size.

Symptoms

Usually the first symptom noticed by a pregnant woman is a missed menstrual period. Nausea and vomiting ("morning sickness") are also common symptoms of pregnancy.

The nine months of pregnancy are usually thought of medically as three three-month periods, or trimesters. During the first trimester, the woman may experience nausea and vomiting, her breasts and nipples will become enlarged, and her waistline may expand. In the second trimester, the uterus expands, abdominal enlargement becomes more apparent,

and the woman can feel the fetus move. Many women feel their best during this trimester. During the last three months, pregnancy tends to become a more cumbersome condition, and the woman may feel tired much of the time. The fetus often "drops" lower in the uterus in the last month.

Prenatal care

Many women wait until they have missed a second period before consulting their doctor. Once the doctor has confirmed the pregnancy, a program of prenatal care will be prescribed for the mother-to-be. Prenatal care consists chiefly of making sure that nothing goes wrong with this completely normal and natural process—in other words, that there are no complications.

Good nutrition is especially important during pregnancy. The body's requirements for calcium and phosphorus, two essential minerals in food, almost double, and there is an increase in the demand for iron and many other elements. Gradual caloric increases are not only allowed but advisable, provided that the additional food does not consist of empty calories, such as excess sugar. Fresh fruits and vegetables and appropriate amounts of high-protein, low-fat foods are good choices. Generally, if the woman was consuming 2,000 calories before pregnancy with no weight gain, she should raise her intake to 2,200 to 2,400 calories in early pregnancy; she may be advised to increase that figure to 2,600 calories by the later stages.

If the fetus' weight is included, most women should gain approximately 23 to 26 extra pounds by the ninth month. This additional weight puts more stress on the back and on the legs, sometimes resulting in such problems as swayback and varicose veins (swollen veins close to the skin surface) in the legs. These conditions can be eased by getting proper rest and exercise and by wearing special hosiery to alleviate or prevent varicose veins.

Once the initial period of nausea and vomiting is over (usually after two or three months), many women increase their caloric intake too much, sometimes in a mistaken attempt to "make up for what the baby is taking." As a consequence, they experience a drastic gain in weight. At the other extreme are those mothers who cannot eat normally because nausea persists throughout

pregnancy. In each of these cases, both the mother and the fetus may suffer. If any sudden weight gain or loss is experienced, the physician should be informed.

Due to either rapid weight gain or inadequate kidney function, some women experience significant swelling in the ankles and lower legs and, to a lesser extent, in the hands and fingers. Under no circumstances should nonprescription diuretics (drugs that increase urinary output) be taken for this condition. The doctor should be consulted.

Proper rest and exercise are important throughout pregnancy. In general, a woman can participate in most, if not all, of the activities and sports she was taking part in before her pregnancy. Her doctor can advise her about any limitations.

Precautions
Many substances and organisms have been found to affect the development and survival of the fetus. It has been estimated that 20 percent of all birth defects are directly related to environmental factors such as drugs, viruses, and vitamin deficiencies. Roughly another 60 percent are caused by the interaction of an environmental

factor and an inherited predisposition. So it is extremely important for every woman who is contemplating pregnancy or who is already pregnant to beware of the possible hazards.

One of the most important aspects of prenatal care is safety in the use of medications and the ingestion of nonfood substances. A pregnant woman (or one who even suspects she is pregnant) should never take a medication without her doctor's approval. This caution includes over-the-counter preparations—even aspirin—as well as prescription drugs. In addition, a woman should not smoke during pregnancy, and she should limit, if not eliminate, consumption of alcoholic beverages. Smoking has been linked to miscarriage (the expulsion of the fetus before it is capable of surviving on its own), low birth weight, and prematurity. Alcohol, too, has been linked to miscarriage, and studies have shown that alcohol can affect the brain of the fetus. Products containing caffeine should probably also be limited. The best guideline to remember is that no drug or nonfood substance can be assumed to be harmless during pregnancy.

The fetus is also susceptible to infections that affect the mother-to-be, especially rubella (German measles) and certain sexually transmitted diseases, such as herpes. A pregnant woman should avoid immunizations with live viruses and postpone travel to foreign countries where infectious diseases are prevalent.

Toxoplasmosis, which is an infection spread by eating or preparing uncooked meat or handling a cat's litter box, presents another risk. The parasite that causes toxoplasmosis is harbored in the bodies of some food animals (pigs, sheep, and cattle) and in the intestinal tracts of cats. A pregnant woman does not have to forgo meat or get rid of her cat. She should, however, be certain to cook meat thoroughly and to avoid emptying or cleaning the cat's litter box.

As the medical profession has learned more about inherited diseases, it has been able to offer genetic counseling to couples concerned about the possibility of having a child with an inherited disease or abnormality. A genetic counselor or specialist in genetic disorders can estimate the likelihood that a couple's offspring will be afflicted with a problem due to an inherited trait or to the age of the parents. For some genetic disorders, tests can determine whether one or both parents are carriers or can detect whether a defect is present in a fetus. However, genetic counseling cannot guarantee the health of a child; it can only be a source of information and advice.

CHILDBIRTH

A normal pregnancy that has run its full course is called a full-term pregnancy—the baby is born after a full gestational (developmental) period of about 40 weeks. If the birth occurs earlier than the 37th week, it is considered premature.

There are three stages of normal labor and vaginal childbirth. During the first stage, contractions of the uterus open the cervix (the neck of the uterus). The plug of mucus that has been sealing off the uterus from the vagina for nine months is expelled. This is often followed by either a slow trickle or a sudden gush of amniotic fluid as the amniotic sac, in which the fetus has been growing, breaks. During this stage, the woman should notify her physician and go to the hospital.

The second stage begins when the cervix is completely dilated (opened). The contractions become much stronger,

accompanied by an urge to bear down and push the baby along the birth canal. A doctor or midwife will instruct the woman to push down only during a contraction so that she conserves her energy and strength. After the baby has emerged, the umbilical cord, which connects the baby to the placenta, is tied and cut.

The baby, who usually gasps and cries on delivery, is immediately checked by the obstetrician or pediatrician. After being cleaned off, the baby may be given to the mother to hold.

Five or ten minutes later, the placenta, or afterbirth, is pushed out by more contractions of the uterus. After this third stage has been completed, the physician will stitch any tears or incisions that were made in the vagina and give the woman medication to stop excessive bleeding.

The entire birthing process can last anywhere from 5 to 24 hours; the average is about 12 hours. Childbirth usually takes longer if it is the woman's first delivery.

In about one out of six pregnancies, vaginal delivery is not possible or desirable, and a cesarean section must be performed. The baby is delivered through an incision in the

495

mother's abdominal wall. (For more information on cesarean delivery, see the next page.)

More and more expectant fathers are taking active roles in the birthing process by attending prenatal classes and participating in the delivery. Most hospitals now welcome fathers into the delivery room so that they can witness the miracle of childbirth and can comfort and support the mother while she goes through labor.

Anesthesia

Although once the norm, general anesthesia is now rarely used during vaginal childbirth because, among other reasons, it slows uterine contractions and causes sluggishness and the possibility of respiratory problems in the baby. Other forms of anesthesia that are used during childbirth include pudendal block; paracervical block; and spinal, epidural, and caudal anesthesia.

In pudendal block, local anesthetic is injected through the wall of the vagina or through the skin of the buttock to reach the pudendal nerve. Blocking this nerve eliminates pain and feeling from the lower part of the vagina, the rear portion of the vulva (the external genitals), and the surrounding skin. It is often used when labor is going well and the mother wants to push. Sometimes this type of anesthesia is used with a paracervical block, in which a local anesthetic is injected around the opening of the uterus.

Various types of spinal anesthesia are used in childbirth. In one method, a solution containing local anesthetic is injected between the fourth and fifth vertebrae of the lower back into the fluid-filled sac surrounding the spinal cord. The heavy solution mixes with the spinal fluid and settles downward, blocking off pain messages from below the waist for about an hour.

Epidural anesthesia is used most commonly and has an effect similar to that of spinal anesthesia. The anesthetic is injected at the same place, but instead of being introduced into the spinal fluid in a single injection, it can be administered over a period of hours through a fine plastic tube with its tip resting against the tough dural membrane covering the spinal cord. The nerves are blocked where they enter the spinal cord, producing a numbing effect. Because the dural membrane is not punctured, the chance of complications is reduced. Caudal anesthesia is the same as epidural except that the tube is introduced at the very tip of the spine (*caudal* comes from the Latin word meaning tail). Because both epidural and caudal anesthesia can slow labor if administered too soon, they are not given until the woman is in active labor.

Cesarean section

Cesarean section is a way of delivering a baby by cutting through the external walls of the mother's abdomen and uterus and removing the baby through these incisions. Cesarean section is performed when a vaginal delivery would cause injury to either the mother or the baby.

In the United States today, about 10 to 20 percent of births are by cesarean section. While cesarean delivery is still considered major surgery, the availability of antibiotics, improved anesthetic techniques, and blood transfusions has made cesareans much safer than in the past. Nevertheless, the indications for performing a cesarean section and the disadvantages of the procedure should be weighed carefully by the woman and her physician.

Types
There are two main types of cesarean section.

In the *classic cesarean*, an incision is made vertically on the skin of the abdomen, extending from the navel to the pubic bone. A vertical cut is also made directly down the center of the uterus in its thick upper section. This operation is generally used only if the baby is lying in an abnormal position or if the placenta is located in an abnormally low position in the cavity of the uterus.

The *lower-segment cesarean* is the more commonly performed procedure. The incision in the uterus is made in the lower, thinner section. This incision may be either a vertical cut down the middle or a curved, smile-shaped cut near the lower part of the abdomen.

The classic cesarean produces more bleeding than the lower-segment cesarean. Also, the incision is more difficult to repair, and the uterus is more likely to rupture during a future pregnancy.

Reasons
Some of the reasons for a cesarean section include the following:
• To save the baby's life when the umbilical cord (the fetus'

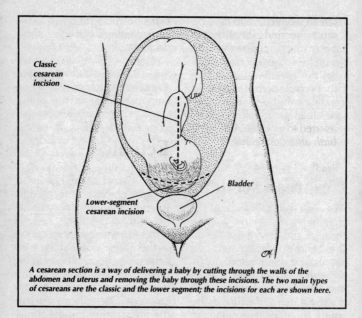

A cesarean section is a way of delivering a baby by cutting through the walls of the abdomen and uterus and removing the baby through these incisions. The two main types of cesareans are the classic and the lower segment; the incisions for each are shown here.

supply line from the placenta) is being pinched off during the birth process, or any other time that the fetus is not receiving adequate blood and oxygen for survival. (These conditions may be indicated by abnormal heart rate patterns during fetal monitoring.)
• To prevent infection of the baby by a dangerous vaginal infection, such as herpes
• To prevent injury to the baby that may result from a breech birth, during which a baby emerges through the vagina buttocks or feet first rather than head first
• To ease the birth or prevent injury when the baby is too large or the mother's pelvis is too small for a vaginal delivery
• To deliver the baby if there is no birth after a long labor
• To facilitate delivery if immediate birth would allow more effective treatment of disease in the mother or the baby
• To be safe if the mother has had a previous cesarean delivery. (The rule used to be that any woman who had one ce-

sarean would have to have cesarean sections for all subsequent births; however, in recent years, many vaginal deliveries have been performed successfully on women who had previous lower-segment cesarean sections. This is often referred to as *VBAC*, or *vaginal birth after cesarean*.)

Disadvantages

Risks of a cesarean section include possible infection, bleeding, and the formation of dangerous blood clots. There is a small chance that the uterus will rupture during a subsequent pregnancy, before or during birth. The mother may be required to stay in the hospital for five to seven days instead of going home with her baby in three days or less. She may not be able to see the baby for a number of hours after delivery if she has undergone general anesthesia. Breast-feeding may be difficult if the mother is being given strong medications to relieve pain, which keep her asleep for long periods of time. There is pain from the abdominal incision, and the mother's activity is restricted once she arrives home. It takes up to six weeks for complete healing of the incision. The expense of the surgical procedure and the

extra hospitalization is also a consideration. However, these disadvantages are relatively unimportant if they save both the mother and baby from suffering severe health problems or even death.

Ectopic pregnancy

An ectopic pregnancy is one in which the fertilized egg develops outside the uterus. Usually it occurs in one of the two fallopian tubes, through which the egg travels from the ovary to the uterus. (In that case, it is also known as a *tubal pregnancy*.) However, on rare occasions, the fertilized egg starts to develop in the ovary, on the cervix (neck of the uterus), or attached to the outside of a nearby organ in the abdominal cavity. (The ovary is not directly connected to the fallopian tube. There is a slight gap between them, which sometimes permits an egg to enter the abdominal cavity.)

Causes

The usual cause of an ectopic pregnancy is an obstruction or narrowing of the fallopian tube that prevents the egg from passing through the tube to the

499

uterus. The obstruction or narrowing is usually the result of inflammation or scarring from an infection, such as gonorrhea, but it may also develop after abdominal surgery or because of a growth, such as a pelvic tumor. Tubal infections can occur after miscarriage or childbirth.

Complications

An ectopic pregnancy can be fatal unless it is promptly treated. The danger of a tubal pregnancy is that it will not be detected until the tube enclosing the enlarging pregnancy has ruptured (broken), causing massive bleeding. When a fertilized egg begins to develop in an area other than the uterus, such as the ovary or the cervix, nearby large blood vessels may be invaded, resulting in massive bleeding.

Symptoms

Symptoms of ectopic pregnancy usually begin two to four weeks after a woman misses her menstrual period. She may be bothered by sharp, continuous pains on one side of her lower abdomen and by slight bleeding from her vagina. When rapid bleeding into the abdomen occurs, which is usually not until after the sixth

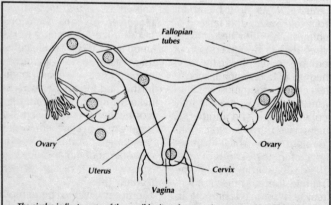

The circles indicate some of the possible sites of an ectopic pregnancy, in which the fertilized egg develops outside the uterus. The most common site is in one of the fallopian tubes, but development in an ovary, on the cervix, or attached to another organ in the abdominal cavity can also occur.

week of the pregnancy, she may experience sudden sharp pains in the lower abdomen, backache, low blood pressure, fainting, and even shock (collapse of the circulatory system).

Diagnosis

The examining doctor may discover a tender swelling on one side of the pelvis. Movement of the uterus during a pelvic examination may cause pain. When ectopic pregnancy is suspected, the patient is generally hospitalized immediately. An ultrasound study may reveal the outline of the expanding mass with no evidence of a pregnancy in the uterus. In most cases, there is slow bleeding from the end of the fallopian tube into the abdominal cavity, which can be detected by inserting a hollow needle through the wall of the vagina beneath the cervix. The diagnosis is confirmed by inserting a laparoscope (a lighted tubelike instrument) through a small incision into the abdominal cavity to inspect the area directly.

Treatment

Treatment for ectopic pregnancy is surgical removal of the embryo and surrounding tissues. When the condition occurs in a fallopian tube, the entire tube may be removed. In some cases, however, it is possible to cut the embryo out, leaving the tube intact.

A woman who has had one ectopic pregnancy has about a 15 percent chance of having a second one. This does not mean that she should not try to become pregnant again; however, when she does try, she should be especially watchful for symptoms of ectopic pregnancy, and when she suspects that conception has occurred, she should see her physician immediately so that the location of the embryo can be determined.

Episiotomy

An episiotomy is a surgical incision into the tissues surrounding the opening of the vagina during childbirth in order to make the delivery easier and to avoid extensive tearing of the tissues. The advantage of the procedure is that it substitutes a controlled surgical incision for excessive stretching and tearing of all the tissues.

Episiotomy is often performed in women who are having their first baby. With subsequent pregnancies, episiotomy may not be necessary, since the tissues surrounding the vagina have often been stretched sufficiently by the first delivery to allow an easy second delivery.

The most common type of episiotomy is an incision made with surgical scissors from the midpoint of the vaginal opening directly down toward the anus. An important risk with this type of incision is that during the birth, the opening might further extend into the anal sphincter (the ring of muscle surrounding the opening from the rectum) or the rectum itself; however, such

a tear can be repaired relatively easily and will eventually heal itself. To avoid the risks of entering the rectum, some physicians prefer the mediolateral episiotomy, in which the incision is made at an angle.

Hyperemesis gravidarum

Hyperemesis gravidarum is excessive vomiting during pregnancy. This type of vomiting is

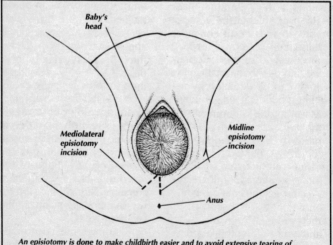

An episiotomy is done to make childbirth easier and to avoid extensive tearing of tissues. The most common type of episiotomy is a midline incision from the midpoint of the vaginal opening directly downward toward the anus. Some doctors, however, prefer an incision at an angle, called a mediolateral episiotomy.

more severe than that caused by ordinary morning sickness, which usually clears up on its own within a few months. In hyperemesis gravidarum, the vomiting leads to starvation, dehydration, and a disruption of the body's chemical balance.

Symptoms include loss of weight, dehydration, and in very severe cases, jaundice. The condition is most often treated in the hospital through the use of antivomiting drugs and intravenous feeding to correct the possible malnutrition, dehydration, and chemical imbalance. A pregnant woman should not treat the vomiting with drugs without consulting her doctor.

Mastitis

Mastitis is an inflammation of the breast, most often caused by bacterial invasion and infection.

Causes
This condition is caused by bacteria normally found on the skin and nipples. The bacteria enter the breast through the nipple and infect the milk glands and ducts. In many cases, the condition occurs on the third to fifth day after the birth of the baby because of the devel-

opment of cracked nipples, through which the bacteria may enter the breast.

Symptoms
Symptoms include pain, swelling, redness, high fever, and a tender lump in the breast. Sometimes the lymph nodes in the armpit next to the breast become tender and swollen. In severe infection, there may be pus in the breast.

Diagnosis
The diagnosis is generally made on the basis of the physical examination and the patient's medical history. If there is a severe infection, signaled by the appearance of pus coming from the nipple, a specimen of the pus can be examined to identify the causative organism.

Treatment
The treatment for mastitis is antibiotic medication to combat the infection. A breast-feeding mother can continue nursing with the affected breast or she may want to expel the milk by hand to prevent painful swelling.

Prevention
A woman who is breast-feeding a baby can reduce the risk of developing mastitis by keeping

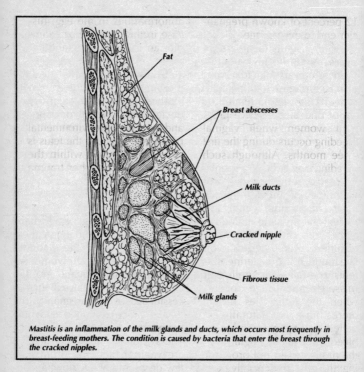

Mastitis is an inflammation of the milk glands and ducts, which occurs most frequently in breast-feeding mothers. The condition is caused by bacteria that enter the breast through the cracked nipples.

her nipples clean and dry between feedings and by wearing clothing that does not rub or irritate the nipples.

Miscarriage

A miscarriage (in medical terms, a *spontaneous abortion*) is the ending of a pregnancy due to the premature delivery of the fetus before the beginning of the 20th week of pregnancy. At that point, the fetus is not developed enough to survive outside the uterus on its own. (After the 20th week of pregnancy, a spontaneous abortion is considered a premature delivery or, if the fetus is dead at delivery, a stillbirth.) Most miscarriages occur within the first 14 weeks of pregnancy. About

12 percent of known pregnancies end in miscarriage.

Types

There are several different types of miscarriages. A *threatened miscarriage* is experienced by about one of every five pregnant women when vaginal bleeding occurs during the first three months. Although such bleeding may indicate a spontaneous abortion, it is rarely more than a threat, and the pregnancy will continue normally. An *inevitable miscarriage* refers to a situation in which bleeding occurs, the cervix begins to dilate (open), but the uterine contents are not yet expelled. A *missed miscarriage* occurs when the fetus dies in the uterus but is not naturally expelled, and the woman has no bleeding or pain to signify that the pregnancy is not progressing; the physician usually diagnoses the condition when the uterus stops enlarging.

Causes

The reason that a miscarriage occurs is not always understood, but it is believed that a fetus is usually aborted because it is not developing normally. Several factors can contribute to a miscarriage, including abnormalities in the father's sperm; abnormalities in the egg; disease in the mother (for example, an infection, a glandular disorder, high blood pressure, kidney disease, or diabetes); uterine abnormalities; the mother's poor nutrition or use of cigarettes, alcohol, or drugs; and exposure to environmental pollutants. Because the fetus is so well protected within the uterus, a fall or other trauma suffered by the mother is rarely, if ever, the cause of miscarriage.

The expulsion of the fetus resulting from an abnormality is thought to be a chance event, not due to a problem or defect in either parent. Of women who miscarry once, most (about 80 percent) have a successful subsequent pregnancy.

Symptoms

The symptoms of miscarriage are vaginal bleeding (from a few drops to a heavy flow) and cramps (either dull and constant or sharp and intermittent) in the lower abdomen or back. The bleeding can start suddenly or follow a brownish discharge. A solid clot of material or tissue may pass from the vagina. If possible, this should be saved for the doctor, who may be able to examine it and confirm that a miscarriage has occurred. A miscarriage can be complete (the uterus expels all the tissue) or incomplete (tissue remains inside the uterus).

A pregnant woman who starts bleeding or experiences pain should contact her physician immediately.

Diagnosis

Depending on the type of miscarriage, diagnosis may be made on the basis of the medical history, physical examination, analysis of any discharge, blood and urine tests (to detect the presence of infection or anemia caused by hemorrhage), or ultrasound studies (to establish the presence or absence of a fetus).

Treatment

There is no medical treatment to stop or avert an inevitable miscarriage. (The drug diethylstilbestrol, or DES, used to be prescribed to deter miscarriages until it was discovered that it had little effect and could cause fetal abnormalities.) The physician generally directs the woman with symptoms to rest in bed and abstain from sexual intercourse.

After an inevitable, incomplete, or missed miscarriage, any remaining fetal or placental tissue must be removed by a surgical procedure known as dilation and curettage, or D&C, in which the physician expands the cervix and gently scrapes out residual material from inside the uterus. Without this precaution, a woman is more susceptible to infections and heavy bleeding.

It is normal for a woman to feel depressed by the loss of the expected child, but it is usually safe for her to attempt to conceive soon afterward (six to eight weeks later) on the advice of her physician.

Prevention

It is advisable for a woman, at the beginning of her pregnancy, to obtain adequate prenatal care and the most up-to-date information on the substances and practices that may contribute to a miscarriage.

Placenta previa

Placenta previa is a condition in which the fertilized egg, or zygote, travels to the lower portion of the uterus and attaches itself to a part of the uterine wall near or even over the uterine opening. As a result, the placenta (a temporary organ in the uterus, which develops during pregnancy to conduct nourishment and oxygen from the mother to the fetus) forms in such a way as to cover all or part of the uterine opening and thus interferes with normal delivery.

There are three types of placenta previa: partial, in which only a portion of the cervix is covered; complete, in which the cervix is completely covered; and low-lying (or marginal), in which the placenta does not cover the cervix, but is close enough to it to potentially interfere with normal delivery. Placenta previa occurs in 1 of every 100 to 500 pregnancies.

Cause

The cause of placenta previa is unknown. Some authorities believe that placental implantation cannot take place on the same part of the uterine wall more than once. If a woman has had several pregnancies, the lower part of the uterus may be the only place left on which the placenta can become implanted.

Symptoms

The major symptom of placenta previa is painless vaginal bleeding. Profuse bleeding may begin as early as the 24th week of pregnancy, with no apparent cause. The blood will be bright red, indicating that it is fresh.

Bleeding occurs as the placenta separates from the wall of the uterus near the uterine opening. In some cases, there is only light blood flow.

Diagnosis

Any vaginal bleeding during pregnancy is abnormal and should, therefore, be reported to the doctor immediately. An ultrasound scan of the woman's abdomen will then be performed.

Treatment

There are two types of treatment: delayed and active. Delayed treatment allows the fetus time to mature. With active treatment, the fetus is delivered by cesarean section as soon as possible.

The degree of vaginal bleeding will usually dictate the type of treatment. If vaginal bleeding is slight, delayed treatment is generally chosen. If vaginal bleeding is heavy, a cesarean section will be performed immediately. Bleeding from placenta previa may be extremely heavy, leading to severe blood loss by the mother. This bleeding stops only after the fetus and placenta have been delivered by cesarean section. If left untreated, both the mother and fetus could die.

Toxemia of pregnancy

Toxemia of pregnancy is a severe condition that sometimes occurs in the last stage of pregnancy and is characterized by high blood pressure, swelling of the extremities (especially the hands, feet, and ankles), and the presence of protein in the urine. If toxemia is left untreated, convulsions and coma can develop. The illness is more accurately called *preeclampsia* before the convulsive stage and eclampsia afterward.

Causes
The causes of toxemia of pregnancy are not clearly understood. Dietary deficiencies may be at the root of some cases. Some types of toxemia may be the result of a deficiency of blood flow in the uterus.

Symptoms
Toxemia of pregnancy is divided into three stages: mild, severe, and full-blown eclampsia. Each stage can be recognized by its own characteristic symptoms. Mild preeclampsia is marked by edema (swelling due to fluid retention), hypertension (high blood pressure), and the presence of protein in the urine. Some of the major symptoms of severe preeclampsia include the following: headache, dizziness, fever, drowsiness, tachycardia (rapid heart rhythm), tinnitus (ringing in the ears), double vision, nausea, vomiting, and scanty or absent urine production. In cases of full-blown eclampsia, convulsions and coma may be followed by severe hypotension (low blood pressure). The condition ultimately leads to death if not given immediate medical attention.

Treatment
Toxemia cannot be completely cured until the woman's pregnancy is over. Until then, treatment includes stimulation of kidney function, control of high blood pressure and convulsions, bed rest, and in severe cases, early delivery of the infant to ensure the survival of the mother.

Prevention
At this time, there is no known preventive measure for toxemia of pregnancy. The first line of defense, though, is the monitoring of all bodily functions in order to spot symptoms as they begin to appear.

CARING FOR YOUR CHILD

Every parent knows the uneasy feeling that comes with the knowledge (or even the suspicion) that a child is sick. Part of the problem is that it can be very difficult to assess the seriousness of a childhood illness. How can you prepare yourself to make the best decisions about your child's health?

First, educate yourself. Carefully read this chapter so that you will know which symptoms to watch for and what to do about them. An informed parent is better prepared to deal with both the major and the minor crises that arise throughout childhood.

Second, trust your instincts. As a parent, you know better than anyone else when your child is not acting or feeling right. Sometimes there are visible signs of illness, like diarrhea and a fever; at other times, a change in your child's behavior alerts you to a problem, even though there are no physical symptoms. If you feel that there is a problem or an emergency situation, act on it.

Third, ask questions. Don't worry that you will inconvenience the doctor or appear stupid if you are uncertain about a diagnosis or plan of treatment. It is the doctor's duty to make sure that you are fully informed about all matters that concern your child's health.

WHEN TO CALL A DOCTOR

Here are some rules of thumb about the need for medical attention for common ailments. Call your doctor if the following situations occur:

- *Fever* is higher than 101°F for more than 24 hours, or a child with a fever looks and acts extremely ill, is difficult to arouse, is incoherent, or is particularly irritable.
- *Common cold* lasts more than ten days or is accompanied by a fever higher than 101°F, a sore throat or puslike nasal discharge for longer than two days, or a persistent cough.
- *Sore throat* is present for more than three days or is accom-

panied by a fever higher than 101°F.

- *Earache* lasts more than one hour, or a child with an earache looks very ill or has a temperature higher than 101°F.
- *Cough* is persistent or short, dry, and sharp, or is accompanied by wheezing, difficulty in breathing, a fever of more than 101°F, or a cold that has lasted more than ten days.
- *Headaches* are frequent and the child appears very ill or a headache awakens a child at night.
- *Stomachache* has been constant for more than two hours or is accompanied by bloody stools or recurrent vomiting of green or yellow material.
- *Vomiting* is accompanied by fever, lasts more than 12 hours, or produces green or yellow material more than twice, or a vomiting child appears very ill or is difficult to wake.
- *Diarrhea* is bloody, lasts more than one day, or is accompanied by vomiting, fever of more than 101°F, or absence of urination for eight hours.

Illness in babies may be a little harder to detect. Call the doctor when an infant

- refuses to nurse or take liquids.
- urinates very little.
- vomits repeatedly.
- becomes extremely fretful or lethargic.
- becomes hoarse, has difficulty in breathing, or has a crowing cry, especially if there is a fever.
- becomes fretful and pulls on his or her ear.
- has a marked increase in bowel movements.
- has blood or mucus in his or her stool.
- displays noticeable protrusion of the fontanelle (soft spot on the head).

Call the doctor if an existing condition is not improving or if you do not know what to do about certain symptoms. Although parents need to use common sense when deciding whether to call the doctor, it is always better to err on the side of caution. A doctor can give directions and reassure you over the telephone.

Respiratory disorders account for almost half of all childhood illnesses. Fortunately, they are easy to diagnose, and the availability of antibiotics makes many respiratory infections fairly simple to cure.

Although children are helpless in the sense that they cannot provide for themselves, they are remarkably tough when it comes to recovering from illness and overcoming physical disorders. This resilience sees them through a time of life when their undeveloped bodies make them vulnerable to mishaps and infections.

MEDICATIONS

Treating a sick child with medication is an example of how parent and doctor must work together in the interest of the child's health. The doctor is responsible for making an accurate diagnosis of the child's condition and prescribing the appropriate drug. It then becomes the parent's responsibility to make sure that the drug is administered correctly.

It has been estimated that in 10 to 30 percent of cases in which medication apparently failed to work, the cause of the failure was improper administration of the medication. Whenever a doctor prescribes a medication for your child, make sure that you understand completely how much to give, how to give it, how often to give it, and for how long.

How much medication to give

The quantity of medication the doctor prescribes for your child is determined by the child's weight and age. Thus, for a given medication, the dosage prescribed for a baby will be much different from that for an adolescent. Make sure that the child takes the complete dose—no more and no less. If the child vomits within 20 minutes of receiving a dose, you can assume that the medication was lost and can give another dose.

Do not use an ordinary kitchen teaspoon when measuring liquid medications; instead, use a specially marked measuring spoon for medication, which should be available from any pharmacy. If your child insists on taking medication from his or her "special" spoon, transfer the medication from the measuring spoon to the child's spoon after measuring.

When to give medication

Medications vary in the amount of time it takes for them to be absorbed by the body. Some medications need to be given at precisely regulated intervals. Therefore, make sure you fully understand the instructions on the label. For example, "four times a day" and "every six hours" do not mean the same thing; the former means that the child should have four doses at fairly equally spaced intervals within the waking hours, whereas the latter means that each dose should be given six hours after the previous one, even if the child must be awakened to do so.

It's also important to give medication for the correct length of time. A common mistake is to assume that because a child acts as if he or she is well, the child is well. The symptoms of an illness can subside long before the illness itself is over; in fact, the healing process may have barely begun. Stopping a child's medication too soon can cause a relapse and complications. For example, streptococcal infections require ten straight days of antibiotic treatment, and stopping too soon can allow disease-causing organisms to flourish again. Therefore, such instructions as "Give for ten full days," "Continue for two weeks," and "Give until finished" should be followed exactly as the physician advises.

How to give medication

Every parent needs to know how to give medication to a child, and every child needs to understand that taking medicine is an unpleasant but unavoidable fact of life. A young child, approached in a reassuring and matter-of-fact manner, will usually accept medication without any trouble.

Liquid medicine can be given directly from the spoon (after careful measurement). An alternate method is to use a non-glass medicine dropper to squirt the liquid slowly into the child's mouth. Be careful not to direct the stream of liquid forcefully against the back of the throat and down the windpipe; instead, it should be released against the inside of the cheek.

If the medicine tastes unpleasant, you can give the child a sweet treat afterward. You may also be able to disguise the medicine in a little applesauce, ice cream, or juice. Be sure, however, to check with your pharmacist first, because some medications should not be diluted or taken with certain kinds of foods or beverages. Also, make sure that the child takes the entire portion.

Do not give pills or capsules to a child under the age of five; the child may choke. If the medication is not available in liquid form, you may be able to crush a tablet or empty the contents of a capsule and mix it with a small quantity of juice or food. Always check with your pharmacist or physician first, though, to be certain that the medication will be effective if given in this way, and always make sure that the child takes the whole dose.

After the age of five or six, your child can probably swallow tablets or capsules whole. You can help the child learn how to do this by practicing when he or she needs a non-prescription remedy such as acetaminophen. Show the child how to put the pill on the back of the tongue and swallow it with a drink or with a spoonful of ice cream, applesauce, or jelly. You can also buy a special glass that delivers the pill into the mouth automatically with the first gulp of liquid. Whenever a child is taking a pill, watch to be sure that the medication goes down smoothly and that the child is in no danger of choking.

Don't encourage a child to take medication by saying that it is candy. Many cases of poisoning have occurred in children who took overdoses of medications that looked or tasted like candy. Many doctors discourage the use of children's vitamin pills that are sweet, brightly colored, or shaped like cartoon characters, believing that such products blur the distinction in the child's mind between candy and drugs.

Apgar score

The Apgar score is a general evaluation of a baby's condition, made soon after birth, to determine immediately whether the newborn needs emergency care. The Apgar score was devised by the late Virginia Apgar, M.D.

Procedure

At one minute and five minutes after an infant's birth, a delivery room nurse, obstetrician, anesthesiologist, or pediatrician rates five factors, using a scale of 0 to 2:

A (Appearance)—A score of 2 is given if the skin is completely pink; 1 if it is pink except for the hands and feet, which appear bluish; and 0 if the entire body appears blue (indicating lack of oxygen).

P (Pulse)—A score of 2 is given for a pulse above 100, 1 for a rate of less than 100, and 0 for no pulse.

G (Grimace, or reflex irritability)—A score of 2 is given if the baby cries vigorously when it is slapped lightly on the soles of the feet, 1 if the baby makes only a grimace or slight cry, and 0 if there is no response.

A (Activity)—An active infant is given a score of 2; an infant who makes some movement of

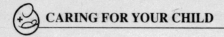

arms and legs is given a 1; and a limp and motionless infant, 0.

R (Respiration)—Strong efforts to breathe, together with vigorous crying, score a 2; slow, irregular breathing, 1; and no breathing, 0.

Scores

Most babies score between 7 and 10 when tested one minute after birth. They are breathing well, crying, pinkish in color, active, and need no emergency measures.

Those babies who score from 4 to 6 usually need help immediately. The throat is suctioned to remove thick mucus, small blood clots, or bits of swallowed membrane (from the amniotic sac that enclosed the baby before birth). Oxygen is sometimes given to assist breathing and restore color.

The baby with an Apgar score of less than 4 is limp, pale, or bluish; may have no heartbeat; and is in grave danger. The throat is suctioned, and the baby is placed on a mechanical respirator, which pumps air in and out of the lungs until the baby can breathe on his or her own.

A second Apgar score is determined five minutes after birth and recorded on the baby's chart beside the first score. The second score is a good measure of the baby's adaptation to the world outside the womb.

Attention Deficit Hyperactivity Disorder

Attention deficit hyperactivity disorder (ADHD) is a nervous disorder that usually affects children. The condition is characterized by very high levels of physical activity, consistently impulsive and immature behavior, and an extremely short attention span. Because of these behavioral patterns, the condition is also known as *minimal brain dysfunction* and, in common usage, *hyperactivity*.

Although ADHD does no physical damage to the body, it can trigger long-lasting social, emotional, and educational problems. Because affected children cannot sit still and concentrate for long periods, they may have trouble with schoolwork. They often appear to be immature, uncoordinated, and boisterous and may have trouble getting along with classmates, teachers, and parents; consequently, they often suffer from a poor self-image.

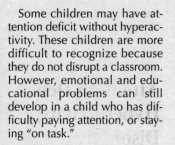

Some children may have attention deficit without hyperactivity. These children are more difficult to recognize because they do not disrupt a classroom. However, emotional and educational problems can still develop in a child who has difficulty paying attention, or staying "on task."

Causes
The cause of ADHD is not known, but several theories have been proposed in recent years. As of yet, none of these theories has been proved or disproved.

The ADHD condition may be the result of a nervous system malfunction or a deficiency of neurotransmitters (chemicals in the brain that transmit impulses between the nerves). According to one theory, based on the supposition that the brain has two systems for responding to situations—one that prompts immediate action and one that encourages hesitation and consideration—the neurotransmitters that control the hesitation response are not working properly in the child with ADHD. In some cases, damage to the fetus during pregnancy or a complication of childbirth may may be responsible for causing a neurologic defect.

ADHD appears to occur more commonly in children of mothers who drank excessive amounts of alcohol or used cocaine throughout pregnancy. It has also been suggested that the additives, preservatives, and colorings found in some processed foods may have a toxic or allergic effect on some children, thus causing ADHD, but no hard evidence is available to support this view.

Symptoms
A variety of symptoms point to ADHD. The child with ADHD is overly active, fidgety, restless, overly talkative or boisterous, impulsive, and seemingly uncoordinated. In school, the child has a very short attention span and seems to forget facts quickly, disrupts the classroom, does schoolwork hastily and incorrectly, skips or adds words when reading, laughs too loud and hard, and prefers to play with younger children.

Diagnosis
There are no specific tests to diagnose ADHD. (Neuropsychiatric tests that measure a child's capability to concentrate are sometimes administered to aid in diagnosis, however.) Symptoms of ADHD seem to be present in all children to some

515

degree, and since ADHD is rather vaguely defined, the symptoms displayed by an individual child should be carefully observed. The quantity, intensity, and duration of these symptoms may single out children with ADHD from others who are merely bored with school or who are having other behavior problems. Care must be taken in diagnosis, since a real danger is that a child will be saddled with the label of hyperactivity not because he or she has an abnormally high energy level but rather because his or her parents or teachers have a very low level of tolerance.

Treatment
Although controversial, drug therapy has proved successful in treating some cases of ADHD. Several stimulant drugs appear to have a calming effect on children with ADHD, because they seem to affect the hesitation response. However, these drugs have been shown to have unpleasant side effects, such as stomach cramps, susceptibility to colds, nervous mannerisms, and stunted growth. Therefore, many children on this therapy are required by their doctors to take "drug holidays" to give their bodies a break from the side effects of the medication.

Special diets that are designed to eliminate all food additives have been prescribed, in keeping with the theory that additives cause ADHD. The findings from studies on this treatment are contradictory. However, many parents report dramatic changes in behavior after this treatment, although part of the change is most likely to be due to the extra attention paid to the child whose meals have to be specially prepared. Parents can help to influence the child's actions by praising or rewarding good behavior and ignoring bad behavior.

Autism

Autism is a form of neurologic disability. The word *autism* comes from the word *auto*, Greek for self, and refers to self-absorption. The autistic child is often wrapped up in his or her own thoughts and may be unable to communicate or relate to others—although there are notable exceptions.

Causes
Although the cause of autism remains a mystery, several reasons for the disorder have been

suggested. Current research seems to indicate that the primary cause of the condition is a problem in the development of the brain. Gender may also be a factor; boys are four times more likely to be affected than girls. There is some evidence for a genetic component as well.

Symptoms
Autism is a collection of symptoms that appears in the first 30 months of life. The disorder encompasses a broad spectrum of severity from mild disability to serious impairment. It is very difficult to characterize the disorder by one set of symptoms as cases vary greatly.

On the severe end, the autistic child is very withdrawn, unaffectionate, and uninterested in people, including siblings and parents. The child may behave as if he or she is alone in the world. There is a speech and language disorder associated with autism: The child may learn to speak late or not at all; if speech develops, it can be odd and limited. Common characteristics of more severe autism include echolalia (repetition of the last phrase or word of everything another person says), a total resistance to change (even something as minor as rearranging the furni-

ture), and the repetition of some simple act, such as rocking or arm-flapping. Approximately 25 percent of all autistic children also experience seizures before their teen years.

Autism does not, however, always manifest itself in such a severe form. Many children affected by the disorder do show interest in other people and do display affection. Cases affect individuals in unique ways.

Diagnosis
In diagnosing autism, the doctor must distinguish it from many other conditions, including deafness or severe hearing impairment and childhood schizophrenia. In general, a multidisciplinary team is usually required for proper diagnosis, rather than just one doctor. The child undergoes neurologic and intelligence testing to determine future learning potential.

Treatment
A child with autism may have to be cared for in an institution or specialized school. Day-care programs are available in some cities, and the trend is to train parents to care for their children at home. The method of treatment often used by professionals, and taught to parents, is known as *behavior therapy*. The

main goals are to limit self-destructive or meaningless actions, to promote language development, and to make the child more social. In behavior therapy, the professional or parent works to develop a close relationship with the child, so that the child will want to imitate the adult.

Because mental development is uneven among cases, individualized education programs are key. Usually the child does best in learning nonverbal skills, and teaching methods have focused on memorization and drills. However, some children with autism grow up to be very verbal—even noted authors. New methods of teaching are always under investigation, and although the disorder never goes away completely, improvement and learning are possible. A majority of those with autism learn to function in family and community settings.

Prevention
Unfortunately, because the cause is unknown, there are no preventive measures.

Cerebral palsy

Cerebral palsy (CP) is a general term to describe various non-progressive disorders of muscle control caused by a period of lack of oxygen to the brain.

Cause
Cerebral palsy is caused by brain or nerve damage that usually occurs before, or around the time of, birth. The damage can result when brain tissue becomes starved for oxygen for any reason. It can result from separation and bleeding of the placenta (the organ that anchors the fetus to the wall of the uterus and provides nourishment) in late pregnancy or from disorders caused by diabetes in the mother. It is characteristic of CP that the neurologic problems are not progressive.

Types
There are four major types of CP: spastic, athetoid, ataxic, and mixed. About 70 percent of cases of CP are the spastic type. Patients with spastic CP move stiffly and with great difficulty, because their affected muscles are constantly tense and tight. One arm and one leg may be affected, or both arms or both legs. Affected extremities appear thin and wasted, are weak, and are likely to twist and jerk. Walking on the toes or with a scissorslike movement is typical. When all four limbs are af-

fected, the mouth, tongue, and palate may also be affected, interfering with speech, eating, and drinking and causing constant drooling.

Athetoid, or dyskinetic, CP accounts for about 10 percent of cases. This disorder, which is caused by damage to the basal ganglia (a mass of nerve-cell bodies at the base of the brain), is characterized by continual slow, twisting movements of the fingers and hands during waking hours. Similar movements of the upper arms or legs and trunk may also occur. There may be sudden, jerky movements as well.

Ataxic CP results from damage to the cerebellum (a portion of the brain crucial to muscular coordination) or the nerves leading from it. The characteristic signs of this type of CP can include weakness, lack of balance and coordination, tremors, difficulty with fine or quick movements, and a clumsy way of walking, with feet wide apart.

Mixed CP occurs frequently. Often, spastic and athetoid types are combined. Ataxic and athetoid types are mixed less often.

Symptoms

Possible signs of CP in a baby include twitching, convulsions, back-arching, muscle spasms, partial paralysis of the face, and very late development of the ability to lift the head, sit, crawl, stand, walk, and talk. Any baby who may have suffered brain damage around the time of birth should be watched carefully for signs of CP (such a baby may have been born nearly lifeless or very small and premature, or may have suffered a severe infection soon after birth). Although it is difficult to diagnose any particular form of CP in the first two years of life, parents should report any suspicion promptly to their doctor.

After infancy, symptoms of cerebral palsy range from simple clumsiness or slight incoordination of muscles to multiple handicaps that prevent normal movement. Frequently, the brain damage that causes CP also causes mental retardation, epilepsy, hearing problems, visual defects, and learning and behavior disorders. However, some CP children are normal except for disordered muscle control.

Diagnosis

Early diagnosis and treatment of CP are essential if a child is to develop as fully as possible. An important part of the diagnostic evaluation is to discover if there is any other reason for the symptoms. A wide range of medical diagnostic studies and psychological tests will be performed.

Treatment
Treatment of a child with CP may involve many different elements, such as speech therapy, physical therapy, special dental care, specially designed clothes, braces, corrective glasses, surgery, a hearing aid, special furniture, and special schooling. Occupational therapy can help the patient in self-care, including dressing and eating. About 50 percent of CP patients have convulsions, which usually can be controlled by anticonvulsant medicines. Ideally, a physician will work with a team of specialists in a hospital or other setting where treatments can be coordinated.

Because CP is a lifelong condition, parents need to learn as much as possible about caring for a CP child. The parents can learn how to continue therapy at home. Every effort must be made to help the child become self-reliant. Parents can often get valuable advice and support from other parents of children with CP and from professionals at the local chapter of the United Cerebral Palsy Association. Therapy for children and adults with CP is provided at rehabilitation centers sponsored by the National Easter Seal Society and by various other agencies.

Prevention
Expectant mothers can guard against CP with good prenatal care, emphasizing adequate diet, rest, exercise, frequent checkups, and avoidance of alcohol, drugs, and infections. During labor and birth, the doctor can keep track of the baby's heartbeat with use of a fetal monitor and, if necessary, operate quickly to save the baby from brain damage caused by oxygen starvation. Expectant mothers with difficult pregnancies should try to have their babies delivered at a hospital with a newborn intensive care unit, directed by a certified neonatologist (a specialist in the care of newborn babies). In such a unit, premature and ill babies can be watched closely and cared for by specially trained nurses and doctors.

Child abuse

Child abuse encompasses all types of mistreatment—physical, emotional, and sexual—that can be inflicted on a child, particularly by a parent, guardian, or other family member. Closely related is child neglect, in which the parent or guardian chooses not to provide for the nutritional, emotional, or physical needs of a child.

Causes

A principal link in the chain of child abuse is the emotional inadequacy of the parent or guardian. Most parents who abuse their children were themselves abused as children. They did not learn how to give or receive affection from their parents and thus find it hard to develop a good relationship with their own children. They often use the same harsh punishment methods—threats, ridicule, and physical violence—that were used on them as children, because they do not know any other way of managing family problems.

Some parents who neglect their children are incompetent because of drug or alcohol abuse, medical or psychological disorders, or severe socioeconomic problems. Parents who do not have a support system of close friends or relatives living nearby may feel isolated and overwhelmed by the constant demands of rearing children. Others who may abuse their children are young parents

with their first child, parents of ill or premature babies who are separated from them shortly after birth, and parents who did not want a child in the first place. Such parents need special attention and support in order to get their families off to a good start.

Symptoms

Physical symptoms of abuse (also known as *battered child syndrome*) include old and new bruises; scars from cuts and burns; serious damage to the eyes, mouth, or internal organs; and X-ray evidence of bone fractures in various stages of healing. When parents cannot give reasonable explanations for the child's injuries, child abuse may be suspected.

Signs of emotional abuse are more difficult to detect. Babies who have been neglected emotionally may appear uninterested in people or even retarded. Another sign in babies is the condition known as *failure to thrive,* which is unexplained lack of growth even though no illness is present. Older children who are excessively well behaved and overly anxious to please adults, but who do not get along well with other children and are mistrustful, may be victims of emotional abuse. At school, they may have trouble with teachers as well as with other children.

Sexual abuse by a parent, older sibling, or other relative is often difficult to detect. There may be no physical symptoms, although venereal disease in a child is grounds for suspicion. The child may be too fearful or too embarrassed to reveal the situation to anyone outside the family.

Outside intervention

When physicians, teachers, or other professionals suspect child abuse, they are required by law in all states to report it to a government social service agency or welfare department. However, punishment of the parents is not the goal of the law. Jailing a parent might injure the child as much as the original abuse. Removing the child from the family may be necessary to protect the youngster from future injury. In most cases, the removal is only temporary. The child may stay in the hospital for a few days while the case is studied and parents are interviewed. In many communities, a team made up of a social worker, a pediatrician, a psychiatrist, and other specialists talk to the child and the parents and develop a long-term treatment plan. This often involves periodic visits by a social worker to the home and psychological help for one or both parents. Practical help, such as day care for small children and household help by a trained homemaker, can ease the burdens on an overworked mother. If there is a local chapter of Parents Anonymous, an organization of parents who formerly abused their children, this may be another source of emotional support.

Prevention

Parents who are afraid that they might abuse their children should talk frankly to their family doctor or a social worker. Joining a support group of other parents may also be helpful.

If a baby is born ill or prematurely and must stay in the hospital after the mother comes home, the parents should visit the baby every day and stay as close as possible so that the baby will not be a stranger when he or she comes home.

Circumcision

Circumcision is the surgical removal of the foreskin, the retractable sleeve of skin covering the glans (the head of the penis). In some religions, the operation is performed as a religious ritual on the eighth day following birth. In hospitals, it is usually done on the day before a baby boy goes home. In any event, if it is to be done for non-medical reasons, it should be done in infancy and not later, when it is a more serious operation and might harm the child psychologically.

During the five-minute operation, which is usually done without anesthesia, the foreskin is carefully cut away. Gauze coated with petroleum jelly is applied to the incision. In most cases, the incision heals rapidly, forming a dry scab that drops off after a few days. Although the incision should be kept as clean as possible (but not submerged in bathwater), no other special care is necessary.

Pros and cons

Routine circumcision for newborns is a controversial issue. The decision about the procedure should be made by the parents after careful consideration.

The operation has become standard in American hospitals in recent decades as a cleanliness measure. In a young boy, the foreskin completely covers the head of the penis and cannot be pulled back very far. If the penis is not kept clean, urine and other substances can cause irritation of the glans and perhaps lead to infection between the foreskin and the glans. However, normal care can prevent this problem. There is some recent evidence that uncircumcised males have a higher rate of bladder and kidney infections as well as an increased risk of penile cancer, but further information is needed before any strong conclusions can be drawn. Even though the foreskin at first cannot be pulled back very far because of bands of tissue that bind it to the glans, it is necessary to wash only the part of the glans that can be uncovered comfortably at any one stage. The bands of tissue gradually dissolve, and by later childhood, the foreskin can be pulled back completely.

Very seldom is there a medical reason to perform a circumcision. It should never be done on the first day of life or if the baby is ill or premature. Furthermore, it should be delayed indefinitely if there is any abnormality of the glans or penis, so that the foreskin can be used later as graft tissue to repair the defect. It should not be done if the mother was taking any medication that promotes bleeding, such as an anticoagulant or aspirin, during pregnancy or is taking such a medication while breast-feeding, nor should it be done if there is any family history of bleeding disorders.

Local infection, which can lead to significant hemorrhage and mutilation, is a risk in circumcision. Many medical authorities feel that there is no absolute medical reason for routine circumcision of newborn boys. Adequate hygiene offers the same advantages as routine circumcision without the risks of the operation.

Parents, therefore, should consider all factors—cultural, religious, and medical—before making a decision about circumcision.

Cleft lip and cleft palate

Cleft lip and cleft palate, a defect in 1 of every 700 to 800 newborns, is characterized by a split running through all or part of the upper structure of the mouth. A cleft lip (or harelip) may be only a small notch near the center of the upper lip, or it may extend into the nostril. A cleft in the palate can be as minor as a split in the uvula (the little projection of tissue that hangs down in the back of the throat), or it may divide the entire soft palate (the muscular tissue that covers the roof of the mouth). In its most severe form, a cleft splits not only the soft palate but the entire hard palate (the bony roof of the mouth) and upper jaw, joining with a cleft lip. The cleft may even divide the palate into three parts, resulting in a split on either side of the nose and leaving the middle section of the upper jaw and gum dangling.

Causes

The formation of a cleft lip occurs in the early stage of pregnancy, soon after the fourth week, when the face starts to form. Bulges of tissue on either side of the face grow toward the midline to form the nostrils and lips. At about the seventh week they normally meet and join; if they do not, a cleft lip is the result.

A failure of development in the eighth week of pregnancy causes cleft palate. The palate is formed from two plates of tissue, which originally are on either side of the developing tongue. As the head and neck grow, the tongue moves downward and the tissue plates move into position and fuse into one—unless there is an error or weakness, which results in cleft palate.

The underlying causes of cleft lip and cleft palate are not fully understood. There is an inherited tendency toward the defects. More than one-fourth of children with cleft lip also have a relative with a cleft. If parents without cleft defects have one child with a cleft, they have a 5 percent risk of having a second child with a cleft; if they have two children with clefts, there is a 12 percent risk of a cleft in future children. Perhaps some difference in the uterus, such as poor blood supply to the fetus, combines with an inherited tendency to produce the error of development. Certain chemicals or medications, alcohol, too many or not enough vitamins, and viral infections have been suggested as possible causes of cleft defects.

Cleft lip and cleft palate are often associated with other birth defects. Of every six children who have a cleft lip, with or without cleft palate, one will have one or more other birth defects. Almost 50 percent of children with cleft palate also have another defect, such as joined fingers or toes, malformed ears, spina bifida, heart disease, or clubfoot.

Treatment
Treatment of a patient with a cleft lip or a cleft palate (or both) requires the services of a specialized team that includes a pediatrician, an orthodontist (a dentist who specializes in the misalignment of the teeth), a speech therapist, a plastic surgeon, a psychologist, an audiologist (a specialist in communication disorders), and an otolaryngologist (a physician who specializes in disorders of the ears, nose, and throat). Treatment may take place at a specialized clinic or hospital center or may be coordinated by a pediatrician.

Before any treatment can begin, however, steps must be taken to permit the child to eat. A cleft lip prevents normal sucking, and a cleft palate allows milk to run out of the nose, often causing choking and vomiting. Special feeding devices are used, such as a nipple with an enlarged flange to cover the cleft or a regular nipple with enlarged holes. A small syringe with a short rubber tube may be used to feed a child with a cleft lip, although sometimes such a child can be

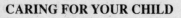

breast-fed. A few days after birth, an orthodontist skilled in cleft palate repair may be able to fashion an appliance that provides a temporary roof for the mouth, enabling regular feeding. At the same time, the appliance prevents the mouth from being distorted before the palate can be closed.

Some surgeons correct a cleft lip in the first few days of the child's life because it will make the baby more acceptable to his or her parents and make it easier to feed the baby by bottle. However, other surgeons delay the operation for 3 months, so that surgery will not interfere with the growing bonds of affection between mother and baby (for one thing, the baby cannot breast-feed for six weeks after the operation) and to rule out other birth defects that might interfere with recovery.

Plastic surgery to correct cleft palate usually takes place in the second year of life. Some surgeons repair the soft palate first, when the child is between 6 and 18 months of age, and the hard palate much later. Although early surgery helps the child's emotional and speech development, some surgeons wait because they are concerned that early surgery may cause distortion of growth in the middle third of the face. While waiting, the child wears an appliance that acts as a roof over the mouth.

The problems created by cleft palate and cleft lip cannot be solved only by surgery. The services of an orthodontist are needed for youngsters with cleft palate, not only to make appliances but to straighten teeth that are poorly positioned. A speech therapist aids the child in developing speech, which is altered because of the missing or inadequate soft palate. A psychologist helps to treat emotional and social problems sometimes caused by being different in speech or appearance. An otolaryngologist should examine the child monthly for middle ear infections, which are common in young children with cleft palates.

Clubfoot

Clubfoot, or talipes, is a common birth defect in which one or both feet are fixed in an awkward, twisted position. The foot resists efforts to stretch or turn it back. In talipes equinovarus, the most frequent form, the foot points down and turns in while the front of the foot curls toward the heel. If not corrected, the condition worsens and interferes with walking. The person seems to walk on the ankle and the outside or inside edge of the foot.

Causes
The cause of clubfoot is unknown. However, there seems to be an inherited tendency for development to be arrested around the ninth week of pregnancy, when the fetus' feet are being formed. Clubfoot may begin as a muscle abnormality. The Achilles tendon is shortened, the ankle and its muscles are deformed, and the heel bone is shortened and flattened to some extent.

Treatment
Correction of clubfoot should begin as early as the first week after birth, when the bones, muscles, ligaments, and tendons are soft and pliable. The correction is usually done in stages. In talipes equinovarus, the first stage is to uncurl the front of the foot away from the heel. The next is to turn the foot so that the sole faces outward. The third stage is to put the foot in a cast with the toes pointing up. This may require surgery to lengthen the Achilles tendon and to free the ankle joint.

Correction generally takes place in a series of small, painless, gradual adjustments. Typically, the doctor flexes and stretches the foot by hand and then fixes it in a cast in a partially corrected position. After a week or so the cast is removed, the foot is manipulated into a better position, and a new cast is applied. Sometimes, instead of making a new cast each time, the doctor places wedges inside the existing cast to adjust the foot. The entire casting process can take three months.

Once the correction has been made, it must be followed up with exercises, devices that hold the feet in place at night while the baby is sleeping, and orthopedic shoes. A night splint (corrective shoes with soles joined by a flat metal bar that keeps the feet in exactly the right position) is often used.

Because clubfoot sometimes recurs, periodic checkups are necessary until the child becomes an adult. However, in most cases the correction is completely successful, and the individual can walk and run normally.

If early treatment does not succeed, or if a child is not treated until the age of nine or ten years, more extensive surgery may be necessary. This

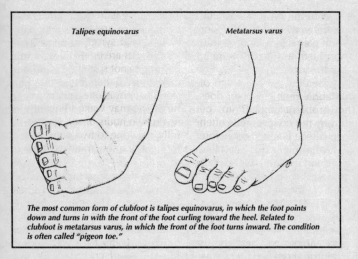

The most common form of clubfoot is talipes equinovarus, in which the foot points down and turns in with the front of the foot curling toward the heel. Related to clubfoot is metatarsus varus, in which the front of the foot turns inward. The condition is often called "pigeon toe."

is followed by several weeks with the foot in a cast. Satisfactory results are usually obtained. The foot is rather stiff, but this does not prevent the individual from engaging in the most active sports.

Related to true clubfoot is a more common condition called *metatarsus varus,* in which the front of the foot turns inward. Also known as *apparent clubfoot* and *pigeon toe,* this is a milder deformity that may not be diagnosed in the first several weeks. Unlike a true clubfoot, the apparent clubfoot can be moved easily into a correct position. It can usually be corrected by manipulation and

exercise, without the need for casts or surgery.

Colic

Colic means different things to different people, but the universal characteristic is crying—not just short periods of fussiness that can be stopped by changing or feeding or cuddling—but long periods of crying with no apparent cause that defy all attempts to stop them.

Causes
It has long been assumed that colic arises from some gastrointestinal disorder. However,

studies have shown no correlation between colic and poor weight gain or excessive vomiting, constipation, or diarrhea. Colicky babies are generally quite healthy, with no sign of nutritional problems. Nor does the problem appear to be hunger; the crying spells often begin after a feeding, not before one. It has been suggested that bottle-feeding is at fault, but breast-fed infants are just as likely to have colic. In some babies with colic, long periods of crying could be related to general irritability, possibly because of immaturity of the nervous system or exceptional sensitivity to the environment. Lactose intolerance, food sensitivities, and allergies have also been suggested as causes of colic.

Symptoms

Colic most often begins when an infant is two to four weeks old. The baby will cry inconsolably for hours each day. These bouts of crying often occur as if on schedule (most often in the late afternoon or early evening). The colicky baby pulls his or her legs up, clenches his or her fists, screams, and turns red. The baby may nurse briefly but then stop to continue crying. The abdomen may be distended as if with gas, and the baby may even pass gas frequently. Generally, there are no other gastrointestinal symptoms; bowel movements are normal, and the baby does not spit up any more than most babies. The baby's sleep pattern is often disrupted; he or she may wake frequently (every two hours or so), cry fretfully, take one to two ounces of formula or a few minutes at the mother's breast, fall into a fitful sleep, and then awaken to repeat the sequence.

Diagnosis

Before assuming that your baby has colic, check for other possible causes of crying, such as pain from an open diaper pin or discomfort from being overheated, constipated, hungry, or wet. See whether your baby responds promptly to talking and cuddling—a baby in pain can be distracted, but only temporarily. Also, check for signs of illness: Colic is not associated with fever, diarrhea, vomiting, cough, a runny nose, or reddened eyes.

Your pediatrician will want to rule out more serious causes of crying before assuming that your baby is suffering from colic. Signs of illness, such as sores in the mouth or gastrointestinal or urinary tract problems, will be sought.

Treatment

If the colic seems to be due, at least in part, to an accumulation of gas in the abdomen, be careful not to overfeed the baby and be sure to burp him or her thoroughly after feedings. If you are bottle-feeding, check the nipple hole; if it is too large or too small, the baby may be swallowing too much air. A warm hot-water bottle on the abdominal area may relieve some discomfort.

If the colic seems to be due to irritability, it might be helpful to restrict visitors and to keep the home environment as peaceful as possible. Some researchers believe that overly sensitive babies may be upset by an atmosphere charged with too much noise, too much activity, and too much emotional stress.

Congenital hypothyroidism

Congenital (present at birth) hypothyroidism is a condition that leads to defective physical and mental development because of a deficiency of thyroid hormone. If untreated, a person born with congenital hypothyroidism grows to a maximum height of three or four feet and has a large, flat, broad head; short forehead; puffy, wide-set eyes; broad, short, upturned nose; thick lips; large tongue protruding from a drooling mouth; narrow chest; potbelly; swayback; rough skin; dry hair; and severe mental retardation.

Causes

Iodine is necessary for the body to produce thyroid hormone, and foods obtained from the ocean are the best sources of iodine. Before the widespread use of iodized salt, hypothyroidism was much more common in inland areas, where foods naturally contain little iodine.

Congenital hypothyroidism can result from a defect in the development before birth. The thyroid gland may be missing or underdeveloped, possibly because of a lack of iodine in the mother's diet during pregnancy. In rare cases, congenital hypothyroidism is caused by an inherited absence of a chemical needed to produce thyroid hormone.

When hypothyroidism first appears in children more than two years of age it is usually due to an inflammation of the thyroid gland resulting from an immune disorder. It can also be caused by certain diseases of the pituitary gland or hypothalamus.

Symptoms
The first symptoms of untreated congenital hypothyroidism usually appear between the ages of three and six months or whenever the mother stops breastfeeding (breast milk contains tiny quantities of thyroid hormone). The baby is "too good," in the sense that he or she seldom cries (when the baby does cry, it is a strange, hoarse cry), sleeps more than normal, is inactive, and thus is easy to care for. This behavior is a result of the baby's lack of thyroid hormone (which regulates the rate of body processes) and increasing mental retardation. The baby's movements are slow and awkward, and the child has feeding difficulties, is constipated, and develops jaundice. The stomach protrudes, and a hernia may develop at the navel.

These symptoms are followed by the appearance of the characteristic facial features: the thick tongue, which interferes with breathing; the wide-set eyes; the turned-up nose; and the dull expression, indicating mental deficiency. The baby's heart beats slowly, resulting in poor circulation and cold skin. The hair is dry and dull. Teeth come in late and decay easily.

The child in whom symptoms of hypothyroidism first appear after the age of two is typically short and fat, with short legs and arms and a head that appears too large. Sexual development in an older child may be delayed.

Diagnosis
Early diagnosis is now much more common since all states began to require that every newborn be tested for thyroid hormone level.

Diagnosis of congenital hypothyroidism may require not only a blood test to determine thyroid hormone levels but also a nuclear medicine study after the administration of radioactive iodine to evaluate thyroid function. Special X-ray studies may also be used to detect delayed development of the skeleton, and an electrocardiogram (which measures the electrical impulses generated in the heart) may be ordered to reveal heartbeat patterns.

Treatment
Treatment for congenital hypothyroidism is lifelong replacement of thyroid hormone with a synthetic substitute, ideally starting at birth. Those who

receive the hormone before the age of three months usually develop normally. Children born without a thyroid gland are more at risk than those whose thyroid gland works poorly; if not treated by three months of age, they will be mentally retarded even though their growth is corrected.

Prevention

Pregnant women can help prevent congenital hypothyroidism in their offspring by eating a well-balanced diet that includes iodine-rich foods, such as fish and seafood, and by using iodized salt. At birth, every child's blood should be tested for thyroid hormone level.

Croup

Croup is a condition marked by a hoarse, barking cough that sometimes follows a cold or fever in very young children, most commonly those younger than two years of age. A croup attack may occur only once, or it may linger or reappear after it seems to have gone.

Causes

Croup is usually caused by a viral infection of the larynx (voice box). The characteristic barking cough is produced when air forces its way through the child's swollen larynx. The air passageways in a child's throat are extremely narrow; when an infection causes swelling, there is little room left for air to pass through, and breathing can be severely hampered as a result. Also, the windpipe and the bronchi (the main breathing tubes that connect the windpipe and the lungs) may become blocked with mucus, further impairing breathing.

Symptoms

The identifying symptoms of croup are a deep, barking cough and breathing difficulties, especially when inhaling. Sometimes a fever and hoarseness are also present. The child may gag while coughing, causing vomiting, which usually relieves the cough somewhat. The coughing attack often occurs in the evening and usually lasts less than an hour.

Symptoms that indicate a worsening condition include blue skin and lips, drooling, and extreme exhaustion. When the croaking sound continues while the child is inhaling, a condition called *stridor* has developed. If any of these symptoms occurs, or if there are severe breathing difficulties, medical help should be obtained immediately.

Diagnosis

The emphasis in diagnostic evaluation is on establishing that the difficulty in breathing is actually due to croup and not to epiglottitis, a life-threatening emergency condition in which the inflamed epiglottis (the lid-like structure covering the opening to the windpipe) swells and rapidly causes complete obstruction of the airway. Epiglottitis is usually caused by bacteria, most often *Hemophilus influenzae,* and is associated with sudden onset of high fever (up to 104°F) and drooling. This is an important diagnostic clue to help doctors differentiate between epiglottitis and viral croup.

Choking on a foreign object may also resemble croup, because both conditions share the symptom of frantic efforts to breathe. An X-ray examination may be performed to rule out this possibility.

Treatment

Croup can usually be treated at home. The first step is calming the child. The barking cough, especially when accompanied by difficulty in breathing, can frighten the child, and this fear can only aggravate the symptoms. Sometimes the child can be told to imagine a relaxing scene or can listen to a calming bedtime story; a relaxed child will respond much better to home remedies.

The goal is to relieve the cough by reducing the inflammation and swelling in the larynx. This can be accomplished by breathing in moist air from a humidifier or vaporizer, by leaning over a pan of hot water with a towel draped over the head, or by sitting in a steamy bathroom with a hot shower running. Moist air reduces the swelling and makes breathing easier. Of course, precautions should be taken to protect a young child from being scalded while taking part in these treatments, and the child should never be left alone.

Drinking extra fluids (not milk or orange juice) at room temperature is also recommended. Cough medicine will not help (and may even harm) a child with croup, nor is it advisable to put a spoon or any other object into the mouth in an attempt to aid the breathing. In a severe case, a physician may administer drugs to control the inflammation in the throat; also, antibiotics can sometimes control the infections connected with croup.

Prevention
It is not known why some children develop croup after a cold or fever and others do not; therefore, there is really no way to prevent croup.

Gilles de la Tourette syndrome

Gilles de la Tourette syndrome is a neuromuscular disorder marked by intense tics (twitchy, repetitive movements of certain muscles). It occurs most often in boys, and it generally begins around the age of seven or eight years. At first the tics are simple: facial twisting, blinking, grimacing, shoulder shrugging, or twitching. Later the tics progress to vocal tics and may be accompanied by psychological problems.

Causes
The cause of Gilles de la Tourette syndrome is unknown. It is still disputed whether the disorder is of physical or psychological origin. Familial incidence ranges from 35 to 50 percent.

Symptoms
The symptoms of Gilles de la Tourette syndrome are at first limited to the muscles in the face, head, neck, and shoulders. Often, the first symptom is a characteristic breathing noise from the larynx (voice box), as if the patient were barking, wheezing, or gasping for air. As the tics spread to the shoulders and arms, there are shoulder shrugs and twitches, as well as neck and arm twists. Vocal tics, such as grunting, snuffing, shouting, and barking sounds, then begin to develop. As the vocal symptoms worsen, the patient typically begins to exclaim in a loud voice using words or phrases with obscene meanings ("swear words"). Echolalia (repetition by the patient of words that have just been said to him or her) may occur. The patient may also seem to fixate on a word or phrase and repeat it over and over with increasing speed. Often, too, the individual will spasmodically and automatically repeat or mimic the actions of those nearby.

The symptoms of Gilles de la Tourette syndrome tend to come and go, especially as the patient approaches puberty and adulthood. Tics that are very violent during waking hours often stop during sleep. Some tics are intensified by emotional upheavals. The tics of Gilles de la Tourette syndrome, unlike those of most neuromuscular disorders, are often suppressed in school or social settings and expressed more often when the patient is alone or with family members. In some cases, the tics can be controlled voluntarily by the patient. The excessive swearing, however, occurs only in the presence of others; some patients attempt to cover it up by coughing, thus developing another tic. Often symptoms decrease in adult life and disappear, only to return during a period of emotional stress. Mental activity remains normal.

Diagnosis
Diagnosing Gilles de la Tourette syndrome is difficult, since symptoms in the early stages often resemble common childhood tics. Also, early- and middle-stage symptoms are difficult to distinguish from those of certain brain conditions. However, Gilles de la Tourette syndrome can be diagnosed with some assurance as the course of the illness unfolds.

Treatment
Gilles de la Tourette syndrome can be treated with medica-

tions, starting with small doses and increasing the dosage until the tics are controlled. Often a combination of drugs is used. Group psychotherapy can be helpful in some cases. In extreme cases, leukotomy (surgical interruption of white nerve fibers of the frontal lobe of the brain) may be considered. There are no known preventive measures.

Hyaline membrane disease

Hyaline membrane disease (HMD) is a respiratory distress syndrome that occurs in premature infants who do not have fully functioning lungs. It is one of the leading causes of illness and death in premature infants.

Cause
The cause of HMD is the inability of the immature lungs to produce enough pulmonary surfactant, which is a chemical in the alveoli (the tiny air sacs in the lungs) that keeps them expanded. Without adequate surfactant, the alveoli tend to collapse when the infant exhales. As a result, the lungs do

not expand completely, and the blood passing through them cannot obtain enough oxygen to sustain life.

Symptoms

The symptoms of HMD are easily observable. The skin is bluish due to lack of oxygenation of the blood, and there are other symptoms of oxygen deprivation—irregular heartbeat; rapid, labored, and shallow breathing; flaring of the nostrils; grunting when breathing out; and edema (swelling of tissues due to fluid accumulation).

Treatment

Treatment of HMD is aimed at maintaining adequate oxygen levels. Until the lungs can sufficiently oxygenate the blood, oxygen must be provided in such a way as to prevent damage to the infant. An oxygen face mask is often used to provide warmed, moisturized oxygen. In more severe cases, a ventilator is necessary.

Great strides in the treatment of HMD have been made in the last few years. An artificial surfactant (a lubricant for the lungs) has been produced that, when administered via the baby's trachea (windpipe), markedly relieves the baby's respiratory distress. Because of

the availability of a synthetic surfactant, the rate of death from HMD has dropped dramatically in the last few years.

Either the condition will clear up as the lungs develop and begin to produce their own natural surfactant or the infant will not survive.

Prevention

The best preventive measure is to guard against premature birth. Women should be carefully monitored during the last weeks of pregnancy for any signs of premature labor.

If the mother is diabetic, the fetal lungs may not be fully formed until the 40th week of pregnancy, and HMD is possible until then.

Hydrocephalus

Hydrocephalus (sometimes inaccurately referred to as "water on the brain") is an abnormal accumulation of cerebrospinal fluid within the cavities (hollow spaces) of the brain.

Normally, cerebrospinal fluid is secreted in the cavities of the brain and absorbed by a membrane that lines the cavities. If the membrane does not absorb the fluid or if the fluid is blocked, it builds up in the cav-

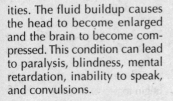
ities. The fluid buildup causes the head to become enlarged and the brain to become compressed. This condition can lead to paralysis, blindness, mental retardation, inability to speak, and convulsions.

Cause

Hydrocephalus is usually the result of a brain infection or a malformation in fetal development. Although the baby's head may not appear abnormally large at birth, it expands rapidly from month to month; if untreated, the child usually dies by the end of the second year. If the blockage is only partial, the child may live for a number of years or may even live a normal life span.

Although hydrocephalus is usually a congenital condition, it can occur later as a result of an infection or tumor.

Symptoms

When hydrocephalus occurs in an infant, the loosely connected bony skull plates pull apart to accommodate the swelling. As a result, the head becomes greatly enlarged. In addition to having an oversized head, the child with hydrocephalus may have an abnormally enlarged forehead and swollen or enlarged blood vessels in the scalp.

Diagnosis

Diagnosis is accomplished through the use of X rays and computed tomography or magnetic resonance imaging (MRI). If infection is suspected, samples of the blood and cerebrospinal fluid will be examined.

Treatment

Surgery can make it possible, in some cases, to bypass the blockage or obstruction, causing the fluid buildup to escape through other exits. Often, the insertion of a small tube connecting a brain cavity with the abdomen or a major blood vessel will allow the fluid to drain. As the child grows, the tube may become blocked, again allowing pressure to build in the brain. If this happens, the tube must be replaced, or the blockage removed. When surgery is successful, the probability of mental retardation is greatly reduced, and the prospects of normal physical and intellectual development are increased.

Immunization

Immunization is the means of producing immunity, or resistance, to a specific disease. Immunization can provide protection against measles, mumps, rubella (German measles), hepatitis B, some types of meningitis, polio, pertussis (whooping cough), diphtheria, Hemophilus B, and tetanus, all of which can cripple or kill.

Every child should receive injections of the combined diphtheria-tetanus-pertussis (DTP) vaccine at 2, 4, 6, and 18 months of age. Every child should also receive a dose of the oral polio vaccine (OPV) at 2, 4, and 18 months of age. Every child should receive injections of the vaccine against *Hemophilus influenzae* type B (Hib), the most common cause of bacterial meningitis in children. The recommended schedule for Hib vaccination depends upon the brand of vaccine used. For example, one brand of the vaccine should be given at 2, 4, and 12 months of age; another should be given at 2, 4, 6, and 15 months of age. The physician who performs the initial vaccination can tell you which schedule applies to your child. At 15 months, a child should receive the combined measles, mumps, and rubella (MMR) vaccine and a test for tuberculosis (TB). DTP and OPV boosters should be given around the time of school entry (when your child is four to six years old). A measles booster should be given when your child is 11 or 12 years of age, and anyone between 4 and 21 years of age should receive a measles booster during a measles outbreak. A diphtheria and tetanus toxoids (DT) booster shot should be given between 14 and 16 years of age, and a tetanus booster should be given every ten years. A person with a high-risk wound, such as penetration into the foot by a rusty nail, should receive a tetanus booster if more than five years have elapsed since the last booster. The initial hepatitis B booster is given soon after birth, with two boosters given in the first six months of life. The American Academy of Pediatrics recommends the varicella (chicken pox) vaccine for all children, adolescents, and young adults who have not already been infected with chicken pox. A single dose should routinely be given between 12 and 18 months of age. This immunization can be given at the same time as the child's first MMR (measles, mumps, rubella) vaccination. Older children may be immunized at the earliest convenient opportunity, also with a single dose. Individuals over the age of 13 who have not been immunized previously and have no history of varicella infection should receive two doses of the vaccine four to eight weeks apart. Once immunized, most individuals are protected from the chicken pox.

Immunization and testing schedule

Hepatitis B	Soon after birth; two boosters during first 6 months
DTP	2, 4, 6, 18 months
OPV	2, 4, 18 months
Hib	2, 4, 6, 15 months or 2,4, 12 months
MMR	15 months
TB test	15 months
Varicella	12–18 months
Measles booster*	11–12 years
DT booster	14–16 years
Tetanus booster	Every 10 years

*If there should be a measles outbreak, any person between 4 and 21 years of age should receive a booster.

If the family does not have a physician, immunizations can usually be obtained through the local public health department. If a child has an acute illness with fever, immunization should be delayed.

Nephrotic syndrome

Nephrotic syndrome is a kidney disorder in which the glomeruli (tiny clumps of blood vessels that filter the blood to produce urine) do not work properly. The defective glomeruli allow proteins, most notably albumin, to escape from the bloodstream and seep into the urine while letting fluid that should be eliminated as waste accumulate within the tissues.

Causes
Nephrotic syndrome is caused by other diseases that affect the kidneys, including some strep infections. The syndrome, in turn, creates vulnerability to other infections, including peritonitis (inflammation of the lining of the abdominal cavity).

Symptoms
As a result of fluid accumulation, the body gradually swells

539

(a condition called *edema*), becoming especially bloated around the face, abdomen, and ankles. The child may urinate very little (approximately one-fifth of the normal amount).

Diagnosis
If initial blood and urine tests point to nephrotic syndrome, the doctor will order more tests and possibly a kidney biopsy.

Treatment
The condition can be controlled with proper medical care, usually in a hospital, where medication (diuretics to eliminate excess fluid and steroids to control inflammation) and diet can be carefully supervised. Symptoms are likely to clear up after a few weeks.

Patent ductus arteriosus

Patent ductus arteriosus is a congenital (present at birth) heart disorder in which the ductus arteriosus, an extra blood vessel present in the fetus that allows the blood to pass from the pulmonary artery (which conveys blood from the heart to the lungs) to the aorta (the main blood vessel that conveys blood from the heart to the rest of the body) fails to close after birth. During the growth and development in the uterus, the fetus is immersed in amniotic fluid, and the lungs are not used. The blood bypasses the lungs through the ductus arteriosus, and the fetus receives oxygen from the placenta.

If the ductus arteriosus remains open after birth, some blood is rerouted from the aorta back through the lungs. As a result, less oxygen-rich blood can be supplied to the tissues throughout the body, and the work of the left side of the heart (which pumps blood from the heart to the rest of the body) is increased.

Cause
In most babies, the duct begins to close before birth and is completely closed by the age of three months. The reasons for this normal closure (and for failure to close) are poorly understood.

Symptoms
Patent ductus arteriosus occurs more often in female infants. If the ductus is small, there are often no symptoms. A large ductus may produce a heart murmur, hypertension, and growth retardation.

Treatment
Patent ductus arteriosus can be treated with medication if diagnosed early. Prenatal tests have become available recently for diagnosis if the condition is suspected. After birth, the condition can be corrected by tying off the duct in a simple surgical procedure.

Phimosis

Phimosis is a constriction of the foreskin (the skin fold over the head of the penis), which prevents it from being drawn back over the glans (head of the penis).

Causes
Phimosis is either congenital or acquired. The acquired form of phimosis is usually caused by an infection involving the inner aspect of the foreskin and the glans itself.

Phimosis also allows debris to accumulate between the foreskin and the glans, providing a breeding ground for bacteria.

Symptoms
If infection becomes established, ulcers (open sores) may appear on the glans, and the lymph nodes in the groin may swell.

Diagnosis
The condition will be apparent on physical examination of the child. If infection is suspected, cultures may be performed.

Treatment
The definitive treatment for this condition is circumcision (the surgical removal of the foreskin). If, for some reason, circumcision must be delayed, there must be careful attention to keeping the area clean and free from infection until the procedure can be performed.

Pinworms

Pinworms are parasites that can infect the gastrointestinal tract and occasionally other sites, such as the female reproductive tract. These worms are tiny (about one eighth to one half of an inch in length).

Cause
The usual cause of the infection is eating food contaminated with fertilized oxyurid eggs. Contamination results from contact with infected feces. Eggs can survive for two or three weeks.

After being ingested, the eggs hatch and release their larvae (an immature form of the worm)

541

into the upper portion of the small intestine. The larvae mature as they pass through the first part of the large intestine. After mating, the adult male worms die, and the females migrate down the large intestine and lay their eggs around the anus. The eggs are transferred by the child's hands from the anus to the mouth, and the cycle continues. Pinworms can be transmitted to other children and adults in the same manner. Also, the hatched larvae can migrate back through the anus and into the bowel.

Symptoms
Many children who have pinworms do not have obvious symptoms. Symptoms that may occur are itching and inflammation around the anus. Worms can also cause irritation, inflammation, and obstruction in the appendix. In girls and women, pinworms can work their way into the vagina and urethra (the passageway from the bladder to the outside) and cause inflammation or infection.

Diagnosis
Aside from noting the symptom of itching, diagnosis can be made by identifying the eggs or worms through a microscope. The physician will usually place a piece of clear adhesive tape against the child's anus. The eggs will adhere to the tape, which is then placed under a microscope for examination.

Treatment
Treatment of pinworms is not difficult. Usually one dose of the drug pyrantel pamoate is sufficient. Other medications are also available. In addition, all members of a family should be treated simultaneously, and their bedclothes, towels, and underwear should be laundered at the same time. The eggs around the anus should be removed by cleaning the anal area thoroughly at the time of treatment. Reinfection is common, and when symptoms develop, another course of treatment is necessary.

Prevention
It is important to teach children clean eating habits, to encourage them to wash their hands frequently, and to be alert and avoid other children who may be infected.

Reye syndrome

Reye syndrome is a relatively rare condition in which encephalitis (inflammation of the brain) is associated with liver damage due to the collection of fatty deposits in that organ. It strikes children and adolescents (most commonly, children between the ages of 5 and 11 years), often while they are recovering from a viral infection, such as influenza or chicken pox.

Reye syndrome is a serious disease that requires immediate treatment. Brain damage, coma, or death can result if it is not diagnosed and treated quickly. It is fatal in about 25 percent of cases.

Cause

The exact cause of Reye syndrome is not known, but since it almost always follows a viral infection, scientists suspect that the virus combines with an unknown substance in the body to produce a toxin. Use of aspirin during a viral illness increases the risk of Reye syndrome. Thus, physicians caution parents not to give aspirin products to their children during chicken pox, influenza infections, or any illness associated with a high fever.

Symptoms

The symptoms of Reye syndrome are sudden vomiting, abnormal sleepiness or hyper-activity, and confusion. Convulsions and coma may occur as the disease progresses.

Diagnosis

Early diagnosis is crucial for treatment of the condition. Reye syndrome is diagnosed by careful observation of the symptoms, testing of a sample of cerebrospinal fluid (the clear fluid of the central nervous system, which is produced in the brain), blood tests to determine the presence of liver damage, and tests of the blood sugar level, which is often low in young children with this disease.

Treatment

There is no known cure for Reye syndrome. Treatment consists of helping the child to weather the first few days of the illness, maintaining normal blood sugar levels, and reducing pressure on the swollen brain. Usually, if the child survives for three or four days, the symptoms will subside and recovery will follow.

If the blood sugar level is low, a normal concentration is restored with the intravenous administration of glucose (a form of sugar). Increased pressure on the brain from the swelling is also reduced with medication.

543

Prevention

An association has been established between aspirin use during and immediately after viral infections (particularly chicken pox and influenza) and Reye syndrome. It is therefore strongly recommended that aspirin not be given to a child or adolescent with such an infection. A doctor can suggest an aspirin substitute if needed for discomfort or fever. Sponge baths may also be helpful in reducing fever.

Scoliosis

Scoliosis is a curvature of the spine. There is usually a main curve in one direction and an upper curve or lower curve, or both, to compensate for it in the opposite direction.

Before the age of three years, boys are more likely to be affected, developing an upper curve to the left and a lower curve to the right. Between the ages of four and ten years, boys and girls are affected in equal numbers, and the direction of curvature varies. Most prevalent is the adolescent form, usually affecting girls between the age of ten and the time their skeletons mature. Most often, the upper spinal area (behind the chest) curves to the right, with compensating curves to the left in the lower neck area and in the small of the back.

Severe, untreated scoliosis can cause diminished lung capacity, back pain, spinal arthritis, and disease of the cartilage disks between the vertebrae.

Causes

Scoliosis can result from unequal leg lengths, or it may be due to defective development of the vertebrae (the bones of the spine) while the fetus was growing in the uterus. Paralysis of the trunk muscles on one side of the body caused by polio, cerebral palsy, or muscular dystrophy; tilting of the pelvis due to hip disease; or deformities of the spine caused by rickets or rheumatism can also lead to scoliosis. Scoliosis with no known cause, the most common kind, is called *idiopathic*.

Symptoms

Parents should be alert for the signs of scoliosis. At first the child may appear to have an uneven hemline, unequal pant legs, or one hip higher than the other. To make a preliminary assessment, ask your child to stand up straight with his or her shirt off while you observe from

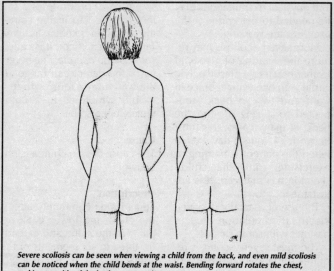

Severe scoliosis can be seen when viewing a child from the back, and even mild scoliosis can be noticed when the child bends at the waist. Bending forward rotates the chest, making one side of the back more prominent.

the rear. Notice if one shoulder is higher than the other or if one shoulder blade sticks out. When the child's arms hang loosely at the sides, notice if one arm hangs farther away from the body than does the other. See if one hip appears higher or more prominent than the other. See if the child seems to tilt to one side. Finally, you should ask your child to bend forward, arms hanging in front and palms together at the level of the knees. A hump on the back at the ribs or near the waist may also be a sign of scoliosis.

Diagnosis

If you have any suspicions of scoliosis, report them to your child's doctor, who will give the child a similar checkup and, if necessary, take X rays or refer you to an orthopedic surgeon to confirm the diagnosis.

Treatment

Treatment of scoliosis may involve only exercises if the curvature is mild. Sit-ups, exercises to stretch the spine, and breathing exercises may strengthen the muscles of the trunk enough to correct the situation. X rays

545

and physical examinations may be needed to determine if the exercises are working.

More severe scoliosis may require the wearing of a special leather brace or a plastic pelvic girdle with one vertical brace in front and two in back, connected to a ring around the neck. In many cases, this must be worn 24 hours a day, except when the patient is bathing or exercising, until the child's skeleton has matured. It is adjustable for growth.

The use of specially designed electrical stimulation devices has met with some success.

The most severe scoliosis requires spinal-fusion surgery, in which certain vertebrae are fused together, with stabilization provided by metal rods, cable, or staples. Checkups are needed after surgery to make sure that the correction is being maintained.

Spina bifida

Spina bifida is a congenital (present at birth) defect of development, marked by defective closure of some of the vertebrae (the bones of the spine) that normally encase the spinal cord. If the meninges (the membranes that cover the brain and spinal cord) protrude as a sac through the gap in the spine, the condition is known as *spina bifida cystica;* if not, it is called *spina bifida occulta.* The severity of the defect can range all the way from a form with few visible symptoms to a completely open spine.

Cause
The cause of spina bifida is unknown.

Description
Spina bifida commonly affects the chest and lower back regions of the spine and extends for three to six segments of the spinal column. If there is a sac, it may collapse while the child is still in the uterus, but it fills with cerebrospinal fluid soon after birth. If the sac is not covered with skin, it can rupture, perhaps leading to meningitis (inflammation of the meninges).

Spina bifida can be accompanied by varying degrees of paralysis, depending on the extent of involvement of the spinal cord and its nerve roots. The paralysis can lead to orthopedic problems, such as clubfoot and dislocated hip, and may also affect the sphincters (closure muscles) of the bladder and rectum, resulting in genitourinary disorders. Abnormal curvature of the spine can hinder surgical closure. Hydrocephalus (accumulation of cerebrospinal fluid within the skull) also accompanies many cases of spina bifida.

Diagnosis

Diagnostic evaluation of the condition begins with X rays of the spine, skull, hips, and lower extremities. Urine tests are also necessary. The need for further tests depends on the extent of the defect. Such tests may include a computed tomography scan (see Chapter 24) and an evaluation of the cerebrospinal fluid.

Treatment

Treatment requires an extensive evaluation of the child's condition by several physicians, including neurosurgeons, urologists, orthopedists, and pediatricians. In some cases, social service workers and psychiatrists will work with the parents. Closure of the defect ensures a better outcome. Long-term survival and quality of life depend on the type and extent of the spinal defect, other defects present, the infant's health, and treatment resources. In addition to surgical closure of the spine, the infant may need additional surgery. The most common complications are

loss of kidney function, clubfoot, dislocation of the hip joints, scoliosis (curvature of the spine), pressure sores, and muscle spasms.

Prevention

Prenatal diagnosis through amniocentesis is growing progressively more accurate but does not, as yet, expand treatment options. Research has shown that lack of folic acid before and during pregnancy increases the risk of spina bifida. All women who plan to become pregnant should make sure that their intake of folic acid is adequate, either through diet (green, leafy vegetables) or vitamin supplements.

Strabismus

Strabismus is commonly referred to as "squint-eye" or "cross-eye." Technically, the term refers to a deviation in which one eye is not parallel with the other.

Causes

In most cases, strabismus is congenital (present at birth), although it can result from later injury to one eye or impaired vision because of disease. The cause of congenital strabismus is unknown, but the effect is generally paralysis or malfunction of the tiny muscles that control the movement of the eyes.

Symptoms
Symptoms of strabismus include obviously crossed, wandering, or squinting eyes, although in some cases lack of parallelism of the eyes is so subtle that it can be detected only by special testing.

Diagnosis
Complete evaluation of the eyes is essential to rule out more serious eye or nervous disorders and to determine how best to correct the strabismus. Such an evaluation is usually performed by an ophthalmologist (a physician who specializes in eye disorders).

Treatment
If muscle imbalance alone is responsible, the strabismus can usually be treated easily with corrective glasses or contact lenses. Eye exercises are effective in many less severe cases. Surgical restoration of the muscle balance can be performed in more extreme cases. Permanent visual loss can result if strabismus is not treated properly by the time the child is four to six years old.

Sudden infant death syndrome (SIDS)

Sudden infant death syndrome (also called *crib death*) is the unexplained and sudden death of a baby—often, the baby is perfectly well when put to bed but dies silently during sleep. In the United States, SIDS is second only to accidents as a cause of death in infants from two weeks to one year of age, causing 8,000 to 10,000 deaths per year. Most deaths from SIDS occur in the third or fourth month of life, with higher death rates for boys, children of teenage mothers, infants from poor families, and babies who were born prematurely. Cigarette smoking by the mother during pregnancy appears to be one of the biggest risk factors for SIDS, and the use of drugs such as cocaine or heroin during pregnancy also places the child at increased risk. More deaths from SIDS occur in winter than in summer.

Causes
Sudden infant death syndrome was once mistakenly believed to be the result of accidental smothering in the bedding of

the crib. It is also not attributable to clogging of the airways by vomited food, to bottle feeding, or to any other cause that parents could prevent. Some investigators believe that a combination of conditions is necessary to trigger SIDS, including a narrowed and inflamed airway, temporary airway obstruction, chronic oxygen deficiency, and irregular breathing, leading to a spasm of the trachea (windpipe) and death. There is now evidence that a baby sleeping on his or her stomach is more likely to die from SIDS. Therefore, it is recommended that babies be put to sleep on their sides or backs.

Counseling for parents
Parents who lose a child to SIDS are totally unprepared for the death and usually have overwhelming guilt feelings—that something they did or did not do caused the death of their child. An autopsy will usually prove that the death was not the parents' fault. Doctors and nurses who take the time to discuss the death fully with the parents can be very helpful. So can another parent who has lost a child to SIDS. There are now many local chapters of the National Sudden Infant Death Syndrome Foundation and the

International Council for Infant Survival, both of which can be valuable sources of counseling and information.

Undescended testes

Undescended testes is a condition in which one or both of the testes (male sex glands) do not descend into the scrotum (the sac between the legs that normally contains the testes) but remain in the abdomen, where they developed before birth. This condition is also called *cryptorchidism* or *cryptorchism* and is not uncommon.

If the testes do not descend, they often degenerate or atrophy (shrink) and thus do not secrete the male sex hormones that they ordinarily supply. This, in turn, can cause the elimination or suppression of the development during puberty of secondary male sex characteristics such as body hair, heavier musculature, deepening voice, and so forth. Damaged sperm, or insufficient production of them, can also result from undescended testes, especially if the situation is still present in adolescence or adulthood. If one testis is damaged but the other has descended and is normal, sexual development will be normal.

Causes

The causes of this condition are not clearly understood. It is conjectured that a membrane in the abdomen gets in the way of normal testicular positioning. If only one testis is undescended, the problem is most likely mechanical in nature; if both are involved, the underlying cause may well be hormonal.

Treatment

Treatment for this condition is controversial. In deciding on treatment, three important considerations must be kept in mind: the potential lack of fertility if the testes do not descend, the likelihood that they will descend without intervention, and the risk that the undescended testes will become cancerous. Hormone therapy is sometimes an effective treatment, but in many cases in which it has apparently been successful, some doctors think that the testes would probably have descended by themselves anyway. Surgery to bring the testes into the scrotum is usually successful if done before the age of five years. The doctor can sometimes cause the testes

to descend by manipulating the tissues around them.

A boy with an undescended testis is at increased risk for cancer of the testes even if the testis is brought down surgically. All boys who have had an undescended testis should be taught to examine their testes for lumps on a monthly basis.

Prevention

There is no known means of preventing undescended testes.

CANCER

Cancer describes a broad group of diseases in which certain body cells grow out of control.

RISK FACTORS

Who is most likely to develop cancer? This question is very difficult, if not impossible, to answer. There are, however, certain risk factors that increase the possibility that a person will develop cancer. Among these risk factors are age (as a rule, the older the person is, the higher his or her risk of getting cancer), family history (for example, if a mother or sister had breast cancer, the risk of developing breast cancer is increased), and environmental and other factors.

The rapid increase in cancer rates during this century has been blamed largely on the environment. Polluted air and water, food additives and colorings, and changes in diet from "natural" to "processed" foods all have been implicated as possible causes. Cigarette smoking has been shown con-clusively to be a cause of lung and other related cancers.

WARNING SIGNS

Often a patient is the first to suspect cancer. This is why it is important to learn some of cancer's most common warning signs. Some of these signs may include:

- A change in bowel or bladder habits
- A sore that does not heal
- Unusual bleeding or discharge
- Thickening or lump in the breast or elsewhere
- Indigestion or difficulty in swallowing
- An obvious change in wart or mole
- A nagging cough or continued hoarseness

The chances of cure are greatest if cancer is discovered at an early stage. Women should learn to perform a breast self-examination to detect suspicious lumps as early as possible. Many physicians recommend that men learn to con-

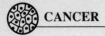

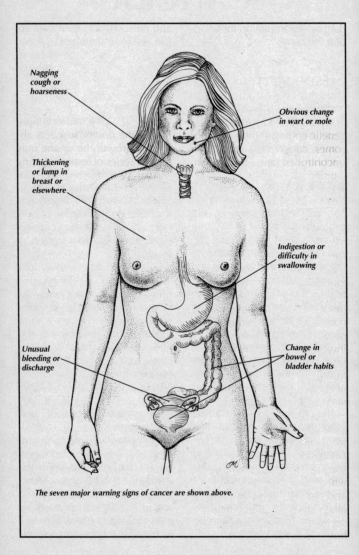

Nagging cough or hoarseness

Obvious change in wart or mole

Thickening or lump in breast or elsewhere

Indigestion or difficulty in swallowing

Unusual bleeding or discharge

Change in bowel or bladder habits

The seven major warning signs of cancer are shown above.

duct self-examination for testicular cancer.

CAUSES AND TYPES
Unlike normal cells, which grow and reproduce in the orderly manner dictated by the genetic coding in their chromosomes, cancer cells grow at an uncontrolled rate—taking over, causing the death of, or replacing normal cells. As the disease progresses, cancer cells often travel through the circulatory system to start growth in other parts of the body; this process is called *metastasis*.

A tumor is an abnormal tissue growth. A tumor may be either *malignant* (cancerous) or *benign* (noncancerous). A benign tumor commonly grows within a self-produced capsule and does not invade or kill surrounding tissue or spread throughout the body. Malignant tissues may grow out of control, quite often spreading to other parts of the body.

Over the years, more than 200 types of cancer have been identified. There are three basic categories of cancer: carcinoma (cancer of the epithelial cells, which line the body's organs and secrete mucus, among other functions), sarcoma (cancer of connective tissue, such as bone, fat, tendons, cartilage, and muscle), and fluid cancers (for example, leukemia). Some cancers may fall into more than one category.

DIAGNOSIS
Following a physical examination, if the doctor suspects abnormal growth, he or she may order a series of tests, including special X-ray examinations (for example, computed tomography scans, in which successive X rays at slightly different levels are used to create a three-dimensional image of a structure), nuclear medicine scans (in which radioactive substances are used in the imaging process), ultrasound scanning (a technique that uses sound waves to create images of internal structures), magnetic resonance imaging (in which a strong magnetic field is used instead of X rays), cytologic tests (microscopic examination of cells), and various laboratory evaluations. The doctor may also order a biopsy (removal of a small tissue sample for microscopic examination) to determine the cell type of the suspected growth and whether it is benign or malignant.

A physician may also recommend a specialist with expertise in treating the specific type of

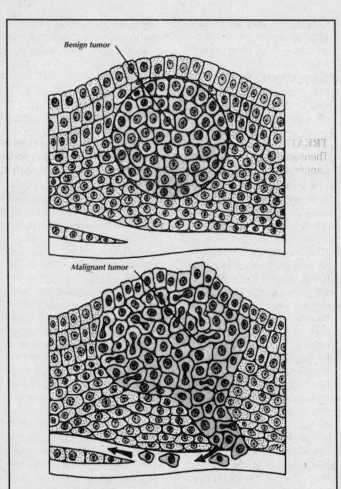

A tumor is an abnormal tissue growth. A benign tumor is noncancerous and does not metastasize; it commonly grows within a self-produced capsule. Malignant tumors are cancerous, however, and often spread to other parts of the body.

cancer. This may be an oncologist (cancer specialist), a cancer surgeon, a radiation oncologist (radiologist who uses radiation to treat cancer), or a hematologist (specialist in blood diseases).

TREATMENT

There are many ways of treating cancer. Many treatment protocols have been developed that are effective in certain types of disease. Cancer therapy often includes surgery to remove the cancer, to clear obstructions of vital passageways caused by the cancer, or to cut nerves sending pain messages to the brain; chemotherapy (use of powerful drugs to kill cancer cells); radiation therapy (use of radioactive materials in the form of energy beams or radioactive implants to destroy cancer cells); and immunotherapy (use of naturally occurring substances to increase the activity of the body's immune system). Combinations of therapies are often used.

Surgery

Surgery is the most commonly used method of dealing with cancers that develop into tumors. If cancer is contained in one area, surgery can sometimes completely eliminate it.

New surgical techniques are expanding the range of tumors that can be safely removed. Furthermore, if the surgeon is able to remove only a section of the tumor, the reduced tumor can often be successfully controlled with chemotherapy or radiation therapy.

More precise surgical techniques mean that surgery today is often less disfiguring than in the past. In addition, new developments in skin grafting make it possible to begin reconstructive work on patients— for instance, those with cancer of the head and neck—simultaneously with the cancer surgery.

Sometimes surgery is performed on a patient even though it is known that surgery will not cure the cancer. The removal of a tumor may simply make the patient more comfortable. In other cases, nerve pathways to the pain center in the brain may be cut. Certain noncancerous growths are sometimes removed because they may develop into cancer or because they are exerting pressure on adjacent anatomic structures (which may lead to functional problems).

Chemotherapy

Chemotherapy (the treatment of cancer with drugs) has gradu-

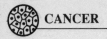

ally become more widely used. Many kinds of cancer can be effectively treated with chemotherapy alone. Anticancer drugs are also often used as a supplement to primary treatment, such as surgery. Once surgery has reduced a cancerous growth, chemotherapy can often eliminate it. Chemotherapy has proved effective against some forms of cancer that formerly were almost always fatal, in particular, Hodgkin disease (cancer of the lymph system), acute lymphocytic leukemia (a blood disease predominantly of children), and cancer of the testes.

Most cancer drugs attack any rapidly reproducing cells in the body, whether they are cancerous or not, producing some of the side effects of chemotherapy. Destruction of normal cells that reproduce frequently, such as those in the digestive tract, the hair follicles, and the bone marrow, can lead to nausea, hair loss, and lowered red blood cell count.

Usually, several drugs used to treat the cancer are administered in combination. If the cancer does not respond to the drugs, or if resistance to a medication develops, another combination of several medications may be tried.

Radiation therapy

Radiation destroys the ability of cells to divide. Cancer cells are far more susceptible to radiation than normal cells, although not all cancers respond to radiation. Like surgery, radiation therapy is usually a localized treatment, directed at a particular cancer site. Radiation treatment may also involve implanting a radioactive object directly into a tumor, destroying it from within. Radiation can be used before surgery to reduce a tumor to operable size, and frequently a patient receives radiation after surgery to destroy any cancer cells that might remain near the cancer site. Some tumors can be treated by radiation alone.

Radiation therapy is continually being refined. Drugs have been discovered that make cancer cells more sensitive to radiation. Different forms of radiation are being tested on resistant cancers. In addition, radiation today can be directed more precisely, and in stronger forms, with little harm to surrounding tissue. However, there are still side effects, including loss of appetite, nausea, and temporary hair loss. It is not certain how dangerous it is to be treated with radiation, which is itself carcinogenic;

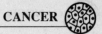

however, it is generally considered that a cancer in the body is far more threatening than the future effects of radiation.

Immunotherapy

The goal of immunotherapy is to enable the patient's body to produce substances that resist the growth of cancer. The theory behind immunotherapy is that cancer develops when, for some reason, the body fails to destroy abnormal cells. Immunotherapy for the treatment of cancer is still in the experimental stage.

PROGNOSTIC FACTORS

A number of prognostic factors (factors that predict length of survival) are important in cancer cases. Most important are the stage and the type of the disease. The earlier the stage of the disease (that is, the earlier in its course it is diagnosed) the better the prognosis is. The type of tumor is also important, since the various types respond differently to treatment. Furthermore, more than one type of cancer can occur within a specific organ. For example, all lung cancers do not involve the same kind of cell. Age and overall physical condition are also important in determining

whether or not the patient will be able to win the fight against cancer.

Bladder cancer

Bladder cancer is the most common cancer of the urinary tract. It occurs most often between the ages of 50 and 70 and is the fourth leading cause of cancer death among men. Four times as many men as women are afflicted.

Bladder cancer has been connected with exposure to a number of carcinogens. Bladder cancer may result because the urinary tract comes into contact with so many foreign substances due to its excretory function. For many years it has been known that those who work with aniline dyes have a high incidence of cancer of the bladder. Bladder cancer is also associated with exposure to tar from tobacco smoke and with schistosomiasis (infestation with a tropical parasite).

Blood in the urine is usually the first symptom of bladder cancer. In addition, urination may be difficult, painful, and frequent. The appearance of blood in the urine may be intermittent, and if this symptom disappears, a doctor is some-

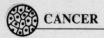

times not consulted. However, anyone with blood in the urine should consult a doctor since, in the early stages, this disease may be curable, and treatment is far more difficult later. If the symptoms suggest bladder cancer, a cystoscopic examination may be ordered. With the patient under local or general anesthesia, a lighted tubelike instrument called a *cystoscope* is passed into the urinary tract through the urethra (the passageway from the bladder to the outside), so that the interior of the bladder can be examined. This instrument can also be used to obtain a biopsy specimen (a small sample of tissue for laboratory analysis) of a suspicious growth.

Treatment of bladder cancer depends on how far advanced the disease is. A small tumor can sometimes be completely removed with a cystoscope. More advanced cases are treated with surgery or radiation or a combination of the two. In certain cancers, chemotherapeutic agents are instilled directly into the bladder.

Bone cancer

This rare form of cancer is most common in those between the ages of 5 and 20. Predisposing factors include bone diseases, bone fractures, and exposure to radiation. Bone cancer is more common as a secondary condition—the result of another cancer that has spread to the bones from another site.

Brain cancer

Any tumor in the brain, whether cancerous or not, is very dangerous. Because the brain occupies an enclosed space within the skull, even a small tumor that weighs only a fifth of a pound can cause crowding sufficient to bring on death. Brain cancer is most often the result of metastasis from other cancer sites, particularly the breast, lung, and skin.

Symptoms of brain cancer are of two kinds. Increased pressure in the skull can cause seizures, headaches, nausea, forgetfulness, and personality changes. However, symptoms may also arise in the part of the body controlled by the area in the brain that is affected by the cancer. For instance, coordination, vision, or strength of limbs may be affected.

In the past, brain tumors did not respond well to treatment, largely because diagnosis could not be made until late in the development of the disease. Recently, however, diagnostic techniques have improved. The computed tomography (CT) scanner produces a three-dimensional image of the brain that can show the size and location of a tumor and can be used to monitor the progress of treatment. Magnetic resonance imaging is also used.

Surgery is the primary treatment for brain cancer. It is often not used, however, when cancer is present in multiple areas or when the tumor originated in another organ. Surgery in the brain is a delicate procedure; often, a tumor deep in the brain cannot be totally removed without risking impairment of body function. However, new techniques in brain surgery—sometimes with the use of a microscope—permit treatment of tumors once considered inoperable. Radiation therapy and chemotherapy are often used after surgery, although the sensitivity of brain tissue demands that these be administered cautiously.

Breast cancer

About one woman in eight will develop breast cancer at some time in her life; one woman in 28 will die from the cancer. (Breast cancer is the most common cancer of women, but lung cancer is the leading cause of cancer-related deaths in women.) The high-risk group includes women over 35, women who have never had children or who had a child for the first time after the age of 30, and women who began menstruation early or who experienced late menopause. Breast cancer also occurs with greater frequency in women who have already had breast cancer. The most important risk factor for breast cancer is family history, however, especially if a woman's mother or sister have been diagnosed with breast cancer.

Self-examination of the breasts can often lead to early detection. All women should perform these examinations monthly at the end of the menstrual period. About 90 percent of all breast tumors are discovered by self-examination. The recommended technique for breast self-examination is shown in the illustration in this section.

If a lump is discovered in a breast, the doctor will probably order an X-ray examination of the breast, known as a *mammogram*. (The American Cancer Society recommends yearly

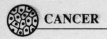
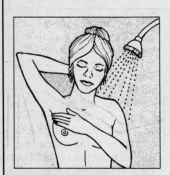

In the shower, examine each breast with the opposite hand while keeping the other hand overhead. Having wet, soapy skin may make it easier to feel lumps.

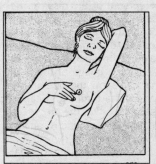

Lie flat on your back with a pillow under your left shoulder and your left hand under or over your head. Using your right hand, gently feel your left breast for lumps or hard areas. Examine your right breast in the same manner.

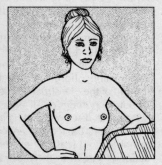

Stand in front of a mirror, with hands resting on hips. Examine breasts for swelling, dimpling, bulges, and changes in skin.

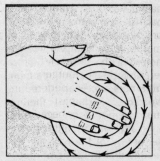

Make rotary motions with the flat pads, not tips, of the fingers moving in concentric circles inward toward nipple. Feel for knots, lumps, or indentations. Be sure to include the armpit area.

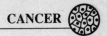
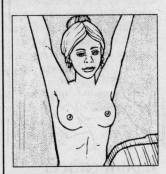

Standing in front of a mirror, with arms extended overhead, examine breasts for changes. This position highlights bulges and indentations which may indicate a lump.

Squeeze nipples gently to inspect for any discharge. Report any suspicious findings to your doctor.

mammograms for women older than 50 years of age.) The doctor may also take a biopsy specimen from the lump to test for the presence of cancer. If cancer is identified, surgery will probably be performed. Women with breast cancer often dread surgery because of the disfigurement that can result; however, surgery for a breast tumor is often less extensive today than in the past. At one time, all breast cancer patients received a radical mastectomy (removal of the breast, underlying chest muscles, and lymph nodes in the armpit). Now it is known that in many

cases the removal of the breast, or even the tumor alone, may be equally effective. In addition, there are techniques for reconstruction of the breast after surgery and for rehabilitation of muscle tone in an arm that has been weakened by surgery. In some cases, radiation therapy and chemotherapy will be used after surgery to destroy remaining cancer cells.

Cervical cancer

The cervix is the lower part of the uterus (womb), which extends into the vagina. Cancer of

561

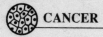

the cervix is the second most common cancer among American women. The death rate from this disease has decreased 50 percent over the last 50 years, largely as a result of early diagnosis. Early cervical cancer has no symptoms but can be detected by means of a Pap smear. A Pap smear is performed routinely in a doctor's office by scraping the surface of the cervix. The collected material is then tested for indications of cancer. Today, two out of three cases of cervical cancer are detected with this test before symptoms occur.

You are more likely than most women to develop cervical cancer if you have had a sexually transmitted viral infection, such as genital warts or herpes; if you began having sexual intercourse before the age of 18; or if you have had many sexual partners. A particularly aggressive type of cervical cancer appears in women who are HIV positive.

If a Pap smear indicates the possibility of cervical cancer, a biopsy of the affected area will probably be performed. Treatment depends on how far the disease has advanced; early forms are almost always curable by surgery. If a patient still hopes to bear children, and the

cancer is in an early stage, this surgery can sometimes be put off until after children have been born. However, this is possible only if the disease does not seem to be progressing, and the cancer must be monitored carefully during this phase. The uterus should be removed eventually.

Colon cancer

Every year, many Americans die of cancer of the colon and rectum. About half of all cases of cancer of the colon can be cured by surgery, and early detection can greatly improve this percentage. A simple test for occult (not visible to the naked eye) blood in the stool can indicate whether further tests should be made for the presence of this type of cancer. Everyone who is older than 50 years of age or who has chronic digestive problems should have this test regularly. Cure is twice as likely if the disease is discovered before symptoms occur. Periodic screening with a flexible sigmoidoscope is also recommended for men and women older than 50 years of age.

Symptoms of cancer of the colon include a change in bowel movements, bleeding from the rectum, pencil-thin stools, and abdominal discomfort not eased by bowel movement. If colon cancer is suspected, the physician will probably perform a rectal exam to search for unusual growths. If further examination is necessary, the doctor may introduce a proctosigmoidoscope (a lighted, tubelike instrument) into the colon through the anus. This instrument permits examination of the inside of the colon and can also be used to obtain a biopsy specimen.

Surgery is the usual treatment for cancer of the colon. If the cancer is near or in the rectum, the surgeon may remove all of the rectum and create an artificial rectum, or colostomy, in the lower abdominal wall. A colostomy is covered with a bag to collect waste material. Colostomy is not automatically done for any colon cancer. The type of operation performed is dictated by the size and location of the tumor.

Leukemia

This is a disease that originates in the bone marrow, the site of blood cell production. The term *leukemia,* which is derived from Greek words that mean literally "white blood," refers to the presence of excessive numbers of white blood cells, especially immature and poorly functioning forms of these cells.

The symptoms of leukemia are caused by the impairment of normal blood cell functions. The primary role of white blood cells is fighting infection. Since many of the white blood cells present are immature, they function poorly and infections are common. Other blood cell types normally present in bone marrow (red blood cells, which carry oxygen throughout the body, and platelets, which are needed for blood clotting) may be crowded out by the cancerous leukemic cells. As a result, symptoms of deficiency of these cell types are often evident in leukemia patients. Symptoms include poor blood clotting ability (due to a shortage of platelets) and fatigue resulting from anemia (due to decreased numbers of red blood cells). Other symptoms are easy bruising, bleeding from the gums, blood in the stools, fever, and frequent infections. The spleen and lymph nodes are usually enlarged.

Leukemia is often treated first with intensive chemotherapy to kill the cancer cells. The patient may appear to become even more ill during treatment be-

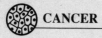

cause of the side effects of the cancer-fighting drugs. After this initial phase, radiation and additional drugs may be administered. Bone marrow transplants are now often used.

Leukemia is the most common form of cancer in children. In recent years, the outlook has improved dramatically for children with this disease. Twenty years ago, nearly all children who suffered from leukemia died. Today, the life spans of many have increased.

Liver cancer

Liver cancer usually is caused by the spread of cancer cells from another site in the body. However, cancer that originates in the liver can sometimes be traced to environmental carcinogens. It is known that anyone who has worked with vinyl chloride, a chemical used in plastics manufacturing, has a higher risk of this disease. It also appears that cirrhosis of the liver (a disease in which normal liver cells are replaced by fibrous tissue) may cause an individual to be more susceptible to cancer of the liver. People who are chronic carriers of the hepatitis B virus may be at higher risk of liver cancer as well.

Symptoms of liver cancer may resemble the signs of a peptic ulcer—aching or burning pain in the upper abdomen, nausea, and vomiting. A swollen or hardened liver often indicates to the doctor the need for further investigation.

If this form of cancer is diagnosed early and is confined to the liver, it can be treated surgically, but most often the prognosis is not good.

Lung cancer

Cigarette smoking is generally accepted as the major cause of lung cancer. Lung cancer is the leading cause of cancer death in men, and in recent years the incidence of lung cancer in women has been growing, probably as a result of the increase in the number of women who smoke. The incidence of lung cancer is also increasing among nonsmokers.

Those who smoke and are over 45, or who have a family history of lung cancer, should be on the lookout for symptoms, since the early signs—a persistent cough or lingering respiratory discomfort—can be very mild. Later, coughing will increase, as will chest pain and shortness of breath, and blood

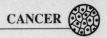

may be found in the sputum (the material coughed up from the lungs).

If it is relatively confined, a cancerous tumor in the lung is usually removed surgically. It is sometimes necessary to remove an entire lobe of the lung. Because lung cancers are usually not detected until they are well advanced, surgery alone may not be able to eliminate them, and radiation and chemotherapy may be used in combination with or in place of surgery.

In recent years, the deadliest form of lung cancer, small-cell carcinoma (also called *oat-cell carcinoma*), has yielded to a new drug therapy that has produced remission (absence of symptoms) in some patients. Unfortunately, the remission is often not permanent.

Lymphoma

This cancer attacks the lymphatic system, particularly the lymph nodes and the spleen. These organs manufacture lymphocytes (cells that protect the body against infection).

The first symptom of lymphoma is usually a swollen spleen or swollen lymph nodes in the neck, armpits, or groin.

Fever and sweating are later symptoms. If these symptoms persist, a doctor should be consulted. If the doctor suspects cancer, a biopsy of the enlarged organ will probably be ordered.

There are two major forms of lymphoma: Hodgkin disease and non-Hodgkin lymphoma. In recent years, there have been dramatic strides in the treatment of Hodgkin disease. In the early stages, radiation alone can be very effective. Later in the course of the disease, more extensive radiation or a combination of radiation and chemotherapy may be required.

Treatment of non-Hodgkin lymphoma is much the same as that of Hodgkin disease. In the past, this form of lymphoma was usually discovered too late for treatment, but recent advances have made long periods of remission possible in many cases.

Ovarian cancer

This is the most dangerous form of cancer of the female reproductive organs, because it is so difficult to diagnose in its early stages. Women older than 50 years of age have a higher incidence of the disease, as do childless women and those with

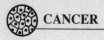

a family history of ovarian cancer and breast cancer.

Symptoms may include pelvic discomfort, constipation, abdominal swelling, and irregular menstruation. Diagnosis is often not possible without an exploratory operation known as a *laparotomy,* in which a surgical incision is made in the abdominal wall. Laparoscopy, in which a lighted tubelike instrument is inserted through a small incision in the abdominal wall, has become a very useful tool in detecting ovarian cancer. Sometimes removing only one ovary is sufficient, but usually it is necessary to remove both ovaries and the uterus.

Prostate cancer

After lung cancer, this is the most common cancer among men. African American men have a higher incidence of prostate cancer than any other group in the world. In general, it is more common in men over 55. Cancer of the prostate (a male sex gland that lies at the base of the bladder) can develop very slowly, often producing no symptoms until the disease is far advanced. Sometimes a routine rectal examination discloses a lump in the prostate. (During a rectal exam, the doctor inserts a gloved, lubricated finger into the rectum and feels the prostate for hard or lumpy areas.) The rectal examination should be included in medical checkups of all men older than 40 years of age.

Your doctor may also order a test to measure substances called prostate-specific antigen (PSA). The level of PSA in the blood rises in men who have prostate cancer. The test is often performed annually in men older than 50 years of age.

When symptoms occur, they are usually the result of enlargement of the prostate, which causes difficult urination or blood in the urine. In cases in which prostate cancer is discovered before it has begun to spread, the cancer can frequently be cured by surgery or radiation. When the disease has spread, usually only its symptoms are treated as they occur.

Skin cancer

About 300,000 cases of skin cancer are discovered every year. Its incidence increases every year (particularly among women), perhaps because people currently are getting more exposure to sunlight. The ultraviolet rays of the sun are a major cause of skin cancer. Fair-skinned people have less melanin (a protective substance in the skin) than dark-skinned people do and are therefore more susceptible to the effects of these rays. Skin cancer can also result from prolonged exposure to certain chemicals, such as arsenic compounds. Burn scars and skin diseases sometimes develop into cancer.

Symptoms of skin cancer are a change in the surface of the skin, a wound that does not heal, and a sudden major change in a wart, mole, or birthmark. All such suspicious signs should be examined by a doctor.

Most skin cancers are highly treatable. Some can be removed in a doctor's office or an outpatient clinic. But since some forms of skin cancer can spread throughout the body, it is important that they be treated early. The most dangerous skin cancer, malignant melanoma, can metastasize through the lymph and vascular systems.

Skin cancer is an unusual form of cancer in that it can be prevented easily. Fair-skinned people and anyone with a family history of skin cancer should avoid exposure to the sun. Additionally, everyone who spends time in the sun should apply a protective sunscreen to exposed portions of the body. It is important that children, whose skin is more sensitive, be protected against the sun. The use of certain drugs, such as barbiturates, antibiotics, and birth control pills, can increase the sensitivity of the skin.

Stomach cancer

The incidence of stomach cancer has decreased by 50 percent in the last 25 years. A change in diet may account for this. Stomach cancer is more common in men than in women and usually occurs between the ages of 50 and 70. The high-risk group includes those with a history of pernicious anemia or alcoholism and those who choose a diet rich in smoked, pickled, or salted foods.

The symptoms of stomach cancer are similar to those of a peptic ulcer (heartburn and abdominal discomfort), which makes diagnosis more difficult. It may not be until the disease is well advanced that the identifying symptoms of bloody stools or vomit appear. A special X-ray study may be obtained after the patient swallows barium (a contrast substance that coats the lining of the stomach), which

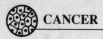

CANCER

allows irregularities in the stomach (such as the presence of a tumor) to show up on X-ray films. If a tumor is identified, a flexible, lighted, tubelike instrument called an *endoscope* may be inserted down the throat into the stomach to examine the tumor more closely and perhaps obtain a biopsy specimen.

Surgery is the most effective treatment of this disease, but only about 10 percent of victims survive more than five years after diagnosis. Surgery is most useful when the tumor has not begun to spread. It is sometimes necessary to remove all or part of the stomach. After such surgery, the patient will require a modified diet.

Uterine cancer

This disease is most common in women older that 50 years of age. Especially susceptible are women who have never given birth, those who are obese or diabetic, and those who suffer from high blood pressure. Women who have taken the female hormone estrogen without progesterone are probably at higher risk than those who have not.

Vaginal bleeding after menopause is the most common symptom of uterine cancer. If a Pap smear shows no abnormalities, a minor surgical procedure known as *dilation* and *curettage (D&C)* may be performed. This involves scraping the interior walls of the uterus to examine the tissue for cancer. If cancer is identified, a hysterectomy (surgical removal of the uterus) is usually performed. Cancer of the uterus is harder to detect than that of the cervix.

Vaginal cancer

Once confined to women older than 50 years of age, vaginal cancer has begun to appear in women between the ages of 17 and 20. The mothers of most of these young women took artificial estrogens, particularly diethylstilbestrol (DES), during pregnancy to prevent miscarriage. A woman whose mother took artificial estrogens during pregnancy should have a Pap smear twice a year. (A Pap test involves scraping the surface of the cervix and testing the collected material for signs of cancer.) Symptoms of vaginal cancer include vaginal pain and bleeding. The disease is usually treated with radiation and surgery.

HEREDITY AND INHERITED DISEASES

To understand how some disorders can be passed from one generation to another, one must first understand the role played by the genes in determining the form and function of each cell in the body.

The genes are the basic units that determine the hereditary characteristics of an organism. Genes, which are composed of molecules of deoxyribonucleic acid (DNA), can be thought of as chemical instructions. Each gene, by virtue of the particular structure of its DNA molecule, contains the code for a specific trait, determining both what a cell is and how it works (as if a computer program not only told the computer what to do but helped to form the machine itself).

Within each cell, thousands of genes are linked in a specific order, like beads on a necklace, to form structures called *chromosomes,* which are, in effect, continuous strands of DNA. It has been estimated that each cell contains about five feet of coiled DNA strands and that each strand is made of about 100,000 genes.

The particular composition of the genes and their arrangement on the chromosomes are what constitute the genetic blueprint for each individual. Cells that develop into liver tissue, rather than blood cells or nerve fibers, for example, do so because that is what their genetic coding dictates. In this way, the cells of the body are programmed to create a person with a certain color of eyes and hair, as well as the thousands of other characteristics that make each human unique.

Sex cells

Each cell in the human body contains 46 chromosomes. The only exceptions are the sex cells (the ovum and the sperm) each of which contains only 23 chromosomes. When these sex

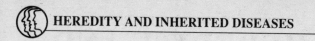

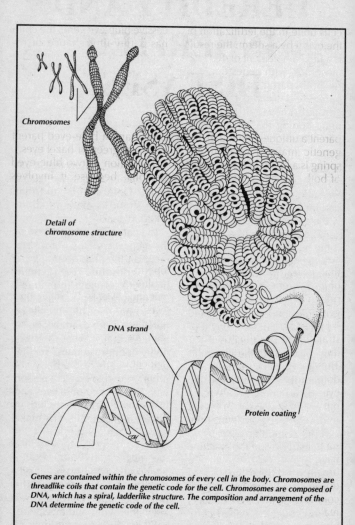

Chromosomes

*Detail of
chromosome structure*

DNA strand

Protein coating

Genes are contained within the chromosomes of every cell in the body. Chromosomes are threadlike coils that contain the genetic code for the cell. Chromosomes are composed of DNA, which has a spiral, ladderlike structure. The composition and arrangement of the DNA determine the genetic code of the cell.

cells unite in the fertilization of the ovum by a sperm, the result is a full complement of 46 chromosomes, with genes donated by both parents. Since each parent contributes only 23 chromosomes (half of the genetic coding that makes each parent a unique individual), the genetic makeup of their offspring is a blend of components of both parents' genetic material.

Dominant and recessive traits

The traits that genes give rise to may be either dominant or recessive. A recessive gene is one that produces a certain trait only if its effects are not overridden by those of a dominant gene.

Eye color provides a relatively straightforward illustration of how inheritance of traits works. The gene for brown eyes is dominant; the gene for blue eyes is recessive. The child of a brown-eyed parent who has two brown-eye genes and a blue-eyed parent (who must have two blue-eye genes) will have brown eyes because the brown-eyed parent has only dominant brown-eye genes to contribute to the child's genetic makeup. However, if the brown-eyed parent has a dominant brown-eye gene and a re-

cessive blue-eye gene, the child has a fifty-fifty chance of receiving a blue-eye gene from each parent and thereby having blue eyes. (Actually, inheritance does not always work with such textbook simplicity—sometimes the child of a brown-eyed parent and a blue-eyed parent will have green or hazel eyes.)

The union of two blue-eyed persons, because it involves only recessive blue-eye genes, will always produce blue-eyed offspring.

The offspring of two brown-eyed persons who each have a recessive blue-eye gene have a one-in-four chance of receiving a blue-eye gene from each parent and, as a result, having blue eyes. (This final combination illustrates how recessive genes can be present but unsuspected, allowing a trait to appear unexpectedly after skipping generations.)

Mutation

Genes are normally transmitted unchanged from one generation to the next. Sometimes, however, mutations occur— that is, the structure of the gene itself is changed, perhaps due to the effect of a toxic substance, an infection, or exposure to radiation. Offspring that receive a mutated gene will exhibit a characteristic that is not present in either parent.

The discovery of the structure of the DNA molecule opened a new era in medical research. Scientists in the new field of genetic engineering are exploring ways of artificially creating mutations in genes so that someday it may be possible to correct the errors in genetic coding that are responsible for causing various disorders.

Genetic counseling

As the medical profession has learned more about inherited diseases, it has been able to offer genetic counseling to couples concerned about the possibility of having a child with an inherited disease or abnormality. A genetic counselor or specialist in genetic disorders can estimate the likelihood that a couple's offspring will be afflicted with a problem due to an inherited trait or to the age of the parents. For some genetic disorders, tests can determine whether one or both parents are carriers or can detect whether a defect is present in a fetus.

Celiac disease

Celiac disease, or celiac sprue, is a chronic disorder of the small intestine caused by sensitivity to gluten, a protein found in wheat and rye and, to a lesser extent, in oats and barley. The disorder causes poor absorption by the intestine of fat, protein, carbohydrates, iron, water, and vitamins A, D, E, and K. Removal of gluten from the diet normally brings improvement.

Causes

The basic cause is probably an inherited defect found mostly in people of northwestern European ancestry. It affects 1 person in 300 in western Ireland, and approximately 1 in 5,000 in the United States. Celiac disease is twice as likely to affect women as men.

One theory about celiac disease holds that the body reacts to gluten and its derivative gliadin as if they were viruses or bacteria. When food containing gluten reaches the portion of the small intestine called the *jejunum,* antibodies in the intestinal wall are stimulated. In the process, for some unknown reason, the intestinal villi (hairlike projections through which nutrients from the intestine are absorbed into the bloodstream) are destroyed. Destruction of the villi is almost total in the jejunum, less so in the rest of the small intestine. Poor absorption of food and water is the result. Another theory states that gluten and gliadin act directly on the intestinal wall as toxins (poisons). One or both of these theories may be correct.

Symptoms

Symptoms of celiac disease may begin in infancy when the child starts eating wheat cereal or other foods containing gluten. The child does not thrive, suffers painful bloating in the abdomen, and passes pale, foul-smelling, bulky stools. Failure to absorb enough iron produces anemia (deficiency of oxygen-carrying red blood cells). Poor absorption of protein may cause edema (swelling of body tissues). There is little fat on the body. Growth may be stunted, signs of vitamin deficiency appear, and softening of bones may produce bone deformities and fractures. Sometimes the symptoms disappear in adolescence and reappear in adulthood.

Adults with celiac disease have many of the same symptoms, including bulky, foul-smelling stools, weight loss, vitamin deficiencies, edema, anemia, and bone pain. The disease can also cause strange sensations (burning, pricking,

tickling, or tingling) in the hands and feet, dry skin, eczema, acne, cessation of menstruation, mood changes, and irritability. The disease may appear for the first time as late as age 60.

Diagnosis

The most definitive test for celiac disease is microscopic examination of a piece of tissue taken from the wall of the small intestine. The sample is taken with the aid of a flexible tube with a cutting instrument at the tip, which is inserted through the mouth into the intestine. The specimen from a patient with celiac disease has almost no villi, and the surface is alternately flat and bumpy, with a disorganized network of blood vessels. Various blood tests taken after the patient has eaten specific substances reveal how well the intestine has absorbed these substances. In addition, blood tests may reveal low levels of protein, calcium, potassium, and sodium. Tests of stools reveal excess fat.

Treatment

The primary treatment of celiac disease is to remove all gluten from the diet, which is easier said than done. Hot dogs, ice cream, commercial soups and sauces, candy bars, and all kinds of baked goods can be sources of gluten (even small amounts of gluten must be avoided). Many doctors refer the patient to a dietitian for detailed lists of foods to avoid and for advice on following a healthful diet, which should be high in calories and protein and low in fat. Vitamin and mineral supplements are given as needed. In stubborn cases, a cortisone drug may be given, which will often result in improvement.

The outlook is good for most patients. Recovery is most dramatic in children. In severe cases, complete return to normal bowel function and normal absorption may take months or may never occur. For that reason, and to rule out other diseases of nutritional deficiency or poor absorption, it is best to see a doctor as soon as symptoms appear. This is one inherited ailment that is almost completely treatable.

Cystic fibrosis

Cystic fibrosis is a serious hereditary disease characterized by abnormal secretions that affect many parts of the body, but primarily the lungs, pancreas, and digestive tract.

Cause

Cystic fibrosis is caused by an inherited defective gene. This defective gene is recessive, meaning that it must be inherited from both parents for the child to suffer from the disease. If the gene is received from only one parent, the child is a carrier but will not get the disease. About 5 percent of the white population in the United States are carriers; the incidence in the black and Asian populations is much lower. Approximately 1 in every 400 marriages involves two carriers. A child of two carriers has a 25 percent chance of getting the disease, a 50 percent chance of being a carrier, and a 25 percent chance of being completely free of the defective gene.

The defective gene causes the exocrine glands to release abnormal mucus, sweat, and other secretions. (Exocrine glands are those that release their secretions through ducts, rather than directly into the bloodstream.) The most serious effects of cystic fibrosis occur when the mucous glands release thick, gummy mucus rather than the normal clear, free-flowing fluid. This thick mucus accumulates in the glands, causing swelling, form-

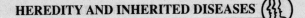
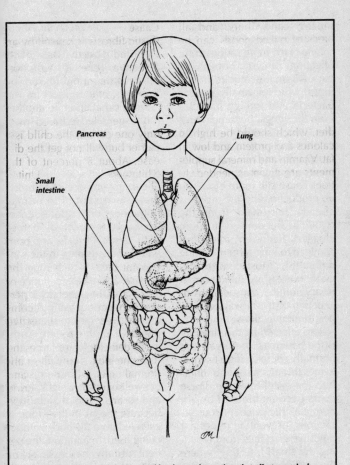

Cystic fibrosis is a disease characterized by abnormal secretions that affect many body parts, particularly the lungs, the pancreas, and the intestinal tract. In the lungs, thick mucus hampers breathing and promotes infection. Thickened secretions can obstruct the ducts in the pancreas and block the passage of pancreatic digestive enzymes into the small intestine.

ing cysts, and, most important, blocking various ducts.

One of the more serious complications of cystic fibrosis occurs when the mucus in the lungs, which normally sweeps bacteria and foreign particles from the lungs, becomes thick and sticky, accumulating in the airways and creating a breeding ground for infection, rather than preventing it. Consequent infections cause still more mucus to be produced, and the airways, already narrowed from the swelling, become even more clogged. Recurrent infections can lead to long-term breathing difficulties. Most deaths from cystic fibrosis are due to respiratory failure caused by obstruction of the airways and by persistent infections.

Also affected by this disorder is the pancreas, the organ that normally secretes digestive enzymes through a series of ducts into the small intestine. These ducts become blocked by abnormally thickened mucous secretions, preventing important digestive enzymes from reaching the small intestine, where they are needed to digest fats.

Reproductive tract secretions are also thickened. In women, an overabundance of mucus in the cervix may block the passage of sperm, making it diffi-cult to become pregnant. About 98 percent of male patients are sterile, because the ducts through which the sperm normally travel are blocked by thickened mucus.

Heat exhaustion is another problem related to this disease, because of the large salt loss due to excessive sweating.

Symptoms
The symptoms of cystic fibrosis may show up at birth or may not appear until adolescence. About 10 percent of babies with cystic fibrosis are born with a mucous plug in their intestinal tract, which must be corrected surgically.

Because the pancreas is prevented from releasing the enzymes necessary to digest fat, digestive problems are common, and stools are large and foul smelling. Typically, children afflicted with the disease eat well but gain weight slowly and show signs of malnutrition because the fat in their food is excreted from the body without being used. In addition, the patient usually has excessively salty sweat, a chronic cough accompanied by mucous discharge, and rapid and difficult breathing. Patients frequently experience fatigue and muscle cramps from salt loss. Sinusitis (inflammation of the air-filled cavities in the facial bones), nasal polyps (growths in the nose), and a barrel-shaped chest from overinflated lungs may also develop.

Because many of these symptoms are also indications of less serious disorders, cystic fibrosis often remains undiagnosed or undetected for some time while the disease progresses.

Diagnosis

Diagnostic evaluation usually includes a physical examination, medical history, chest X ray, and a sweat test. (Most cystic fibrosis patients have excessively salty sweat, although the salt level does not indicate the severity of the condition.) Tests of the patient's stool and digestive juices can show how well the pancreas is functioning.

Treatment

Although cystic fibrosis cannot be cured, its symptoms can be relieved to some extent. Dietary management is extremely important; patients are advised to reduce the fat in their diets, to eat nutritious foods with high amounts of essential minerals and vitamins, to take salt tablets, and to take pancreatic enzyme tablets to aid digestion of fats. The risk of respiratory infections can be reduced by means of antibiotics, aerosol mists, appropriate vaccinations, and postural drainage (in which the patient is positioned so that gravity can be used to help clear mucus from clogged lungs). A regular program of exercise may also be useful.

Prevention

There is no means of preventing cystic fibrosis today. Researchers continue to look for a reason why the defective gene causes mucus to become abnormal, as well as for a way to identify carriers of the gene. One new test measures certain chemicals present in the amniotic fluid (the liquid that surrounds a fetus in the womb), so that an unborn baby with the gene can be identified.

Down syndrome

Down syndrome is a congenital (present at birth) disorder characterized by varying degrees of mental retardation and a variety of physical abnormalities.

Cause

Normally, each cell in the human body has 46 chromosomes; the cells in someone with Down syndrome, however, have 47. In ways that are as yet unknown, the presence of the extra chromosome causes all of the unusual characteristics of Down syndrome. In 95 percent of cases, the condition is called trisomy 21 (because the extra chromosome is attached to the 21st pair of chromosomes), and the mistake in genetic coding is one that apparently could happen to anyone.

Symptoms

Down syndrome is marked by a number of physical characteristics: somewhat slanted eyes in small sockets (which is why it used to be called *mongolism*); a small, short head, flattened in back and front; a nose flattened at the bridge; a thick tongue; short hands, feet, neck, trunk, arms, and legs; a single, rather than a double, crease across the top of the palm; flabby arms and legs with poor muscle tone; a wide gap between the first and second toes; and generally retarded physical development.

A child with Down syndrome may have a poorly functioning thyroid gland (which regulates metabolism, the rate at which the body uses energy) and pituitary gland (which regulates other glands, including those responsible for growth, matura-

tion, and reproduction). Children with Down syndrome are at much higher risk of developing leukemia, and approximately one-third of them are also especially susceptible to infection.

Education

Characteristically slower than other children to walk, talk, and learn, youngsters with Down syndrome benefit from "early intervention" programs designed to help them develop their abilities as much as possible. Such programs are frequently available from the time the mother and baby leave the hospital after the birth. A number of organizations exist to promote such programs and assist parents in developing their child's potential.

The degree of retardation that accompanies Down syndrome ranges from mild to severe (the average IQ is about 50), and the extent to which an individual will be affected is not predictable at birth. Some children with Down syndrome attend special education classes in public schools; others attend special schools for the mentally retarded. As adults, some may be able to live independently and work in the community. Depending on the degree of re-

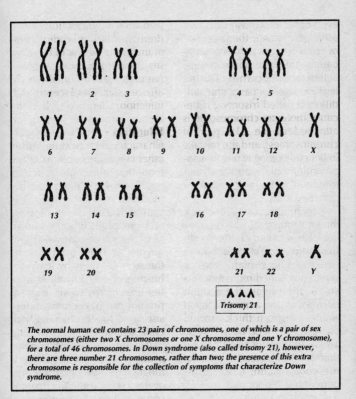

The normal human cell contains 23 pairs of chromosomes, one of which is a pair of sex chromosomes (either two X chromosomes or one X chromosome and one Y chromosome), for a total of 46 chromosomes. In Down syndrome (also called trisomy 21), however, there are three number 21 chromosomes, rather than two; the presence of this extra chromosome is responsible for the collection of symptoms that characterize Down syndrome.

tardation that is present, others will require more supervised living arrangements and may be able to hold simple, routine jobs.

Prevention

Prospective parents can reduce their chances of having a child with Down syndrome by start-ing their families early. At age 20 a woman's risk of giving birth to a child with Down syn-drome is only 1 in 2,000 live births, but at age 35 the risk is 1 in 300, at age 40 it is 1 in 100, and at age 45 it is 1 in 40 live births. The age of the father also has some bearing on the risk, but not as much as the age of

579

the mother. Diagnosis of Down syndrome can be made between weeks 16 and 18 of pregnancy through a procedure called *amniocentesis*. During amniocentesis, the doctor will insert a needle through the mother's abdominal wall and into the uterus. A sample of the amniotic fluid is then drawn into a syringe, grown on a special culture plate, and analyzed to see if there are abnormal chromosomes.

A technique used to check the chromosomes of the growing fetus is called *chorionic villus sampling*. This procedure, performed during the eighth or ninth week of pregnancy, involves the removal of a small portion of the placenta by a small instrument inserted through the woman's cervix. Tissue that is obtained can be immediately evaluated for the presence of chromosome abnormalities.

Hemophilia

Hemophilia is a sex-linked hereditary bleeding disorder in which the clotting mechanism of the blood does not function properly. Blood normally contains several factors that enable clotting to occur. These are des-ignated coagulation factors I through XIII. In the most common form of hemophilia—classic hemophilia, or hemophilia A—factor VIII is deficient. In this case, factors I through VII function adequately, but the clotting process is interrupted by a lack of sufficient amounts of factor VIII. Hemophilia B is the other common form of hemophilia, although it occurs significantly less often than hemophilia A. Hemophilia B is caused by a deficiency of factor IX. Hemophilia B is also known as *Christmas disease*.

Cause

Hemophilia is inherited as a sex-linked recessive trait—a woman can pass on the defective gene for the trait without being affected herself. The gene that causes the disorder appears on the X chromosome, which is the female sex chromosome. (Men have one X chromosome and one Y chromosome, whereas women have two X chromosomes.) If a woman has one defective X chromosome, the presence of her other, normal X chromosome ensures that she will not suffer from the disease herself. However, she can pass on her defective X chromosome to her sons, who will have the disease because they do not have a normal X chromosome to counteract the defect. If she passes the defective chromosome to her daughters, they, too, will be carriers but will not have the disease. A male hemophiliac passes his defective X chromosome to his daughters, making them carriers. However, he passes on only his normal Y chromosome to his sons, who therefore will not have the disease (unless their mother is a carrier). Although the condition appears almost exclusively in men, a woman can be a hemophiliac if her mother is a carrier and her father is a hemophiliac (in such a case, she inherits two defective X chromosomes).

Symptoms
Although affected individuals are born with the disease, the onset of symptoms is variable. Milder cases may not be readily apparent. The symptoms of hemophilia usually become evident during early childhood. When a cut in the skin occurs or an injury is suffered, the bleeding may be substantial and prolonged. In severe cases, spontaneous internal bleeding may occur without any obvious cause. Blood may appear in the urine due to internal bleeding. Pain is also a symptom when

the bleeding occurs internally, between muscles and into joints. The course of the disease may result in irreversible damage to the joints, which, in turn, results in greater pain and in limitation of movement.

Diagnosis
If a child has any of the symptoms of hemophilia, or if there is a family history of hemophilia, a physician should be consulted. The physician will order laboratory tests to establish the diagnosis. The most common test for hemophilia is determination of the partial thromboplastin time (PTT), which indicates how long it takes for the blood to clot. Additional laboratory tests may be ordered in certain cases.

Treatment
Treatment of hemophilia has recently undergone dramatic changes. An important breakthrough has been the development of factor VIII replacement therapy. One therapy, cryoprecipitate, is prepared from donated blood plasma (the fluid portion of blood, which contains more factor VIII than whole blood does). The plasma of an individual donor is quickly frozen by a special process and then slowly

thawed, so that the portion rich in factor VIII can be separated out. This portion can then be prepared later for intravenous administration. Cryoprecipitate has the disadvantage of having to be stored and prepared in a hospital. Also, since cryoprecipitate is produced from the plasma of a single donor, the amount of factor VIII present in a given preparation is variable.

Treatment of hemophilia A has been further advanced by the development of a process of rapid freezing and dehydration (removal of water) of plasma, called *lyophilization*. Freeze-dried concentrates are prepared and packaged so that they can be readily dissolved by a simple mixing procedure. (This process is similar in concept to the preparation and use of freeze-dried coffee.) This concentrate, which quickly stops bleeding, is particularly efficient for home use in comparison with cryoprecipitate therapy.

There is a drawback, however, to the use of freeze-dried concentrate: the increased likelihood that an infection or infections will be transmitted to the hemophilia sufferer. Whereas the cryoprecipitate is prepared from the blood plasma of a single donor, the concentrate is prepared from the plasma of thousands of donors. The recipient of concentrate is therefore placed at increased risk of infection compared with a recipient of cryoprecipitate. Hepatitis (a serious infection of the liver), for example, may be transmitted in blood products, and the virus that causes acquired immunodeficiency syndrome (AIDS) is carried in bodily fluids. Both of these diseases have developed in a number of hemophilia patients who were treated with concentrate. (New blood-testing procedures have now reduced this risk, however.)

Treatment of hemophilia B involves the use of fresh or stored plasma. Concentrate is also available for hemophilia B and is known as *prothrombin complex concentrate*.

Prevention

There are no preventive measures for hemophilia. Genetic testing can now identify carriers of hemophilia with considerable accuracy.

Huntington chorea

Huntington chorea (also known as *Huntington disease*) is an inherited degenerative nerve disorder that seldom becomes apparent before early middle age (age 35 to 50). It is characterized by disorganized body movements and mental deterioration. It is thought that Huntington chorea is the result of a disturbance in the part of the brain that automatically regulates voluntary movements.

Cause
The condition is transmitted as a dominant genetic trait from a parent who has the disease. There is a 50 percent chance of a child's inheriting the disease from an affected parent. Since the symptoms of Huntington chorea usually do not appear until the victim is between 30 and 50 years of age, a person with a family history of the disease lives through the years of adolescence and early adulthood in dread of reaching the middle years, when the symptoms may begin. Even more tragic, a person who is unaware of a family history of Huntington chorea may have children before discovering that he or she has the disease.

Symptoms
The first symptoms of mental deterioration are usually personality changes—obstinacy,

moodiness, lack of interest in surroundings, and inappropriate behavior may be displayed. It should be noted, however, that all of these symptoms can also be due to psychological or other disorders that have nothing to do with Huntington chorea.

The symptoms of Huntington chorea are accompanied by irregular, jerky movements that begin in the arms, the neck, and the face. They may start as fidgeting and gradually develop into facial grimaces, halting speech, irregular movements of the torso, and muscle contractions in the neck that cause the head to be held to one side.

In advanced cases of Huntington chorea, a wide stance will be adopted in an attempt to maintain balance. The gait will become prancing, as control of the legs deteriorates. As the disease progresses, the victims usually become paranoid, walking ability is lost altogether, swallowing becomes difficult, and dementia (loss of intellectual capabilities) increases.

Treatment
No treatment has yet been found to control the symptoms or halt the disease. However, the body movements may be controlled somewhat by drugs,

most notably haloperidol and chlorpromazine. There is no known treatment for the mental degeneration that accompanies the physical symptoms.

Prevention

There are no preventive measures for Huntington chorea, other than advising affected patients not to have children.

Muscular dystrophy

Muscular dystrophy is the general term for a group of rare diseases in which the body's muscles weaken and waste away. Muscular dystrophy almost always strikes in childhood and is usually inherited. Duchenne muscular dystrophy, which is usually inherited through the mother, is considered to be the most common form of the disease.

The disease is progressive; that is, it becomes gradually worse once it takes hold. In severe forms of muscular dystrophy, the child must use a wheelchair to get around by the age of 11 or 12. Scoliosis (curvature of the spine) may also be caused by the disease. Severe cases can be fatal, often when

the patient is a young adult. Pneumonia is sometimes a fatal complication because of weakening of the muscles involved in breathing.

Muscular dystrophy is sometimes confused with multiple sclerosis, which is a disease of the nervous system that can ultimately result in spasticity and paralysis. There is no deterioration of the nervous system in muscular dystrophy.

Symptoms

Symptoms of muscular dystrophy vary. Muscles usually begin to weaken first in the hips, legs, and shoulders. A child of four or five who waddles from side to side, who has difficulty standing up properly, or who falls frequently should be examined by a physician. The child may also have difficulty in standing up straight or raising an arm high above the head.

Parents should not be overly concerned about the natural awkwardness that occasionally overtakes the older toddler. However, a child near five years of age who consistently has problems with muscular coordination should be checked.

Diagnosis

The diagnosis of Duchenne muscular dystrophy is rarely made

efore the age of three. The disease does not affect each gender equally: It is most commonly seen in boys.

The physician may want to obtain a muscle biopsy specimen (a small tissue sample) to confirm a diagnosis of muscular dystrophy. The biopsy can usually be done on an outpatient basis in a hospital or in a physician's office.

Treatment

There is no treatment for the disease, but an exercise program designed by a physical therapist may be helpful. The patient's diet should be regulated so that he or she does not become overweight; excess weight only taxes the child's weakening muscles.

Prevention

Because muscular dystrophy is an inherited disease, women in the family of an affected child should be tested to see if they are carriers (they can pass on the disease to their children).

Phenylketonuria

Phenylketonuria (PKU) is a disorder characterized by the presence of increased amounts of certain amino acids in the blood and urine. (Amino acids are the chemical building blocks of protein.) The condition is caused by the inability to convert phenylalanine (an amino acid essential for optimal growth in infants and for maintenance of nitrogen balance in adults) into tyrosine (another amino acid). Excess phenylalanine is normally eliminated from the body by conversion to tyrosine. In PKU, this mechanism does not work, permitting an accumulation of phenylalanine. The result is mental retardation in infants or young children if the disorder is untreated.

Cause

Phenylketonuria is hereditary and is found in most population groups, although it is very rare in Jewish and black children. The incidence in the United States is about 1 in every 16,000 live births.

Diagnosis

Early diagnosis of PKU is essential because symptoms are usually not obvious in a newborn infant. Therefore, screening tests are now mandatory for all babies born in the United States and Canada. Sometimes, infants with PKU will have nervous system disorders, very light coloring of the skin and hair, eczema (a skin disorder), and a musty odor. Older children may be extremely hyperactive. The light coloring is often an early clue to the disease; the infant's skin, hair, and even eyes will be lighter than those of other members of the family.

Treatment

Treatment of this disorder within the first few days after birth is essential if mental retardation is to be prevented. Treatment consists of limiting the child's phenylalanine intake so that the essential amino acid requirement is satisfied without any excess. This can be done by feeding the infant special formulas with little or no phenylalanine. Milk is a protein food rich in phenylalanine, so it must be avoided. When it is time to introduce solid foods into the infant's diet, low-protein natural foods, such as fruits, vegetables, and certain cereals, are usually permitted.

Early diagnosis and treatment can enable the child to develop normally and to lead a normal life. If PKU is not diagnosed in the first few days of life, extreme hyperactivity, seizures, and mental retardation usually occur. Treatment and special diet is continued throughout the child's life.

Sickle-cell anemia

Sickle-cell anemia is an inherited blood disorder, occurring almost exclusively in black people, in which the normally round red blood cells are transformed into crescentic, or sickle-shaped, cells that are less able to transport needed oxygen. The disease is chronic, marked by fatigue, breathing difficulty on exertion, swollen joints, attacks of extreme illness, complications from other diseases, and shortened life. In the past, half of all victims died by the age of 20 and few survived past 40. With new technology and forms of treatment the outlook is much better, but sickle-cell anemia remains a chronic debilitating disease.

Cause

The deformation of the red blood cells occurs because of the presence of defective hemoglobin (the iron-containing compound in the red blood cells that carries oxygen). It occurs when part or all of the body is not getting enough oxy

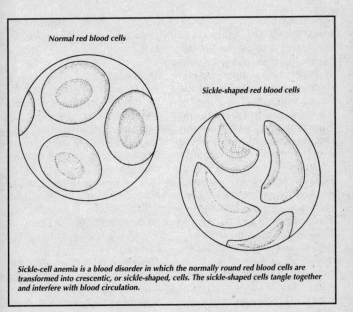

Normal red blood cells

Sickle-shaped red blood cells

Sickle-cell anemia is a blood disorder in which the normally round red blood cells are transformed into crescentic, or sickle-shaped, cells. The sickle-shaped cells tangle together and interfere with blood circulation.

gen. Because of their hooked shapes, the blood cells tend to tangle together and pile up, temporarily clogging tiny blood vessels and slowing circulation. Tissue formerly nourished by the clogged blood vessels becomes starved for oxygen and may die. The anemia (deficiency of red blood cells) that results from the accelerated breakdown of defective red blood cells not only weakens the body but increases oxygen deficiency, which results in more "sickling" of the cells.

The disease occurs in about 1 of every 330 African Americans. About one in ten is a carrier of the defective gene for sickle-cell anemia but has no symptoms and is not affected by the disease. However, if two carriers conceive a child together, the risk that their child will be afflicted by sickle-cell anemia is one in four. The risk that the child will also be a carrier is one in two. Both the carrier state and the active state of the disease can be established by a routine blood test.

587

Symptoms

In half the victims, symptoms of sickle-cell anemia begin between the ages of six months and two years. Among the first signs is unusual swelling of the fingers and toes. The bones of the hands and feet thicken, and clumping of sickle cells may affect the bone marrow, where new blood cells are produced.

Youngsters are especially subject to "sickle-cell crises," marked by severe pain in the abdomen, joints, bones, and muscles due to lack of oxygen. These crises may last from four days to several weeks and commonly occur eight to ten times a year before the age of ten. (They may occur less often in later years, however.) Signs of a sickle-cell crisis include paleness of the lips, tongue, and palms; lack of energy; sleepiness and difficulty in awakening; irritability; pain; and a temperature of 104°F (or a temperature over 100°F that lasts for at least two days).

Thickening of the heart muscle, enlargement of the heart, liver, and spleen in children, heart murmurs, and gallstones are common. The heartbeat is usually rapid. Children with the disease are usually small for their age. Adults may have narrow shoulders and hips, a barrel chest, a curved spine, long arms and legs, and an elongated skull.

Treatment

At present, there is no cure for the disease. Treatment includes giving painkillers, making the patient as comfortable as possible, and treating problems as they occur. These problems include severe anemia, which may require a blood transfusion, and frequent infections, which occur because of immune-system impairment.

Prevention

Avoiding cold, fatigue, and other stress may help to reduce the number of sickle-cell crises. Screening programs are available for those who wish to know whether they carry the gene for sickle-cell anemia. Those who have the gene can obtain genetic counseling. There is no risk of disease in offspring if only one parent is a carrier, but each child will have a one-in-two chance of being a carrier.

Tay-Sachs disease

Tay-Sachs disease is a hereditary metabolic disorder that

chiefly afflicts infants of eastern European Jewish descent. This disease is fatal, usually by the age of four years. It is marked by retarded development, loss of vision, and paralysis.

Cause

The disease is caused by a deficiency of a certain digestive enzyme. This deficiency results in the accumulation of fatty acids in the brain.

Symptoms

The symptoms of Tay-Sachs disease in an infant are most often noted after four to six months of normal development. A previously well infant begins to lose motor coordination skills and to exhibit loss of interest in his or her surroundings. As Tay-Sachs disease becomes more advanced, seizures occur, and the head becomes considerably enlarged.

Diagnosis

The physician may notice poor muscle tone and an exaggerated startle response to sound. A distinctive cherry-red spot may be seen in the retina of the eye. The diagnosis is confirmed with special blood tests.

Diagnosis of the disorder can be made before birth by amniocentesis, a procedure in which a small amount of amniotic fluid (the fluid in the sac surrounding the fetus in the uterus) is removed via a needle inserted through the mother's abdomen and tested.

Treatment

There is no known cure or treatment for Tay-Sachs disease.

Prevention

There is a blood test that helps identify carriers of the defective gene. (A carrier has the gene but does not have the disease.) This test is especially recommended for all Jews of reproductive age. If two carriers have children, each child conceived has a one-in-four chance of having the disease. It is, therefore, a good idea for carriers to seek genetic counseling before starting their families.

INDEX

INDEX

INDEX